Fundamentals of

Applied Pathophysiology for Paramedics

Fundamentals of
Applied Pathophysiology for Paramedics

EDITED BY

Ian Peate, OBE FRCN EN(G) RGN DipN(Lond) RNT Bed BEd (Hons) MA(Lond) LLM

Editor in Chief, *British Journal of Nursing*; Consultant Editor, *Journal of Paramedic Practice*;
Consultant Editor, *International Journal for Advancing Practice*; Visiting Professor, Northumbria University;
Visiting Professor, St Georges University of London and Kingston University London;
Professorial Fellow, Roehampton University; Visiting Senior Clinical Fellow, University of Hertfordshire

AND

Simon Sawyer PhD BPara BPsychMan/Mar GCHPE

Director of Education, Australian Paramedical College; Adjunct Senior Lecturer in Paramedicine, Griffith University,
Queensland, Australia

WILEY Blackwell

Registered Offices
John Wiley & Sons, Inc., 111 River Street, Hoboken, NJ 07030, USA
John Wiley & Sons Ltd, The Atrium, Southern Gate, Chichester, West Sussex, PO19 8SQ, UK

For details of our global editorial offices, customer services, and more information about Wiley products visit us at www.wiley.com.

Wiley also publishes its books in a variety of electronic formats and by print-on-demand. Some content that appears in standard print versions of this book may not be available in other formats.

Library of Congress Cataloging-in-Publication Data

Names: Peate, Ian, editor. | Sawyer, Simon, editor.
Title: Fundamentals of applied pathophysiology for paramedics / edited by
  Ian Peate, Simon Sawyer.
Description: Hoboken, NJ : Wiley-Blackwell, 2024. | Includes index.
Identifiers: LCCN 2023047914 (print) | LCCN 2023047915 (ebook) | ISBN
  9781119862802 (paperback) | ISBN 9781119862819 (adobe pdf) | ISBN
  9781119862826 (epub)
Subjects: MESH: Pathologic processes–diagnosis | Paramedics |
  Physiological Phenomena | Emergency Treatment
Classification: LCC RC67 (print) | LCC RC67 (ebook) | NLM QZ 140 | DDC
  616/.047–dc23/eng/20231201
LC record available at https://lccn.loc.gov/2023047914
LC ebook record available at https://lccn.loc.gov/2023047915

Cover Design: Wiley
Cover Images: © Brian Jackson/Adobe Stock Photos; Anatomy Insider/Adobe Stock Photos

Set in 9.5/12.5pt Source sans pro by Straive, Pondicherry, India
Printed and bound by CPI Group (UK) Ltd, Croydon, CR0 4YY
C9781119862802_040324

To all those health and care professionals all around the world who worked tirelessly during the COVID-19 pandemic

Contents

x

Contributors

George Bell-Starr FdSc MCPara
George began his career in paramedicine studying at the University of Worcester before starting with South Western Ambulance Foundation Trust as a newly qualified paramedic in 2017. He has continued to study, focusing particularly on clinical reasoning. His key areas of interest include mentoring, developing paramedic practice and frailty. In late 2020, he began training as an advanced practitioner in primary care within the Mid-Dorset Primary Care Network.

Carl Clare RN DipN MSc (Lond) PGDE (Lond)
Carl began his nursing a career in 1990 as a nursing auxiliary. He later undertook three years of student nurse training at Selly Oak Hospital (Birmingham), moving to the Royal Devon and Exeter Hospitals, then Northwick Park Hospital, and finally the Royal Brompton and Harefield NHS Trust as a resuscitation officer and honorary teaching fellow of Imperial College (London). Since 2006, he has worked at the University of Hertfordshire as a senior lecturer in adult nursing. His key areas of interest are long term illness, physiology, sociology and cardiac care. Carl has previously published work in cardiac care, resuscitation and pathophysiology.

Neil Coleman MSc
Officer in the National Ambulance Service, Ireland
With a wealth of experience spanning over two decades in the National Ambulance Service, Neil is an Advanced Paramedic, Assistant Professor at University College Dublin, and former soldier and firefighter. Neil has actively contributed to the development and presentation of courses from entry-level first aid to the accreditation of a BSc programme. He has overseen several large-scale medical education programmes, including International Trauma Life Support, the Advanced Paramedic Programme (Ireland), and served as the Global Education Manager for a European-based College. Neil is dedicated to advancing healthcare education to ensure a lasting impact on the profession and the training of future paramedic professionals.

Sadie Diamond-Fox MCP ACCP (mFICM) BSc (Hons) RN PGCAHP NMP (V300) FHEA
Sadie qualified as an adult nurse in 2008 and has since worked in various critical care departments. She progressed to her current advanced practice roles, which include advanced critical care practitioner, assistant professor in advanced critical care practice (FHEA) and regional advancing practice supervision and assessment lead for Health Education England. Sadie is also currently a second-year PhD candidate. She has an extensive teaching portfolio spanning multiple disciplines within postgraduate healthcare education, making a wide range of contributions at local and international levels. Her key areas of interest are postgraduate healthcare education, acute, emergency and critical care, physiology and pharmacology, advanced-level practice and simulation and virtual reality education modalities.

Terry Dore MSc PGDip HPE PGDip AP PGCert
Terry worked for 20 years in Dublin Fire Brigade as a firefighter/paramedic and progressed to advanced paramedic after study at University College Dublin (UCD). He subsequently undertook a research MSc at UCD and a BSc (Hons) in paramedic studies in University of Limerick. He studied at the Royal College of Surgeons in Ireland and gained a postgraduate diploma in health professions education, becoming a clinical educator. He currently teaches advanced paramedic practitioners for the National Ambulance Service in Ireland and has recently begun an MSc in health, safety, and human factors at the Technological University Dublin. He has a keen interest in prehospital research and wishes to progress evidence-based prehospital practice. Terry is certified with both the Health and Care Professions Council and the Pre-Hospital Emergency Care Council as a paramedic and advanced paramedic in the United Kingdom and Ireland, respectively.

Sarah Eastwood (nee Lumley) BHSc (Hons) BNurs (Hons) PGradDip
Sarah began her paramedic career with Queensland Ambulance Service in Brisbane in 2012 while studying a double degree in paramedicine and nursing. Sarah then moved to Cairns upon qualifying as an advance care paramedic. Sarah undertook her postgraduate qualifications in paramedic science through Monash University and then completed her training as a critical care paramedic in 2021. Sarah also works as a flight care paramedic with the Queensland Ambulance Service. After working casually as an academic for Central Queensland University, Sarah recently accepted a lecturer position, where her main areas of interest are electrophysiology and clinical education. This is Sarah's first published writing.

Derek Fox MSc EMS
Derek is employed as a district officer/advanced paramedic and has been a member of Dublin Fire Brigade for 32 years. He currently holds a diploma in emergency medical technology from North-eastern University in the USA. He also holds a Graduate Diploma in Emergency Medical Science and a Masters (MSc) in emergency medical science, both from University College Dublin, giving him advanced paramedic status in Ireland. He is currently a facilitator and a national examiner for the Pre-Hospital Emergency Care Council. He has been involved in the training and 'on road' supervision of advanced paramedics and paramedics for Dublin Fire Brigade and emergency medical technicians for a private company.

Alexandra Gatehouse MCP ACCP (mFICM) Bsc (Hons) Physiotherapy NMP (V300)
Alex graduated from Nottingham University in 2000 with a Bsc (Hons) in physiotherapy. Following junior rotations in the Newcastle Hospitals NHS Foundation Trust she specialised in respiratory physiotherapy in adult critical care, also working in New Zealand. In 2012, she trained as an advanced critical care practitioner, completing a Masters in clinical practice in critical care and qualifying in 2014. Alex subsequently completed her non-medical prescribing qualification and continues to rotate within all of the critical care units in Newcastle Upon Tyne, also enjoying teaching on the regional transfer course. She is a co-founder of the Advanced Critical Care Practitioner Northern Region Group and is a committee member of the North East Intensive Care Society. Alex has presented abstracts at the European Society of Intensive Care Medicine and the North East Intensive Care Society conferences.

Ashley Ingram BSc (Hons) MCPara
Ashley began his career with South Western Ambulance Foundation Trust as an ambulance care assistant. Over the space of seven years, he worked his way up to a registered paramedic, training while working full time. He worked as an ambulance paramedic for three years, during which time he took a keen interest in palliative and end-of-life care. He has recently embarked on a primary care role as a frailty practitioner. Working within a multidisciplinary team, he focuses on admission avoidance with patients who reside in care homes in Dorset, UK. He looks forward to developing this role in the future.

Noleen P. Jones RN RNT Adv Dip in Leadership and Management BSc Nursing Med FHEA
Noleen's nursing background is mainly in critical care, where she worked for 26 years. During that period, she additionally held the posts of senior sister and lead nurse for education and training before moving onto clinical practice development for the Gibraltar Health Authority. This role enhanced her interest in education. She increasingly taught on the pregraduate nursing programmes, leading on to her undertaking a teaching and learning course and moving into teaching fulltime. Noleen is also a basic life support and moving and handling instructor for the organisation. Noleen is Principal Lecturer (Ag) at the Gibraltar Health Authority School of Health Studies. Noleen teaches in the BSc and diploma and access (adult) nursing courses at the University of Gibraltar. Her key interests include cardiac and respiratory care, simulation and teaching practice skills.

Kylie Kendrick BNurs BSc Paramedicine Registered Paramedic GC.paramedicine MPH PhD(C) FHEA
Kylie joined Rural Ambulance Victoria in 2008, working as a clinical mentor until transitioning into higher education. Kylie has undertaken a Master's in public health. Her research investigated the sleep health in undergraduate students. She has now transitioned to a PhD, where her research remains relevant to sleep health, although she has moved to the paramedic cohort. Kylie has undertaken a variety of roles in higher education, including programme development and accreditation, and has received citations for outstanding contributions to student learning through innovative practice.

Ian Macleod BParamedicSc DipVET Dip WHS

Ian is a career paramedic with 20 years' experience in a range of operational contexts and leadership roles. He has a strong passion for facilitating quality training and development for students and colleagues. Ian lives in South Australia with his supportive paramedic wife Stacey and 10-year-old stepson Levi. In addition to paramedicine, Ian works in mines and industrial fire and rescue and training content writing, and is an accredited rock-climbing guide. While currently engaged as a remote area paramedic in outback South Australia, Ian is completing a Master of Medical and Health Science through research, concentrating on virtual reality as a pedagogical platform for mass casualty triage training. He retains a strong interest in emergency and disaster management. At home, Ian has an extensive LEGO collection, enjoys four-wheel-driving, camping and trailbike riding.

Tom E. Mallinson BSc (Hons) MBChB PGCHE MRCGP MCPara MCoROM FHEA FAWM FRGS

Tom initially trained as a paramedic with the University of Hertfordshire and the London Ambulance Service NHS Trust before completing his medical degree at the University of Warwick. He is currently a prehospital care doctor and rural GP in Scotland. Tom is also Co-Director of Prehospital Care with BASICS Scotland and a lecturer in remote paramedic practice for the College of Remote and Offshore Medicine, Malta.

Tim Millington BSc (Hons) Paramedic Science BSc (Hons) Physiology/Pharmacology MSc Advance Clinical Practice

Tim began working as a paramedic at Doncaster Ambulance station in 2009.He went on to establish himself in a busy emergency department in Rotherham, working throughout the COVID-19 pandemic as an advanced clinical practitioner and non-medical prescriber. He is presently a PHD candidate with the University of Hertfordshire. He has a research interest in resuscitation and has published work in the *Journal of Paramedic Practice*. He is also an experienced advanced life support instructor with the Resuscitation Council UK. He currently works as a consultant paramedic practitioner with the Yorkshire Ambulance Service NHS Trust and an advanced clinical practitioner in emergency medicine with Rotherham Hospital Foundation Trust.

Ian Peate OBE FRCN

Ian began his nursing career at Central Middlesex Hospital, becoming an enrolled nurse practising in an intensive care unit. He later undertook three years of student nurse training at Central Middlesex and Northwick Park hospitals, becoming a staff nurse and then a charge nurse. He has worked in nurse education since 1989. His key areas of interest are nursing practice and theory. Ian has published widely. He is editor in chief of the British Journal of Nursing, founding consultant editor of the Journal of Paramedic Practice and consultant editor International Journal for Advancing Practice. Ian was awarded an OBE for his services to nursing and nurse education and was granted a fellowship from the Royal College of Nursing. Ian is visiting professor at Northumbria University, St George's University of London and Kingston University London, professorial fellow Roehampton University and visiting senior clinical fellow at the University of Hertfordshire.

Rory Prevett GDip BSc (Hons) Dip NQEMT AP

Rory began his prehospital paramedic career in 2004, becoming a firefighter/paramedic with Dublin Fire Brigade. He later undertook a postgraduate diploma with University College Dublin to become an advanced paramedic, winning the Pantridge Award for academic excellence. With a keen interest in education and training, he became an instructor for International Trauma Life Support, Ireland, and a member of the teaching faculty for International Trauma Life Support Dublin Fire Brigade/Royal College of Surgeons in Ireland. He has a deep interest in airway management. He has in the past sat on the statutory regulator (PHECC) Medical Advisory Committee and was a prehospital governance assessor for Pre-Hospital Emergency Care Council. He currently holds the position of Chief Practitioner for the Order of Malta Ambulance Corps, Ireland, and was previously the clinical manager for Medicore Private Ambulance Service, Dublin.

Liam Rooney BSc (Hons) GDip Dip NQEMT-AP

Liam has worked as a firefighter/paramedic since 2007, when he completed his Diploma in Emergency Medical Technology – Paramedic with the Royal College of Surgeons, Ireland. In 2016, he completed a BSc (Hons) in Paramedic Studies at the University of Limerick, winning the Graduate Entry Medical School Award for overall performance. In 2017, he undertook a graduate Diploma in Emergency Medical Science through University College Dublin. Liam currently practices as an advanced paramedic with Dublin Fire Brigade. He joined the faculty of DX2 Institute of Pre-Hospital Education in 2017, where he delivers multiple courses in prehospital education, and is also a tutor at University College Dublin. He has a keen interest in geriatric medicine and pain management in dementia patients.

Simon Sawyer PhD, BPara, BPsychMan/Mar, GCHPE

Simon has worked as an advanced life support paramedic in Victoria, Australia, since 2012. He began designing and teaching paramedic programmes as a lecturer at Monash University in 2015. Simon holds an adjunct senior lecturer position with the Paramedicine Department at Griffith University, where he studies family and domestic violence, paramedic education and paramedic wellbeing. Simon completed a PhD on the paramedic response to family violence and teaches paramedics how to respond to patients experiencing family and domestic violence. Simon is currently the Director of Education at the Australian Paramedical College and still works as a paramedic.

Melanie Stephens BSc (Hons) MA PGCAP PhD

Melanie commenced her career at Manchester Royal Infirmary in 1991 as a registered general nurse and is currently a senior lecturer in adult nursing within the School of Health and Society. Melanie is a health and social care researcher with specific research interests in pressure redistributing properties of seating, tissue viability, and interprofessional working and learning. She has undertaken research to provide an evidence base for products used in the 24-hour management of pressure ulcers and affective domain development of student nurses. Melanie co-led an amendment to the UK Tissue Viability Society seating guidelines with service users and is using this work to impact policy and practice. She is currently leading a feasibility study on the impact of interprofessional student training care homes on residents, care home staff and students. Experienced in mixed methods of enquiry, working with practitioners and commerce to develop research for the use in the clinical environment.

Scott Stewart PhD(VU) MBus(VU) DipHealthSci(AOTC) DipEd(Monash) BSc (Monash) MACPara Registered Paramedic

Scott dabbled in zoology before working as a biology and maths teacher in a secondary school and then joining Ambulance Victoria in 1992. Scott's Master's research evaluated customer satisfaction in ambulance services while his PhD focused on the teaching of evidence-based practice. He has lectured in paramedicine at Monash University, Victoria University, St George's University of London and is currently paramedicine national professional practice lead and senior lecturer at the Australian Catholic University. Scott was involved in the Gibraltar Ambulance Service transitioning to paramedic level and was a consultant for the South East Coast Ambulance Service, UK, on the development of a critical care paramedic level. He is currently engaged in developing the Timor-Leste ambulance service. Scott is a member of the Global Paramedic Higher Education Council.

Matt Wilkinson BP(H1) PhD(C)

Matt is a practicing emergency paramedic and medical researcher. He is currently a Westpac Scholar and inaugural University of Melbourne MDHS PhD Award recipient, and his undergraduate thesis won a University Medal and Best Presentation at two international medical conferences. As well as working clinically, he also tutors Indigenous undergraduates. He lives on the Sunshine Coast with his partner and their beautiful golden retriever puppy (called Waffles).

Aimee Yarrington FCPara BSc (Hons) MSc

Aimee has been a qualified midwife since 2003. She has worked in all areas of midwifery practice, from high-risk consultant-led units to low-risk stand-alone midwife-led units. She left full-time midwifery practice to join the ambulance service, starting as an emergency care assistant and working her way up to paramedic, while always keeping her midwifery practice up to date. She has worked in several areas within the ambulance service, including the emergency operations centre and the education and training department. Her work towards improving the education of prehospital maternity care has led to her being awarded a fellowship award from the College of Paramedics. Aimee strives to improve the teaching and education for clinicians dealing with prehospital maternity care.

David Yore GDip Dip NQEMT P

David has a background in paramedicine and more recently in education and training. He has developed a keen interest in research and professional development. He began working in the field in 2016 and has since progressed to work in a statutory emergency ambulance service following the completion of a diploma in paramedical science from University College Cork, Ireland. David is undertaking a Master's in specialist paramedic practice and hopes to continue his research, particularly in the areas of paramedicine and prehospital care.

About the Editors

Ian Peate OBE FRCN

Ian began his nursing career at Central Middlesex Hospital, becoming an enrolled nurse practising in an intensive care unit. He later undertook three years of student nurse training at Central Middlesex and Northwick Park hospitals, becoming a staff nurse and then a charge nurse. He has worked in nurse education since 1989. His key areas of interest are nursing practice and theory. Ian has published widely. He is editor in chief of the British Journal of Nursing, founding consultant editor of the Journal of Paramedic Practice and consultant editor International Journal for Advancing Practice. Ian was awarded an OBE for his services to nursing and nurse education and was granted a fellowship from the Royal College of Nursing. Ian is visiting professor at Northumbria University, St George's University of London and Kingston University London, professorial fellow Roehampton University and visiting senior clinical fellow at the University of Hertfordshire.

Simon Sawyer PhD, BPara, BPsychMan/Mar, GCHPE

Simon has worked as an advanced life support paramedic in Victoria, Australia, since 2012. He began designing and teaching paramedic programmes as a lecturer at Monash University in 2015. Simon holds an adjunct senior lecturer position with the Paramedicine Department at Griffith University, where he studies family and domestic violence, paramedic education and paramedic wellbeing. Simon completed a PhD on the paramedic response to family violence and teaches paramedics how to respond to patients experiencing family and domestic violence. Simon is currently the Director of Education at the Australian Paramedical College and still works as a paramedic.

We are delighted to have been asked to edit this new text *Fundamentals of Applied Pathophysiology for Paramedics*. There are 19 chapters in the text, a systems approach has been generally adopted. This textbook offers readers an introduction to pathophysiology related to the paramedic setting in a variety of academic programmes at colleges, universities or a vocational setting. Key disorders are described, together with a number of additional conditions that provide information on diseases with distinguishing features for each.

The *Fundamentals of Applied Pathophysiology for Paramedics* has been written by experienced clinicians and academics, primarily for the student undertaking programmes of study that are related to paramedic practice, with the aim of making the subject understandable, stimulating and related to your work as a paramedic. The human body has an amazing capacity to respond to illness in a number of physiological and psychological ways; humans are able to compensate as a result of the changes that occur due to the disease and pathophysiological processes, and the impact that they can have on a person. The *Fundamentals of Applied Pathophysiology for Paramedics* can assist in developing the paramedic's critical thinking, encouraging innovation and creativity related to the health and wellbeing of the people to whom you offer care and support. Critical thinking and clinical reasoning will lead to correct clinical judgements and practice; they are fundamental requirements in paramedicine.

Pathophysiology addresses the cellular and organ changes occurring when disease is present, as well as the impact that these changes can have on a person's ability to function. When there is an interruption to normal physiological functioning (e.g. illness), this becomes a pathophysiological issue. It has to be remembered that normal health is not and will never be exactly the same in any two people, because of this the term 'normal' has to be treated with caution. An understanding of pathophysiological 'normal' and 'abnormal' can assist when helping the patient in a competent, compassionate, safe and effective manner. The *Fundamentals of Applied Pathophysiology for Paramedics* is a foundation text, helping the reader to grow personally and professionally concerning the provision of care. It is primarily intended for those who come into contact with people who may present with physical health problems in various settings. The text focuses on the adult person. Illness and disease are discussed explicitly, highlighting the fact that people do become ill and they do experience disease.

The *Fundamentals of Applied Pathophysiology for Paramedics* considers diseases, their aetiology and acquired diseases. Chapters address signs and symptoms, investigations and diagnosis, with the purpose of revealing the cause of the signs and symptoms to make a diagnosis. Another important part of the pathophysiology is the prescription of any treatment that the paramedic is required to provide and administer. To do this effectively, it is essential that you have a sound knowledge of pathophysiology. Pathophysiology also allows the paramedic to offer a prognosis, referring to a patient's chance of survival or recovery; depending on the disease, the prognosis can be a full recovery, partial recovery, or fatal.

The early chapters help to prepare the reader for some of the more complex discussions that are to follow. Chapters commence and conclude with questions that aim to trigger reflection and encourage further thought. In the snapshots (case studies), pseudonyms are used to maintain confidentiality. Where appropriate, we have included boxed information that will help you when you are offering care and support to people. Red flags are also incorporated; these flags contain significant information warning you to be cautious in your approach. Orange flags alert the reader to psychological considerations and information concerning the management of medicines as related to the chapter. The snapshots generally include data concerning the patient's vital signs, control and dispatch information, pertinent background information, a 'windscreen' report and an ABCDE approach. These elements can help to relate important concepts to care, offering more insight into the patient's condition and therefore to their needs. This approach has been taken to help you to in learn as you apply the concepts being discussed.

We encourage you to ask questions such as 'Why is the patient experiencing this?', 'Why are they, all of a sudden, experiencing this change?', 'What do we need to do to help this patient?', 'Is this an emergency?' and then to go on and answer these questions. When you are able to understand what is going on in a person's body at the cellular level, you will be helped to understand it. Understanding pathophysiology and pathophysiological changes can help you as you respond and react to abnormal changes in patients in a faster, more accurate way. This understanding can make a significant difference in your role as a paramedic and to positive patient care outcomes.

We do not expect you to read the *Fundamentals of Applied Pathophysiology for Paramedics* from cover to cover; you are instead encouraged to dip in and out of it. The aim is to invite you in and encourage you; to stimulate your appetite, so you may read and learn further. We truly hope that you enjoy reading the text and applying it to practice situations. We hope that you will enjoy studying the topics that have been presented so as to encourage you to delve deeper. We also wish to stimulate you with a sense of curiosity with enthusiasm, ensuring that the patient is at the centre of all that you do and that the care you offer is safe, effective and appropriate.

Ian Peate
Simon Sawyer

Acknowledgements

Ian would like to thank his partner Jussi Lahtinen for his ongoing encouragement.

Simon would like to thank Ian for the opportunity to collaborate in this project.

We would like to thank the team at Wiley for their enthusiasm, encouragement and support.

CHAPTER 1

Learning the Language: Terminology

Ian Peate

AIM

This chapter aims to provide insight and understanding with regards to the terminology used in the provision of healthcare related to anatomy, physiology and pathophysiology.

LEARNING OUTCOMES

On completion of this chapter, you will be able to:

- Discuss the terms anatomy, physiology and pathophysiology.
- Describe the prefixes and suffixes used in anatomy, physiology and pathophysiology.
- Explain the directional terms used in medicine.
- Describe the anatomical planes and anatomical regions of the body, and the body cavities.

Test Your Prior Knowledge

1. What do you understand by the term *pathology*?
2. What is the difference between a sign and a symptom?
3. How is the root word altered by a prefix or a suffix?
4. What are the contents of the thoracic cavity?

Introduction

Science, and particularly the provision of healthcare, is replete with Latin and Greek terminology. Latin names are used for all parts of the body and Greek terms are also common (the Greeks are said by many to be the founders of modern medicine). Paramedics and other healthcare staff use pathophysiological concepts as they work with people to whom they offer care and may be experiencing some type of health condition or disease.

Fundamentals of Applied Pathophysiology for Paramedics, First Edition. Edited by Ian Peate and Simon Sawyer.

Red Flag Alert: Jargon

Like any country with its own language, the medical field also has its own jargon. This is important so communication between healthcare professionals can take place quickly and efficiently without the need for too much explanation. It is a specific language that is not just used by paramedics, nurses, doctors and other people who are actively involved in the medical arena but is also important for all others who work in the healthcare arena (e.g. pharmacists, physiologists and dentists). Its correct use can have a significant impact on ensuring the best patient care.

What is important is that we are all speaking the same language; failure to do so or making assumptions can lead to error and mistakes.

Anatomy and Physiology

Anatomy discusses the study of the structure and location of body parts, while physiology is the study of the function of body parts. Both these terms are interlinked. Understanding where the body parts are located can help you to understand how they function. As an example, McGuiness (2021) explains that the various functions of the heart and the four chambers, together with the valves, make up the anatomy. Visualising these many structures can assist in understanding how blood flows through the heart and how the heart beats; this is related to its function and is its physiology.

Anatomy

The Body Map

Learning anatomical terminology is like learning a new language. Developing your learning, understanding more and adding different terms to your vocabulary can help you to talk confidently about the body. The anatomical directional terms and body planes present a universally recognised language of anatomy. When undertaking the study of anatomy and physiology, it is essential that you have key or directional terminology so that you are able to give a precise description as you or others refer to the precise location of a body part or structure.

Reflective Learning Activity

When you are next on placement, identify how many times during a shift you hear the various clinicians describe and discuss the anatomy, physiology and pathophysiology of a patient. Note the terminology being used and how there is a clearer understanding between the team when using one language – anatomical and physiological terminology.

All parts of the body are described in relation to other body parts and a standardised body position known as the anatomical position is used in anatomical terminology. An anatomical position is established from a central imaginary line that runs down the centre or mid-line of the body. When in this position, the body is erect and it faces forwards, with the arms to the side, palms face forwards with the thumbs to the side, the feet are slightly apart with the toes pointing forwards (Figure 1.1).

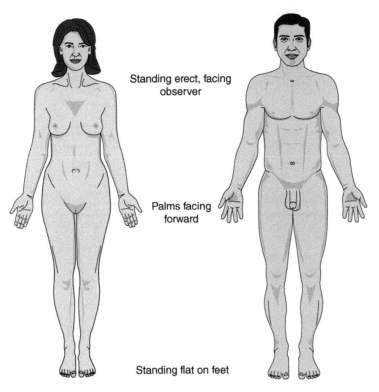

Standing erect, facing observer

Palms facing forward

Standing flat on feet

FIGURE 1.1 Anatomical position.

Orange Flag Alert: Speaking with Patients

While you are encouraged to use the correct anatomical and physiological terminology when conversing with other colleagues, caution must be exercised when speaking in front of and with patients. Paramedics can inadvertently use words and jargon that are strange to patients; they may not realise that the meaning is not clear. While there are some concepts that are familiar and obvious to paramedics, these same concepts may be alien to patients.

Try first to establish what the patient knows and understands before you launch into a discussion that begins at a level that is either too complex or too simple for the patient. Too often, our healthcare environments fail to recognise the needs of people with different levels of understanding about their health. This can mean that patients fail to receive the right care at the right time.

Use of jargon can instil fear, cause confusion and result in poor patient care.

The standard body 'map' or anatomical position (just like a map) is that of the body standing upright (orientated with the north at the top), with the feet at shoulder width and parallel, toes forward (Figure 1.1). Humans are bilaterally symmetrical. The standard position is used to describe body parts and positions of patients irrespective of whether they are lying down, lying on their side or facing down.

As well as understanding the anatomy and the physiology (the structure and function), understanding directional terms and the position of the various structures is also required. Table 1.1 lists common anatomical descriptive terms that you will need to become acquainted with. This list is not exhaustive, you will come across additional terms as you work through the various chapters. Figure 1.2 depicts anatomical positions.

TABLE 1.1   Anatomical descriptive terms.

Anatomical term	Relationship to the body
Anterior	Front surface of the body or structure
Posterior	Back surface of the body or structure
Deep	Further from the surface
Superficial	Close to the surface
Internal	Nearer the inside
External	Nearer the outside
Lateral	Away from the mid-line
Median	Mid-line of the body
Medial	In the direction of the mid-line
Superior	Located above or towards the upper part
Inferior	Located below or towards the lower part
Proximal	Nearest to the point of reference
Distal	Furthest away from the point of reference
Prone	Lying face down in a horizontal position
Supine	Lying face up in a horizontal position

4

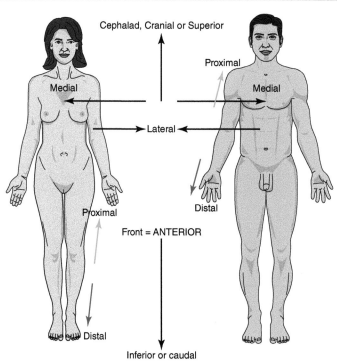

FIGURE 1.2   Anatomical positions.

Snapshot 1.1

You are on a call to a nursing home for a 70-year-old man who is dysphasic.

Pre-arrival Information

The patient is conscious and breathing.

Windscreen Report

The area outside the nursing home looks safe. There is an ambulance parking bay available close to the main door.

Entering the Location

As you arrive, a member of staff greets you; he is waiting at the door. He tells you that the patient was experiencing dysphagia and struggling to swallow his breakfast then he suddenly dropped his spoon. You are told that this is unusual for the patient, as he normally enjoys his breakfast and eats without any assistance.

On Arrival with the Patient

The patient has been put in the left lateral position in the communal dining area with a pillow supporting his head. You explain to the patient what you are doing using terminology that he will understand.

Patient Assessment

General appearance: The patient is alert and conscious, and he appears to be slumped to the left-hand side as if he has a left-sided hemiparesis. He is dysphasic.
Circulation to the skin: pale.
Work of breathing: normal.

Primary Survey

Danger: nil.
Response: alert on the ACVPU (alert, confusion, voice, pain, unresponsive) scale.
Airway: open, clear and patent.
Breathing: rate – appears normal rate (18 breaths/minute); there is no evidence of tachypnoea or dyspnoea. Rhythm – regular. Quality – bilateral equal air entry with chest rise and fall.
Circulation:
- Heart rate feels slightly tachycardic.
- Rhythm – irregular.
- Quality – palpable radial pulse.
- Skin: normal skin temperature, taken with a tympanic thermometer.
- Capillary refill time: two seconds. No evidence of cyanosis.

Disability:
- PEARL: normal pupil size.
- GCS: E4, V3, M6 = 13/15.
- Grip strength: weakness in left-hand side.
- Allergies: penicillin.

Exposure: appropriate for vital signs.

Environment

There is a chair and by patient's front door. Safety reassessed – nil danger.

Reflective Learning Activity

Look through the information provided in Snapshot 1.1 and highlight all of the information that is associated with anatomy, physiology and pathophysiology. Highlight and find the anatomical and physiological terms and determine the meaning.

Anatomical Planes of the Body

A plane is an imaginary two-dimensional surface that passes through the body. There are three planes that are generally referred to in anatomy and healthcare (Figure 1.3).

- Sagittal
- Frontal
- Transverse.

The *sagittal plane*, the vertical plane, is the plane that divides the body or an organ vertically into the right and left sides. If this vertical plane runs directly down the middle of the body, it is known as the midsagittal or median plane. If it divides the body into unequal right and left sides, then it is called a parasagittal plane.

The *frontal plane* is the plane dividing the body or an organ into an anterior (front) portion and a posterior (rear) portion. The frontal plane is often referred to as a coronal plane (the word *corona* is Latin for crown).

The *transverse plane* divides the body or organ horizontally into the superior (upper) and inferior (lower) portions.

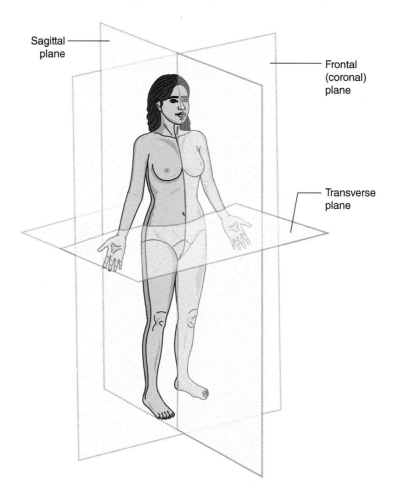

FIGURE 1.3   Anatomical planes.

Anatomical Regions of the Body

The body is divided up into regions, like a map. The anatomical regions of the body refer to a particular area/region of the body, which helps to compartmentalise. The body is divided into:

- the head and neck
- the trunk (thorax and abdomen)
- the upper limbs (arms)
- the lower limbs (legs).

See Tables 1.2–1.5 for a representation of the correct terminology for each region.

Body Cavities

Body cavities are spaces within the body that contain the internal organs (Figure 1.4). The cavity can be filled with air or with organs. Minor body cavities include the oral cavity (mouth), the nasal cavity (nose), the orbital cavity (eye), middle ear cavity and the synovial cavities (these are spaces within synovial joints).
There are two main cavities in the body:

- The dorsal cavity is located in the posterior region of the body.
- The ventral body cavity occupies the anterior region of the trunk.

The dorsal cavity is subdivided into two cavities:

1. The *cranial cavity* encloses the brain and is protected by the cranium (skull).
2. The vertebral/spinal cavity contains the spinal cord and is protected by the vertebrae.

The ventral cavity is subdivided into two:

1. The *thoracic cavity* is surrounded by the ribs and intercostal muscles, the thoracic cavity contains the lungs, heart, trachea, oesophagus and thymus. It is separated from the abdominal cavity by the diaphragm muscle.
2. The *abdominopelvic cavity* contains the stomach, spleen, liver, gallbladder, pancreas, small intestine and most of the large intestine:
   a. The *abdominal cavity* is protected by the muscles of the abdominal wall and partly by the diaphragm and ribcage.
   b. The *abdominopelvic cavity* contains the urinary bladder, some of the reproductive organs and the rectum. The pelvic cavity is protected by the bones of the pelvis.

TABLE 1.2 Anatomical regions of the head and neck.

Anatomical phrase	Area of body related to
Cephalic	Head
Cervical	Neck
Cranial	Skull
Frontal	Forehead
Occipital	Back of head
Ophthalmic	Eyes
Oral	Mouth
Nasal	Nose

TABLE 1.3 Anatomical regions of the trunk (thorax and abdomen).

Anatomical phrase	Area of body related to
Axilla	Armpit
Costal	Ribs
Mammary	Breast
Pectoral	Chest
Vertebral	Backbone
Abdominal	Abdomen
Gluteal	Buttocks
Inguinal	Groin
Lumbar	Lower back
Pelvic	Pelvis/lower part of abdomen
Umbilical	Navel
Perineal	Between anus and external genitalia
Pubic	Pubis

TABLE 1.4 Anatomical regions of the upper limbs.

Anatomical phrase	Area of body related to
Brachial	Upper arm
Carpal	Wrist
Cubital	Elbow
Forearm	Lower arm
Palmar	Palm
Digital	Fingers (also relates to toes)

Physiology

Human physiology is concerned with the study of the function of the body. Anatomy and physiology therefore relate to the study of the structure and the function of the human body.

The human body is organised in a most precise way, whereby atoms combine in appropriate ways forming molecules in the chemical organisation of the body. The molecules combine to form cells, and cells organise themselves collectively as functioning masses that are known as tissues and then organs and systems. Chapter 2 of this text describes cells and the organisation of tissues within the body.

TABLE 1.5 Anatomical regions of the lower limbs (legs).

Anatomical phrase	Area body related to
Femoral	Thigh
Patella	Front of knee
Pedal	Foot
Plantar	Sole of foot
Popliteal	Hollow behind knee
Digital	Toes (also relates to fingers)

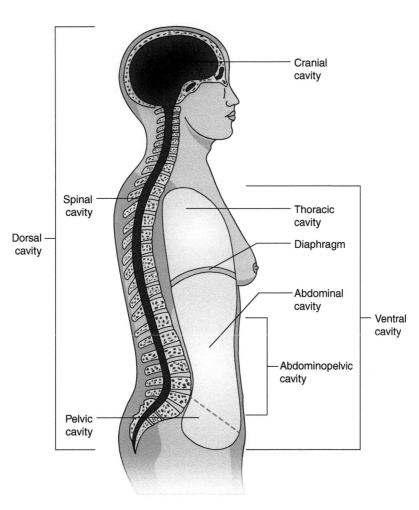

FIGURE 1.4 The cavities of the body.

Terminology

Already in this chapter, you may have come across some complex terms. It is important to learn the language (the terminology) that is used in the provision of healthcare, as it is an important part of safe and effective practice. While it is not a precourse requirement to be proficient in Latin or Greek to learn anatomical terminology before becoming a paramedic, it is essential that you understand and are able to use the terminology effectively.

There are three basic parts associated with medical terms (Table 1.6). The word root is the core of the word. It provides the basic meaning to the subject of the word. Prefixes and the suffixes modify the word. In the word 'hepatitis', for example, the word root is *hepa*, which means liver. When the suffix *itis* (which means inflammation) is added, the word changes and it becomes hepatitis – inflammation of the liver.

A prefix is added to the beginning of the word root and also changes the word. If the root word is *nutrition* and the prefix *mal* (meaning bad) is added, then malnutrition means bad or poor nutrition.

Look at this example:

> Hypothermia
>
> The word root is 'therm' (heat)

Hypo means low (this is the prefix), so hypothermia means low heat. Now take a look at this word: myocarditis – let's break it up:

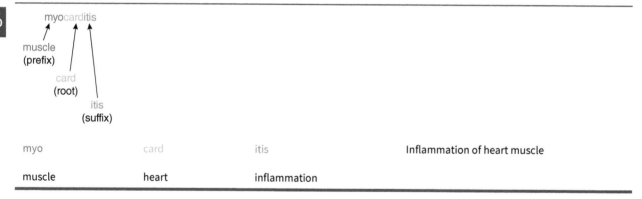

| myo | card | itis | Inflammation of heart muscle |
| muscle | heart | inflammation | |

The prefix can change the word:

> Myocarditis **myo** + carditis = inflammation of heart muscle.
> Endocarditis **endo** + carditis = inflammation of the inner layer of the heart.
> Pericarditis **peri** + carditis = inflammation of the outer layer of the heart.

TABLE 1.6   Basic components.

Component	Description
Word root	This is usually found the middle of the word and this is its central meaning
Prefix	The prefix comes at the beginning of the word and it usually identifies some subdivision or part of the central meaning
Suffix	Comes at the end and modifies the central meaning as to what or who is interacting with it or what is happening to it

The suffix can also alter the word:

Cardiologist cardi + ologist = a practitioner specialising in the heart.
Cardiomyopathy cardio + myopathy = damage to heart muscle.
Cardiomegaly cardio + megaly = enlargement of the heart.

In these examples, the prefix and suffix can change the word but, the root *card* stayed the same.

There are many frequently used prefixes and suffixes; you will already know some of them. See Table 1.7 for a list of some prefixes and suffixes that are used to make up a number of medical terms.

As is the case when learning any language, it can take time to learn all the words and, indeed, the learning will be lifelong. When you are in practice, you will be able to reinforce your learning, using your new vocabulary with confidence. Take your time, seek clarification if needed, and be patient with yourself.

Knowing the various anatomical terms can make it easier to understand the various pathophysiological concepts that can help you provide care that is patient centred, safe and effective.

Pathophysiology

Pathophysiology brings together a blend of pathology and physiology to consider the connection between disordered physiology and disease or illness. Pathology defines the illness itself and physiology examines how these injuries or diseases change natural biological processes. The study of pathophysiology requires the use of clinical reasoning, which is then used to make a diagnosis and prescribe treatment to address the effects of disease. Learning how pathology, physiology and anatomy interconnect can ensure that the care provided is appropriate, safe and effective.

Pathophysiology, according to Singh et al. (2017) is the study of the changes of normal mechanical, physical and biochemical functions, caused by a disease or resulting from an abnormal syndrome. The chapters in this text address these key pathophysiological concepts. Medical terminology is used to express and describe the various pathophysiological concepts.

Pathophysiology is a key component of paramedic practice. It enables the clinician to take on a number of important responsibilities, such as understanding and ordering diagnostic tests, care for and treating people with acute and chronic illnesses, managing medications and managing general health and wellbeing, as well as disease prevention for patients and their families. Paramedics and other healthcare practitioners who can recognise the pathophysiological signs and symptoms of the conditions in those to whom they offer care will be able to provide a higher quality of safer and more effective care. Asking questions such as 'Why is the person experiencing this?', helps to you to understand what is going on in a person's body at the cellular level, thus helping you to understand how to help them.

Pathophysiology is used to understand the progression of disease so as to identify the disease and implement treatment options for patients. Information gathered is used to identify the next course of the disease so that the most suitable course of action can be taken with the patient, with the appropriate care they need provided. The medical procedures and medications that are administered to patients will depend very much on the nature of the disease. The main objectives when understanding pathophysiology are to assist you to:

- Use critical thinking to understand the pathophysiological principles for care provision.
- Analyse and explain the effects of disease processes at a systemic and cellular level.
- Discuss the many variables that may be at play affecting the healing of the organ and tissue systems.
- Analyse the environmental risks of the progression and development of particular diseases.
- Explain how compensatory mechanisms can be used to make a response to physiological alterations.
- Compare and contrast the effects of culture, ethics and genetics and how these can have an impact on disease progression, treatment and health promotion, as well as disease prevention.
- Evaluate and review diagnostic tests and determine whether the evaluation and review have any relationship to the signs and symptoms that the patient is experiencing.

TABLE 1.7   Some prefixes, suffixes, their meaning and examples.

Prefix/suffix	Meaning	Example
a/an	No, not, without, lack of	Anoxia (without oxygen), anuria (without urine), asepsis (without sepsis), asymptomatic (without symptoms)
ab	Away from	Abduction (to move away from the midline), abnormal (away from normal)
ad	Towards	Adduction (to move towards the midline), adrenal (towards the kidney), addiction (drawn towards or a strong dependence on a drug or substance)
aemia	Of blood	Leukaemia (cancer of blood cells), anaemia (lack of red blood cells),
algia	Pain	Cephalgia (headache), mastalgia (breast pain), myalgia (muscle pain)
ante	Before/in front of	Antepartum (before birth), anterior (to the front of the body), anteprandial (before meals)
arthro	Joint	Arthroscope (an instrument used to look into a joint), arthritis (joint inflammation), arthrotomy (incision of a joint)
baro	Pressure/weight	Isobaric (having equal measure of pressure), bariatrics (the field of medicine that offers treatment to people who are overweight), baroreceptor (a sensor reacting to pressure changes)
brady	Slow/delayed	Bradycardia (slow heart rate), bradykinesia (slowness in movement), bradylalia (abnormally slow speech)
cyto	Cell	Leucocyte (white blood cell), erythrocyte (red cell), cytology (study and function of cells)
derm	Skin	Dermatitis (inflammation of the skin), dermatome (a surgical instrument used for cutting slices of the skin), dermatology (the study of skin)
dys	Difficulty/ impaired	Dysphasia (difficulty swallowing), dyspepsia (disordered digestion), dysuria (difficulty in urination)
ectomy	To cut out	Appendectomy (removal of the appendix), mastectomy (removal of the breast), prostatectomy (removal of the prostate)
endo	Inner	Endocardium (lining of the heart), endocarditis (inflammation of the heart), endotracheal (within the trachea)
erythro	Red	Erythrocyte (red blood cell), erythropaenia (reduction in the number of red blood cells), erythema (reddening of the skin)
haem	Blood	Haematogenesis (the formation of blood), haematology (the study of blood), haemarthrosis (bleeding within the joint)
hydro	Water	Hydrophobia (abnormal dread of water), hydrocephalus (accumulation of fluid within the cranium)
hyper	Above/beyond/ excessive	Hypertension (high blood pressure), hyperflexion (movement of a muscle beyond its normal limit), hyperglycaemia (high blood glucose)
hypo	Below/under/ deficient	Hypotension (low blood pressure), hypothermia (low temperature), hypoglycaemia (low blood glucose)

TABLE 1.7 (*Continued*)

Prefix/suffix	Meaning	Example
intra	Within	Intravenous (within the veins), intraocular (within the eye), intracerebral (within the brain)
ism	Condition/disease	Hirsutism (heavy/abnormal growth of hair), hyperthyroidism (overactivity of the thyroid gland)
itis	Inflammation	Appendicitis (inflammation of the appendix), mastitis (inflammation of the breast) myocarditis (inflammation of heart muscle)
osteo	Bone	Osteoporosis, (a condition that weakens the bones), osteopenia (a generalised reduction in bone mass), osteomalacia (pertaining to soft bones)
otomy	To cut into	Tracheotomy (cutting into the trachea), craniotomy (a hole made into the skull), thoracotomy (cutting into the chest)
ostomy	To make an opening (a mouth)	Colostomy (an opening into the colon), jejunostomy (an opening into the jejunum)
micro	Small	Microscopic (so small can only be seen with a microscope), microcephaly (small brain), microsomia (small body)
macro	Large	Macroscopic (large enough to be seen with the naked eye), macrocytic (an abnormally large cell), macroglossia (an abnormally large tongue)
mega/megaly	Enlarged	Cardiomegaly (enlarged heart), splenomegaly (enlarged spleen), hepatomegaly (enlarged liver)
myo	Muscle	Myocardium (heart muscle), myocyte (muscle cell), myometrium (uterine muscle)
neo	New	Neonate (new born), neoplasm (new growth [tumour]),
nephro	Kidney	Nephritis (inflammation of the kidneys), nephrostomy (an incision made into the kidney)
neuro	Nerve	Neuroma (a tumour growing from a nerve), neuralgia (pain felt along the length of a nerve), neuritis (inflammation of a nerve)
ology	Study of	Dermatology (study of the skin), neurology (study of the nervous system), cardiology (study of the heart)
oma	Tumour (swelling)	Melanoma (a cancer of melanocytes), carcinoma (a type of cancer), retinoblastoma (tumour of the eye)
ophth	Eye	Ophthalmology (study of the eye), ophthalmoscope (an instrument used to examine the inside of the eye), ophthalmotomy (an incision made into the eye)
osteo	Bone	Osteomyelitis (bone infection), osteosarcoma (bone cancer), osteoarthritis (inflammation of the joints)
oto	Ear	Otology (the study of the ear), otosclerosis (abnormal bone growth inside the ear)
patho	Disease	Neuropathy (disease of the nervous system), nephropathy (disease of the kidney), retinopathy (disease of the retina)

13

(*Continued*)

TABLE 1.7 (*Continued*)

Prefix/suffix	Meaning	Example
para	Beside/alongside	Para thyroid (adjacent to the thyroid), paraumbilical (alongside the umbilicus)
penia	Deficiency	Leucopoenia (deficiency of white cells), thrombocytopenia (deficiency of thrombocytes)
peri	Around	Pericardium, (the serous membrane around the heart) periosteum, (a covering enveloping the bones), peritoneum (the serous membrane lining the walls of the abdominal and pelvic cavities)
plasm	Substance	Plasma (liquid part of blood and lymphatic fluid), cytoplasm (substance of a cell lying outside of the nucleus)
plasty	Repair	Arthroplasty (surgical repair or replacement of a joint), myoplasty (surgical repair of a muscle)
pneumo	Breathing/air	Pneumonia (a type of chest infection), pneumothorax (a collapsed lung), pneumograph (a device used for recording respiratory movement)
poly	Many/much	Polycystic (many cysts), polyuria (much urine), polyarthritis (arthritis affecting more than four joints)
rhino	Nose	Rhinitis (inflammation of the mucous membrane of the nose), rhinoplasty (surgical repair of the nose)
rrhoea	Discharge	Diarrhoea (frequently discharged faeces), rhinorrhoea (excessive discharge of mucus from the nose), galactorrhoea (excessive production of breast milk)
sclero	Toughen/hard	Sclera (hard/tough layer of the eyeballs), scleroderma (hardening and contraction of the skin and connective tissue), sclerosis (abnormal hardening of body tissue)
sub	Under	Sublingual (underneath the tongue), subarachnoid (underneath the arachnoid [layer of the brain]), submucosa (tissue below mucus membrane)
tachy	Fast/rapid	Tachycardia (fast heart rate), tachypnoea (fast respiratory rate),
toxo	Poison	Cytotoxic (having a destructive action on cells), toxaemia (blood poisoning resulting from the presence of toxins), ototoxic (being toxic to the ear)
uria	Urine	Haematuria (presence of blood in the urine), nocturia (passing urine at night), pyuria (pus in the urine)
vaso	Vessel	Vaso constriction (narrowing of the vessel), vaso dilation (widening of the vessel), vaso spasm (sudden contraction of a vessel)

The Determinants of Health

While it is important to understand the pathophysiological changes that a patient may be experiencing, the healthcare provider must also appreciate the socioeconomic and cultural factors that can impact on patient outcomes. These 'non-medical' factors are as important as to whether the most appropriate test or diagnostic tool is being used or treatment implemented. It is important to understand the molecular and genetic determinants of disease; however, the non-biological factors have the potential to influence interactions with patients and their families.

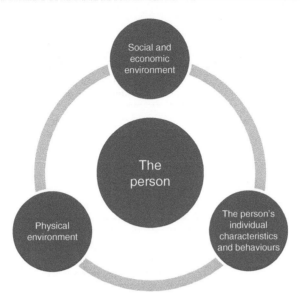

FIGURE 1.5 The determinants of health. Source: World Health Organization (2020).

There are many factors that come together to impact the health of individuals and communities. Regardless of whether people are healthy, health is determined by a person's circumstances and environment. To a large extent, factors such as where we live, the state of our environment, genetics, our income and education level, and our relationships with friends and family all have significant impacts on health. However, the more commonly considered factors, such as access and use of healthcare services may have less of an impact. The social determinants of health are outlined in Figure 1.5. The determinants of health include political, social, economic, environmental and cultural factors, which shape the conditions in which we are born, grow, live, work and age. Creating a healthy population requires greater action on these factors, not simply on treating ill health.

Using a Medical Dictionary, Hints and Tips

Learning to use a medical dictionary and other resources (be these electronic or hard copy) to help find the definition of a term is an important aspect of understanding the correct use of the numerous medical terms. When starting to work with an unfamiliar resource (print or otherwise), spend some time reviewing its user guide. The time spent at this stage can help later when you are looking up unfamiliar terms.

Accuracy in spelling medical terms is extremely important. Changing just one or two letters has the potential to completely change the meaning of a word and the consequences of this can be grave. Some frequently used terms and word parts are confusing because they look and sound alike however, their meanings are very different (Table 1.8). Beware, too, that you may encounter alternative spellings used in the United Kingdom, Australia, Ireland, Canada and the United States.

- If you know how to spell the word:
  - With the first letter of the word, start in the appropriate section of the dictionary. Look at the top of the page for clues (there may be catch words there). The top left word is the first term on the page and the top right word is the last term on that page.
  - Now, search alphabetically for words that begin with the first and second letters of the word you are searching for. Continue looking through each letter until you have found the term that you are looking for.
  - When you think you have found it, be sure to check the spelling, letter by letter, working from left to right. Terms with similar spellings have very different meanings (e.g. prostrate and prostate).
  - When the term has been located, carefully check all the definitions.

TABLE 1.8   Confusing terminology (Stansfield et al. 2015).

Term/word	Means	Comments
arteri/o	Artery	Endarterial means pertaining to the interior or lining of an artery (*end* means within, *arteri* means artery, and *al* means pertaining to)
ather/o	Plaque or fatty substance	An atheroma is a fatty deposit within the wall of an artery (*ather* means fatty substance and *oma* means tumour)
arthr/o	Joint	Arthralgia means pain in a joint or joints (*arthr* means joint and *algia* means pain)
-ectomy	Surgical removal	An appendectomy is surgical removal of the appendix (*append* means appendix and *ectomy* means surgical removal)
-ostomy	Surgical creation of an artificial opening to the body surface	A colostomy is the surgical creation of an artificial excretory opening between the colon and the body surface (*col* means colon, and *ostomy* means the surgical creation of an artificial opening)
-otomy	Cutting or a surgical incision	A colotomy is a surgical incision into the colon (*col* means colon, and *otomy* means a surgical incision)

- If you do not know how to spell the word:
  - Listen carefully to the term and then write it down.
  - If you cannot find the word on the basis of your spelling, begin to look for alternative spellings based on the beginning sound; for example, f can sound like f but, the word may begin with ph (such as pharynx, phlegm), k can sound like k but, the word may begin with ch (cholera for example) or c (crepitus). Psychologist begins with p but, it sounds like it should begin with an s.
- Look under categories:
  - Medical dictionaries may use categories, such as diseases and syndromes, and may group disorders with these terms in their titles: so venereal disease would be found under 'disease, venereal' and fetal alcohol syndrome would be found under 'syndrome, fetal alcohol'.
- Multiple-word terms:
  - When searching for a term that includes more than one word, begin the search with the last term. If you don't find it there, then move forward to the next word. Congestive heart failure, for example, is sometimes listed under 'heart failure, congestive'.

Searching for Definitions on the Internet and Handheld Devices

Internet search engines are helpful resources in locating definitions and details about medical conditions and terms. It is important, however, that you use a site such as the National Institute for Health and Care Excellence (known as NICE) or Scottish Intercollegiate Guidelines Network (known as SIGN), as these bodies are known to be reputable information sources.

Beware of suggested search terms. If you don't spell a term correctly, a website might take a guess at what it is that you are searching for. Be sure to double-check that the term you are defining is the term intended.

Take Home Points

- Use the appropriate anatomical terminology to identify key body structures, body regions and directions in the body.
- A standard reference position for mapping the body's structures is the normal anatomical position.
- The terminology used in anatomy, physiology and pathophysiology can be bewildering; however, the purpose of this language is not to confuse, but rather to increase precision and reduce errors.

- Anatomical terms are very often derived from Greek and Latin words.
- Anatomical terms are made up of roots, prefixes and suffixes.
- Without doubt, it is important to understand the pathophysiological changes that a patient may be experiencing. The paramedic must also appreciate the socioeconomic and cultural factors that can impact on patient outcomes – the determinants of health.
- Learning how to use a medical dictionary and other resources to find the definition of a term is an important aspect of understanding the correct use of the numerous medical terms. The time that is spent at this stage can help later when looking up any unfamiliar terms.

Medications Management: Name Confusion

Recent examples of medicine names that have been confused resulting in medication errors include:

- mercaptamine and mercaptopurine
- sulfadiazine and sulfasalazine
- risperidone and ropinirole
- zuclopenthixol decanoate and zuclopenthixol acetate

Some of these errors could result in life-threatening conditions.
Be extra vigilant when administering medicines with commonly confused drug names to ensure that the intended medicine is administered.

- Human factors can be associated in recognising medications of similar names with similar packaging, such as 500mL bags of fluids (e.g. dextrose 50% and dextrose 10%).
- Adhere to local professional guidance in relation to checking the right medicine.

Summary

Medical terminology may appear intimidating and complicated. A number of terms used in healthcare and medicine are derived from Latin and Greek. To understand the terminology used, it is essential when learning to break it down into its parts. When this is done, you can see how it all fits together – like the carriages of a train. In translating medical terms, it is important to understand the word root. The word root (the foundation of the term) can have a prefix and suffix attached to it.

To communicate safely with other healthcare professionals, it is imperative that there is a consistency in the language being used so as to reduce any risk of confusion. Learning the language requires practice.

It is vital to understand the pathophysiological changes that a patient may be experiencing so as to provide the most appropriate care intervention. It is equally important to have an understanding of the impact of socioeconomic and cultural factors that can impact on patient outcomes – the 'non-medical' factors.

References

McGuiness, H. (2021). *Anatomy and Physiology: Therapy basics*. London: Hodder Education.

Singh, I., Weston, A., Kundur, A., and Dobie, G. (2017). *Haematology Case Studies with Blood Cell Morphology and Pathophysiology*. London: Academic Press.

Stansfield, P., Hui, Y.H., and Cross, N. (2015). *Essential Medical Terminology*, 4e. Chicago, IL: Jones and Bartlett.

World Health Organization (2020). Health impact assessment. https://www.who.int/health-topics/health-impact-assessment#tab=tab_1 (accessed 27 September 2023).

Further Reading

Lysanets, Y.V. and Bieliaieva, O.M. (2018). The use of Latin terminology in medical case reports: quantitative, structural, and thematic analysis. *Journal of Medical Case Reports* 12: 45. http://dx.doi.org/10.1186/s13256-018-1562-x.

Online Resources

Health Information and Quality Authority. Safer better care. www.hiqa.ie (accessed 27 September 2023).
National Institute for Health and Care Excellence. www.nice.org.uk
NHS England (2022). Abbreviations you may find in your health records. https://www.nhs.uk/using-the-nhs/nhs-services/the-nhs-app/abbreviations (accessed 27 September 2023).

Glossary

Acute disease	Sudden appearance of signs and symptoms that last a short time.
Aetiology	Study of the cause(s) of disease and/or injury.
Chronic disease	Develops more slowly, lasting a long time or a lifetime.
Clinical manifestations	Also known as signs and symptoms.
Diagnosis	The naming or identification of a disease.
Exacerbations	Periods when clinical manifestations become worse or more severe.
Iatrogenic	Diseases and/or injury that occur as a result of medical (or paramedical) intervention.
Idiopathic	Diseases with no identifiable cause.
Nosocomial	Diseases that are acquired as a consequence of being in a hospital environment.
Pathology	Study of structural alterations in cells, tissues and organs that help to identify the cause of disease.
Pathogenesis	Pattern of tissue changes that are associated with the development of disease.
Prognosis	Expected outcome of a disease.
Remissions	Periods when clinical manifestations disappear or diminish significantly.
Sequelae	Any abnormal conditions that follow on and are the result of a disease, treatment or injury.

Multiple Choice Questions

1. A vasectomy is:
    a. The surgical removal of the vagal nerve
    b. The surgical cutting and sealing of part of each vas deferens
    c. A medical procedure that causes infertility
    d. A specific test to determine the diameter of a vein

2. Lymphoedema refers to:
   a. Removal of lymph glands in the neck
   b. Removal of lymph glands in the groin
   c. A chronic condition that causes swelling in the body's tissues
   d. Infection of the lymph nodes located in the thorax

3. Abduct:
   a. Is the same as adduct
   b. Means to pull away from the body
   c. Relates to the torso only
   d. Is to pull towards the body

4. What is the difference between the words afferent and efferent?
   a. Afferent means 'bringing to or leading towards an organ or part' and efferent 'conveys or conducts away from an organ or part'.
   b. Afferent means 'conveys or conducts away from an organ or part' and efferent means 'bringing to or leading towards an organ or part'.
   c. Afferent is associated with the kidney only and efferent is associated with the brain only.
   d. None of the above.

5. The term xerosis means
   a. Liver disease
   b. Abnormal dryness, as seen in the eyes, skin or mouth
   c. Excessive and abnormal production of mucous
   d. Depleted production of mucous

6. What are determinants of health:
   a. They are the measures that are used by physiotherapists to determine prognosis
   b. Determinants of health are only applicable in low income countries
   c. The determinants of health include: the social and economic environment, the physical environment and; the person's individual characteristics and behaviours
   d. All of the above

7. The sagittal plane:
   a. Divides the body top and bottom
   b. Divides the abdomen only left and right
   c. Divides the contents of thoracic cavity top and bottom only
   d. Divides the body or an organ vertically into the left and tight sides

8. The word corona is Latin for:
   a. Halo
   b. Neck
   c. Heart
   d. Crown

9. The prefix is added to:
   a. The end of the second letter of a sentence
   b. The beginning of a word
   c. The end of a word
   d. Words beginning with a vowel only

10. Pathophysiology is:
    a. Another term for renal failure
    b. A mental health disorder
    c. The study of functional changes in the body occurring in response to disease or injury
    d. All of the above

19

CHAPTER 2

Cell and Body Tissue Physiology

Terry Dore and Ian Peate

AIM

This chapter aims to provide insight and understanding regarding cells and tissue physiology.

LEARNING OUTCOMES

On completion of this chapter you will be able to:

- Outline the structure and functioning of human a human cell.
- List organelles and describe their function within the cell.
- Explain the transport system within a cell.
- Explain cell mitosis and meiosis.
- Describe the ageing process.

Test Your Prior Knowledge

1. What is the basic structural and functional unit of all living organisms?
2. What are the four primary types of tissue in the human body? Provide examples of each.
3. What is the role of red blood cells in the body, and what is their primary function?
4. What is the difference between voluntary and involuntary muscle tissue, and where can each be found in the body?

Introduction

Understanding of the normal function of the human body necessitates knowledge of the basic building blocks of all tissues. Atoms form molecules, which form into cellular organelles. Cellular organelles form the structures within the cell, facilitating its ability to function by synthesising chemical reactions to produce energy, and producing proteins and

Fundamentals of Applied Pathophysiology for Paramedics, First Edition. Edited by Ian Peate and Simon Sawyer.

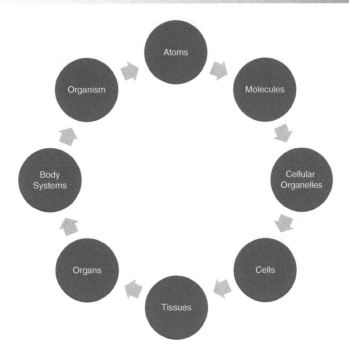

FIGURE 2.1 The cell cycle.

other products to facilitate reproduction. Similar cells form tissues and similar tissues form organs that group together to work as body systems (Figure 2.1).

Cell Anatomy and Function

To understand illness and disease processes, we must understand cellular anatomy and function. All organisms are composed of cells, irrespective of species or size. The constituent parts of cells are similar in all living organisms, such as their chemical composition and the complex biochemical reactions that take place to facilitate their existence. Cells are formed primarily from elements of carbon, oxygen, nitrogen and hydrogen. Cells function independently and collectively as tissue and organs. They are the fundamental structural units of the body that facilitate body function. There may be many cells with very different functions and characteristics (e.g. size, shape or purpose) which share similar traits. This is known as cell theory and stipulates that all organisms are made from cells and their products. Different living organisms share similarities in their cellular characteristics, abilities and structures. Shared cellular characteristics include:

- Cells can carry out active functions.
- Cells need fuel and oxygen to produce energy and take this fuel into the cells via the process of endocytosis.
- Cells can grow and repair themselves if damaged.
- They can engulf and consume bacteria and other pathogens.
- Cells can reproduce themselves via a process called simple fission. This is achieved when full-size cells divide into two, thus replicating themselves, a process that is reproduced many times.
- Cells may be acted upon or stimulated and may cease to function at optimal levels.
- Cells do not always use all the energy they ingest via endocytosis and release what they do not use.
- Cells take in raw material, which is used to store and release energy. This stored energy is used to enable the cell to grow and repair itself.
- At the end of their lifespan all cells will die. Some have a long lifespan and others very short, but all eventually die. When cells die, the organism eventually also dies – this is the circle of life.

Cells have a complex structure, which mirrors the organisms they form, having as many molecules as the human body itself has cells. It has a membrane-bound protoplasm that contains the many living parts of the cell. Within this membrane, organelles perform specific cellular functions to keep the cell alive and to perform its various functions.

The Cell Membrane

The cell membrane or plasma membrane encompasses all the contents of the cell within a flexible bilipid double membranous fold. The flexibility of the membrane allows for rapid change as the cell grows, divides and is imposed upon by adjacent cells. It has a phospholipid bilayer with a hydrophilic (water loving) head and a lipophilic (fat loving) hydrophobic (water hating) tail. The hydrophilic heads face outward peripherally into the extracellular environment and internally to the cytosol. As the heads are hydrophilic, they permit water to move freely into the bilayer, where they encounter the hydrophobic tails sealing the membrane to their free passage.

The membrane is composed of:

- Phospholipids
- Glycolipids
- Cholesterol.

The membrane has proteins expressed on its surface that perform different functions (e.g. anchoring the cell in the extracellular environment), recognition proteins and enzymes. Receptor proteins expressed externally also facilitate ligand gated ion channels, which permit ions to enter and leave the cell. Carrier proteins move solutes such as glucose, sodium, calcium and potassium across the membrane. Specialised channels composed of proteins traverse the central membrane, facilitating the movement of other solutes and water.

The membrane has many embedded proteins, both peripherally and deep within the bilayer, and has specialised channels for both active and passive transport. It offers protection and selectively permits nutrients, waste products, proteins and water into and out of the cell as it is *semi-permeable*. It controls the movement of water into and out of the cell through osmosis. Aquaporins facilitate transport of water through specialist water channels constructed of transmembrane proteins. These channels allow the free movement of water both into and out of the cell to achieve equilibrium. Equilibrium of water molecules is also dependent on the osmolarity, which is in turn dependent on the concentration of all solute particles within a given volume of solvent. Both the solute (dissolved particles) and solvent (water) must be in balance on both sides of the cell membrane and only then is equilibrium achieved. Osmolarity is expressed as osmoles per litre (osmol/l).

Passive Transport

The movement of materials into and out of the cell may occur via passive or active transport. *Passive transport* occurs during processes such as diffusion or osmosis, where substances move down their concentration gradient to achieve equilibrium. Energy is not expended by the cell in diffusion as substances use the intrinsic energy in the concentration gradient for particles to move from high to low concentration. In osmosis, water and any solutes dissolved in it move passively from areas of high to low concentration in the same manner. This process uses the intrinsic energy of the concentration gradient to facilitate equilibrium of both the water and its dissolved solutes until both are in balance.

Active Transport

Active transport encompasses processes such as active transport pumps, *endocytosis* and *exocytosis*. There are substances that may need to move against their concentration gradient from areas of low concentration to areas of high concentration. This may be achieved using active transport, which involves the use of energy from the cell in the form of adenosine triphosphate (ATP). Some examples of active transport are substances such as sodium, potassium, calcium and amino acids moving across the cell membrane both into and/or out of the cell.

Active transport of ions, in particular, uses solute pumps such as the sodium/potassium pump. This sodium/potassium pump moves $3 \times Na^+$ ions out of the cell and simultaneously moving $2 \times K^+$ into the cell – both against their concentration gradients. The energy to move these ions is derived from ATP. The molecule disassociates and loses a phosphate group, liberating energy in a process known as hydrolysis, forming a compound called adenosine diphosphate (ADP). The liberated phosphate molecule is chemically reattached within the cellular mitochondria to reform ADP to ATP.

Active transport may be primary or secondary, with primary transport deriving energy directly from ATP. Secondary active transport does not derive energy directly from ATP but takes it indirectly from active transport of other substances using the stored energy in ionic gradients. Glucose uses the transport of sodium into the cell by 'piggybacking' its entry into the cell via *symport proteins*. The sodium enters the cell using these proteins, which are energised by cellular ATP, and at the same time glucose uses this movement to facilitate its entry across the cell membrane, thus getting a free ride into the cell in the same direction as the sodium. Substances may also piggyback this secondary energy to move in the *opposite* direction, using carrier proteins using the antiport system. Secondary active transport is also known as 'coupled transport' as it couples up with primary active transport to reach its destination.

Endocytosis facilitates the movement of material into the cell across the cell membrane by processes such as:

- *Phagocytosis* – the cell ingests material such as pathogens or debris from dead cells in pseudopods when it encompasses and consumes them. This pseudopod breaks away from the membrane internally to become a phagosome, which is broken down by organelles such as lysosomes.
- *Pinocytosis* – the cell consumes a fluid bolus of extracellular fluid that contains solute material. It uses pseudopods to surround material, which is ingested and breaks from the internal membrane internally to become pinocytic vesicles. These are then broken down further by specialist organelles.
- *Receptor mediated endocytosis* – targets specific material for specialist packaging and ingestion via receptors on the membrane surface, such as low-density lipids.

Exocytosis exports unwanted material and proteins produced for export in other parts of the body out of the cell in vesicles. Hormones or neurotransmitters are other examples of materials synthesised within the cell that are used elsewhere in the body.

The Cytoplasm

The cytoplasm encompasses all the material within the plasma membrane, with the exception of the nucleus. The cytoplasm is home to the cellular organelles, which are suspended in cytosol. Cytosol is the also known as intracellular fluid, and is the area of the cell where all the chemical reactions take place. Cytosol is composed mostly of water, which may constitute 75–90% of its volume and acts as a solvent for both dissolved and suspended substances that facilitate cellular function.

Within the cytosol, there are dissolved ions of potassium, sodium and calcium, which regulate cell function by signalling and osmolar regulation. There are both large and small suspended molecules within the cytosol, with small molecules including amino acids, fatty acids and glucose (substrates used in metabolic function). Larger molecules include nucleic acids and proteins such as enzymes, which act to catalyse metabolic function within the cellular environment. Suspended in the cytosol, there are lipid droplets, which store molecules of triglyceride and granules of glycogen that act as glucose stores.

The Nucleus

The nucleus usually resides in the centre of most cells. It contains most of the cell's genetic material. It is the largest organelle within the cell and, in some cells such as large skeletal muscle cells, there may be more than one nucleus to facilitate the regulation of the large volumes of material found in their cellular spaces. The genetic material in the nucleus is stored

23

within molecules of DNA (deoxyribonucleic acid), which are folded and arranged in chromosomes. The nucleus controls cellular activity and regulates it through gene expression.

All cells in the body have nuclei, with the exception of red blood cells. Red blood cells are produced in the bone marrow and cannot self-reproduce as they lack nuclei, which encode the cells genetic material for the production of new proteins to reproduce themselves. They have a relatively short life span (about 120 days) and senescent red blood cells are destroyed by the action of macrophages during haemolysis. This function occurs predominantly within the spleen, which is a lymphoid organ and is primarily a filter for the blood (Mebius and Kraal 2005).

The nucleus is surrounded by the *nuclear envelope*, which segregates the nucleus within the cellular membrane from the rest of the material within the cytoplasm. This is a double membranous structure that is studded with openings created from proteins called nuclear pores. These regulated openings facilitate the movement of substances across the membrane between the cytoplasm outside and the nucleoplasm inside. Material is moved across this membrane by both diffusion of smaller particles and active transport of proteins and other large particles. The nuclear envelope's outer membrane is continuous with rough endoplasmic reticulum (RER) and has many ribosomes in place to link amino acids together and form proteins.

Nucleoplasm is a jelly-like substance similar to cytoplasm, within which all the contents of the nucleus are suspended within the nuclear envelope. These contents include nutrients, dissolved ions and nuclear material such as nucleoli and chromatin. Nucleoli are spherical and non-membrane-bound. Within them, ribosomal RNA is assembled into RNA subunits to be passed through the nuclear pores for and joined together in the synthesis of proteins. Chromatin is composed of threads of DNA, which coil to form chromosomes. Chromatin contains the cell's genetic material in the form of DNA, which gives specific codes to the cellular ribosomes for specific protein production. This chromatin code facilitates the production of a myriad of different proteins depending on the instructions coded in the DNA it forms.

Cellular Reproduction

Mitosis

Within the body there are *somatic* cells, which reproduce by replication of the parent cell, and reproductive cells or *gametes*. The vast majority of cells are somatic cells that reproduce by cell division, producing a cloned version of their parent cells. During life, these cells must constantly reproduce during tissue growth and to replace dead or damaged cells that no longer serve their functional purpose. Cellular reproduction occurs in the following ways:

- *Mitosis* – *somatic* cells that simply replicate the parent cell asexually, producing an exact cloned copy. Somatic cells are *diploid*, having 23 pairs of chromosomes. When they divide and reproduce, the new cell also has 23 pairs of chromosomes. This reproduction occurs in most mature cells, although some mature cells do not reproduce, such as heart muscle (myocardium) and nerve cells.
- *Meiosis* – division of reproductive cells (known as *gametes*) during which cells reproduce by a process of reduction. The new cell has 23 single chromosomes – half the number of their parent cell.

Somatic cells reproduce via the process of *mitosis* and there are several complex phases through which the cell goes. Cells are constantly growing and dividing to fulfil the body's need for homeostasis. This is known as the *cell cycle*. The cycle occurs during two main stages known as the *interphase* and the *mitotic phase*.

Interphase

During interphase, the cell is preparing to divide. This is followed by the mitotic stage, when the division and replication of the cell occurs. The cell is building up a store of energy to facilitate cellular division. Interphase may be subdivided into G1, S and G2, and takes the longest duration. During G1, the number of cellular organelles increases dramatically, while protein production is stepped up in preparation for cell division. The S phase sees the replication of nuclear material (DNA) in the nucleus in preparation for its division, as the daughter cell will have its own copy of the cell's DNA. The G2 phase sees the cell increase in size, producing more proteins and material in preparation for the division of the cell.

Mitotic Stage

The mitotic stage occurs during when the division of the nucleus (mitosis) and division of the cytoplasm (cytokinesis) occurs. Mitosis is divided into four phases:

1. *Prophase* sees chromatin fibres shorten and condense to form *chromosomes*, which are formed from two identical strands of *chromatids*. The chromatids are held together by a central structure called a *centromere*, with the whole structure being encased in protein complex known as a *kinetochore*. The nuclear envelope dissipates and breaks up, diminishing the nucleolus and leaving the chromosomes within the cytoplasm.

2. *Metaphase* occurs as the 46 chromosomes (23 pairs each with two chromatids) attach to the *mitotic spindle* and line up along the metaphase plate through the cell's midline.

3. *Anaphase* occurs and the chromatids of each chromosome separate at opposite ends of the mitotic spindle. The sister chromosomes are pulled further apart as the microtubules shorten and while the cell starts to elongate prior to the division of the cytoplasm during cytokinesis.

4. *Telophase* sees the reforming of nuclear envelopes and nucleolus reappearing around the 46 chromatids at each end of the cell. Microtubules lengthen and the as the cell deepens prior to separating as cytokinesis (division of the cytosol) occurs. Each separate daughter cell has a complete set of identical chromosomes.

The cells reproducing during mitosis may continue this cycle until the body's needs for growth replacement of dead cells is complete. The cycle is regulated within the body by chemical signals; checkpoints are reached during various stages of reproduction to ensure that there are no errors during each stage before cell division occurs. Cells need time to ingest raw materials and fuel to reproduce two sets of all the organelles and a complete second set of DNA to reproduce a new identical nucleus. When the body has no need to produce new cells, the process of reproduction is halted, and cells remain in a resting state until the cycle is required to start again.

Meiosis

Meiosis is the process of reproduction that occurs in the gonads (testes and ovaries), where cells called *gametes* are produced from *germ cells*. This is a process also known as *reduction division*, where the number of chromosomes is reduced as the cells divide.

The process starts with diploid cells, which produces produce gametes – sperm in males and oocytes in females. There are two stages of division in meiosis – meiosis 1 and meiosis 2. Meiosis 1 produces two haploid cells from homologous pairs (from two sister chromatids). During meiosis 2, both haploid cells divide again producing four haploid gametes (sex cells).

First Meiotic Stage
- Prophase 1: this stage resembles the prophase in mitosis where chromatin fibres shorten and condense to form individual chromosomes. Paired homologous chromosomes line up together, forming a tetrad (four sister chromatids). Crossing over occurs where alleles or segments of genes from the same segment of homologous chromosomes swap randomly, creating infinitely different gene combinations. This results in difference in every gamete, including siblings, which offers genetic variety. The nuclear membrane dissipates, and the centrioles move to opposite poles with spindles fanning out.

- Metaphase 1: homologous chromosomes are aligned at the cell's equator and spindle fibres attach to each one from opposite poles.
- Anaphase 1: homologous chromosomes are separated in each tetrad to different poles.
- Telophase 1: chromosomes from each homologous pair are at separate poles with sister chromatids making up each chromosome. The chromosomes at each pole, although sharing sister chromatids, are no now longer identical due to the sharing of alleles during crossing over. The spindle fibres disappear as the cell splits during cytokinesis and the cell divides, forming two new genetically different daughter cells. Each cell has one set of chromosomes with paired sister chromatids.

Second Meiotic Stage

- Prophase 2: In this phase, unlike in prophase 1, there is no DNA replication before both nuclear envelopes dissipates. Centrioles again move to opposite poles of both cells and spindles spin out.
- Metaphase 2: in both cells, chromosomes again line up at the equator and spindle fibres attach from opposite poles.
- Anaphase 2: sister chromatids now separate into chromosomes and are drawn to opposite poles in both cells.
- Telophase 2: the spindle fibres disappear as both cells split during cytokinesis and the two cells divide, forming four new genetically different daughter cells. Each cell has one set of chromosomes.

Differentiation

Cells within the body have many roles and functions, which necessitates the process of producing specialist cell types. We have looked at the process of cellular reproduction of somatic cells in mitosis and sex cells during meiosis. Some cells develop for specialisation within the body; this process is known as differentiation. Stem cells are cells that can reproduce repeatedly without specialising and have the potential to become any cell. They may divide into identical daughter cells if required or one can develop into partially specialised cells. These partially specialised cells are known as progenitor cells as they are different from stem cells. They specialise because of the activation of genes that may only become active at certain stages in life as the body matures, develops and changes. Some stem cells that were differentiated prior to birth in the fetus or embryo may be used to regenerate tissues in the adult body, such as spinal injuries or even myocardium post injury. There is currently much research into the seemingly endless positive applications of stem cell therapy.

Cellular Organelles

Cellular organelles are specialised structures that are suspended within the cytosol of cell cytoplasm. They have individualised specialist roles within the cell to maintain life, facilitate cell growth and cellular reproduction. They are responsible for cellular respiration, energy generation, protein synthesis, excretion of waste products and transport of material into and out of the cell.

The shape of the cell and anchoring of cellular organelles in situ is facilitated by the *cytoskeleton*. These structures are composed of protein filaments, which extend throughout the cytosol and which are composed of microfilaments, intermediate filaments and microtubules.

Microfilaments usually reside just under the plasma membrane and surround the cell. They are particularly prolific in muscle cells and contain *actin filaments* and *myocin*. Intermediate filaments contain both *keratin* and *neurofilaments* and are composed of a number of different protein subunits, making them thicker than microfilaments. Microtubules are the thickest of type of cytoskeleton filaments and are composed of long tubes of *tubulin protein* subunits.

Centrioles, as mentioned earlier, are structures that assist with cellular reproduction by anchoring chromosomes prior to cytokinesis.

Cilia and Flagella

Cilia are membrane-bound organelles found in many cells. They are hairlike projections that extend from the cell membrane and are motile or moving. This enables them to be effective in cells such as the basement layer of the respiratory tract. Here, these hairlike projections move unidirectionally in a rhythmic manner to help expel debris and foreign matter trapped in mucus. They may also be found in the middle ear and help to enable the movement of fluids across the surface of cells. Flagella have longer structural projections than cilia and when moved rhythmically may enable cells to propel forward, such as sperm cells.

Ribosomes

Ribosomes are protein production facilities. They are found on both RER and freely within the cytoplasm. Ribosomes are composed of ribosomal RNA and link amino acids together to produce specialised proteins. Proteins from ribosomes found in RER produce proteins to be exported out of the cell via exocytosis. Ribosomes that are free within the cytosol produce proteins to be used within the cell itself, such as enzymes to promote metabolic function.

Endoplasmic Reticulum

Endoplasmic reticulum may be found as both RER and smooth endoplasmic reticulum (SER). These structures are a series of membranes which form connected cavities and sacs known as cisternae. They are found throughout the cytoplasm with RER being continuous with the outer membrane of the nuclear envelope, as mentioned earlier. RER is rich in ribosomes and produces a myriad of different proteins depending on the type of cell. The synthesis of proteins such as enzymes, antibodies, phospholipids, blood proteins, hormones and integral proteins occurs within this organelle. These proteins are exported from the cell via exocytosis or stored within the cell's lipid bilayer membrane.

SER is continuous with RER but does not contain ribosomes so it is not engaged in protein production. SER has many enzymes expressed on its surface which act as catalysts for cellular reactions specific to the cell type. Gonad cells synthesise sex steroid hormones. Liver and kidney cells work to deactivate and detoxify the body, while the liver also works to break down glycogen into glucose, synthesise cholesterol and metabolise lipids. Cells in the gastrointestinal tract absorb and transport fat molecules.

Golgi apparatus

The Golgi apparatus is another organelle which resides within the cytosol that synthesises and secretes substances that it modifies post synthesis from the ribosomes. It has a complex structure similar to SER, but it can have up to 20 stacked cisternae, which are far more extensive and produce many different substances. The Golgi transports proteins and lipids through its network of cisternae and further modifies them before they are packaged into vesicles for delivery to targeted destinations, usually outside the cell. It receives lipids and proteins, further modifies them as they move through the structure before packaging them for delivery, almost like a production line. The Golgi apparatus structure sits close to the RER near the nuclear envelope and has a number of distinct geographical locations:

- The *CIS face* is the receiving area for proteins produced by the RER to be further modified.
- The *lumen*, a transit space, is where phosphorylation of proteins occurs after leaving the CIS face.
- The *cisternae*, flattened sac-like spaces, are where carbohydrates are added to proteins to form glycoproteins, or lipids added to proteins to form lipoproteins.
- The *trans* face, the exit, is the area where completed proteins leave the Golgi and where vesicles fuse to receive and transport them.

Vesicles

Vesicles are membrane-bound sacs that detach from the RER to encompass and transport substances between different organelles and out of the cell via exocytosis.

Lysosomes

Lysosomes are vesicles that are membrane bound and originate from the trans face of the Golgi. They have digestive and hydrolytic enzymes and an acidic core, which is maintained by a proton pump (hydrogen ions) in the membrane of the lysosome. These organelles are responsible for many important functions such as:

- Breaking down and digesting molecules imported during endocytosis to release their contents. Endosomes are like the recycling centres of the cell. They have an essential job in breaking down and digesting molecules that the cell brings in from the outside.
- Breaking down and destroying older end-of-life organelles within the cell, which is called auto phagocytosis.
- Breaking down bone, releasing calcium.
- Breaking down stored glycogen.
- Breaking down of products from phagocytosis and release of products from lysosomal digestion, such as amino acids for cellular use.

Peroxisomes

Peroxisomes are membrane-bound vesicles that self-replicate and are smaller in size than lysosomes and contain the enzymes *oxidase* and *catalase*. Oxidase catalyses the removal of hydrogen atoms usually from fatty acids and amino acids creating hydrogen peroxide, which is toxic in the cellular environment. Catalyse then converts hydrogen peroxide into water and oxygen for cellular use.

Mitochondria

Mitochondria are organelles that provide the space for energy production within the cells; they are commonly known as the cell's powerhouse. They are prolific in organs with high metabolic function, such as the liver, kidneys and muscle cells. They have a double membrane surrounding the inner fluid-filled matrix, like the membrane of the cell itself. The outer membrane is smooth and the inner membrane has many folds, called *cristae,* which enlarge the surface area. This is where the cell's energy is created using enzymes that oxidise fatty acids and enzymes of tricarboxylic acid cycle.

The mitochondria are responsible for energy production in the cell. This is also known as *cellular* or *internal respiration,* which comprises *glycolysis*, the *citric acid cycle (Krebs cycle)* and the *electron transport chain.* Mitochondria are constantly moving and can migrate freely through the cells cytoplasm. They have their own primitive RNA and ribosomes. This allows them to enlarge their cristae and to reproduce in times of high energy demand. Energy is released from glucose and other fuel sources by breaking them down in catalysed reactions that are facilitated by enzymes within the cristae. These reactions are specific to maximise energy production, and they produce water and carbon dioxide in addition to energy. The oxidation of metabolites produces energy to attach a phosphate group to ADP, producing ATP, which is made available for cellular energy production.

Body Tissues

Body tissues are composed of similar cells working together to perform specific tasks. The hierarchy of the body will see similar tissues forming organs, which in turn will form body systems. The basic unit of function is the cell, with similar cells forming body tissues. The most common cells composing the body are the following.

- *Epithelial tissue* is found lining body surfaces and internal organs, and most glands consist of it. Epithelial tissue is primarily responsible for protection, secretion, absorption excretion, filtration and diffusion. Epithelium may be classified to include simple, stratified, pseudostratified, cuboidal, columnar, transitional, glandular and squamous.
- *Connective tissue* can be blood, bone, ground substance, cartilage, elastic/fibrous and some adipose tissue. It functions to support, protect, deliver material and give structure to the body.

- *Nervous tissue* may be found in the brain, the spinal cord in the central nervous system, and throughout the body in the peripheral nervous system. It is composed of nerve cells, which have a cell body, axon, dendrite and terminal axon. These cells are responsible for the control of body function. Interaction between the body and the outside world is the facilitated by the nervous system as it communicates through electrical impulses. The nervous system and its components facilitate the human experience, including emotion, environmental awareness, memory and reasoning.
- *Muscle tissues* are composed of muscle cells that facilitate body movement by using their elongated fibres, which can contract. There are three distinct types of muscle cells, which have specialist functions such as cardiac muscle, smooth muscle and skeletal muscle.
- *Skeletal muscle* is under conscious control and is found attached to bones. It has long striations. Skeletal muscles usually work as antagonistic pairs and move by shortening one muscle group as the opposing muscle group relaxes, moving the bones on which they are attached. These muscles are known as *striated voluntary muscle* and include cells that are composed of muscle fibre.
- *Cardiac muscle* is found in the heart and has a rich blood supply to perfuse tissue. During life, cardiac muscle has a high energy output as it is in constant motion. The functioning unit of the heart's muscle cells is myocardium which is cross-striated and is involuntary and not under conscious control. These muscles are also called *striated involuntary muscle*. They are paced by specialist cells which ensure that the contractions are rhythmic and coordinated, maximising their contractile force to eject blood around the body. They cannot divide to replicate, and injury may result in life-changing or life-ending events.
- *Smooth muscle* is also involuntary and is composed of elongated cells, which are spindle shaped. They may be referred to as *nonstriated involuntary muscles*, which can divide as necessary, allowing them to regenerate if they are damaged. Smooth muscle is found in areas that are not in the heart or under conscious control as skeletal muscle. Examples include the walls of hollow internal organs such as the bronchial tree, blood vessels, intestines and uterus. This muscle ensures peristalsis in the gastrointestinal tract, helps to empty the bladder, contract the uterus during childbirth, and contract and relax blood vessels in the maintenance of blood pressure.

The Ageing Process

All humans are subject the ageing process and eventual death. Over time, there is general degradation of cellular material, which eventually causes irreparable damage to cellular function. During cellular metabolic function within the mitochondria, oxygen molecules transport electrons and then bind to hydrogen, creating water as a byproduct. Occasionally, the oxygen fails to bind with hydrogen, creating an unbound oxygen molecule known as a *free radical*. Free radicals may bind with other molecules, such as proteins or lipids, and, in doing so, they damage their structure, potentially creating mutations. As we age, the number of free radicals increases exponentially. During cell replication, the end regions of chromosomes known as *telomeres* shorten with each division cycle, losing small amounts of DNA in the process. There is a finite number of times that cells can replicate prior to critical shortening of the telomeres with subsequent catastrophic loss of genetic material. This may be a causative factor signalling senescence (cellular decline) and shortened telomeres are linked to disease several processes. Shortened telomere syndrome may also be inherited by mutations in genes and cause pathogenic illness such as pulmonary fibrosis, premature emphysema and osteoporosis, and potentially predisposing patients to cancers (Mangaonkar and Patnaik 2018).

Cancers

Cancers are a leading cause of death and can be described as unregulated proliferation of cellular reproduction, resulting in malignant invasive growths. Cancerous growths are a result of genetic mutations, which occur in cells due to several factors, including environmental such as viruses, toxins, radiation or chemicals and inherited factors.

Cellular genetics mutate genes that regulate cell growth, such as tumour suppressor genes, which will further mutate creating malignancies that may be local or in tissue around the body (Hanselmann and Welter 2022). As the causative factors in the creation of cancers are multifactorial, damage to genetic material that promotes repair of DNA may be passed on and inherited by children. Cancer treatments are progressing and may be very invasive such as surgeries, chemotherapy and radiotherapy. These treatments are used in combination or alone, depending on the types of cancers involved and their stage of advancement.

Take Home Points

- Cells are the basic structural and functional units of all living organisms; they can be classified as prokaryotic or eukaryotic. Prokaryotic cells lack a true nucleus, while eukaryotic cells have a well-defined nucleus containing genetic material.
- The four primary types of tissues in the human body are epithelial, connective, muscle, and nervous tissue.
- Epithelial tissue covers body surfaces, lines cavities, and forms glands. It plays a crucial role in protection and secretion. Connective tissue supports and connects different body structures. It includes various types such as adipose, cartilage, bone, and blood. Muscle tissue is responsible for body movement and can be categorised into three types: skeletal, smooth and cardiac muscle. Nervous tissue is essential for communication and consists of neurons and glial cells. Neurons transmit electrical signals.
- Red blood cells (erythrocytes) are specialised for oxygen transport in the blood, and white blood cells (leucocytes) play a vital role in immune defence.
- The extracellular matrix is a significant component of connective tissue, providing support and maintaining tissue integrity.
- The cell membrane (plasma membrane) surrounds the cell, regulating the movement of substances in and out of the cell.
- The nucleus houses the cell's genetic material (DNA) and controls cellular activities. Mitochondria are the powerhouse of the cell, responsible for producing ATP (cellular energy). Ribosomes are involved in protein synthesis, and the endoplasmic reticulum and Golgi apparatus process and transport proteins within the cell.
- Smooth muscle tissue is found in the walls of internal organs and blood vessels, controlling involuntary movements. Cardiac muscle tissue forms the heart and is responsible for pumping blood. It contains intercalated discs for rapid conduction.

Summary

This chapter has looked at the cell and its many constituent parts, which are the building blocks of the body. There are many complicated functions constantly occurring within all cells to facilitate life and our ability to experience the world. The following chapters look in detail at the body's different systems and the specialist tissues that form them. They cover how things work normally and what happens when disease and injury processes occur.

References

Hanselmann, R. and Welter, C. (2022). Origin of cancer: cell work is the key to understanding cancer initiation and progression. *Frontiers in Cell and Developmental Biology* 10: 787995. https://www.frontiersin.org/articles/10.3389/fcell.2022.787995/full.

Mangaonkar, A.A. and Patnaik, M.M. (2018). Short telomere syndromes in clinical practice: bridging bench and bedside. *Mayo Clinic Proceedings* 93: 904–916.

Mebius, R. and Kraal, G. (2005). Structure and function of the spleen. *Nature Reviews Immunology* 5 (8): 606–616: https://pubmed.ncbi.nlm.nih.gov/16056254.

Further Reading

Moini, J. (2020). *Anatomy and Physiology for Health Professionals*. Burlington, VA: Jones and Bartlett.

Nair, M. and Peate, I. (2018). *Fundamentals of Applied Pathophysiology for Nursing Students*, 3e. Oxford: Wiley-Blackwell.

Pilbery, R. and Caroline, N. (2014). *Nancy Caroline's Emergency Care in the Streets*, 7e. Burlington, VA: Jones and Bartlett.

Story, L. (n.d.). *Pathophysiology*, 4e. Burlington, VA: Jones and Bartlett.

Waugh, A. and Grant, A. (2014). *Anatomy & Physiology in Health and Illness*, 12e. Edinburgh: Elsevier.

Online Resources

Khan Academy. Structure of a cell. https://www.khanacademy.org/science/biology/structure-of-a-cell

NHS. Stem cell transplant. https://www.nhs.uk/conditions/stem-cell-transplant/what-happens/

Glossary

Active transport	The process by which substances move against a concentration gradient from an area of low concentration to one of higher concentration.
Adenosine diphosphate (ADP)	Found inside cells, helps to produce ATP during reactions which produce cellular energy and is itself formed from ATP at a later stage.
Amino acid	The building block of proteins.
Carbohydrate	Organic compound composed of carbon, hydrogen and oxygen.
Catalyst	A substance speeding up a reversible chemical reaction. Enzymes are catalysts.
Chemical reaction	A process in which molecules are formed, changed or broken down.
Chromosomes	Tightly coiled chromatin.
Concentration gradient	The gradient demonstrating the difference between an area of high concentration and one of low concentration of a substance.
Cytoplasm	Collective name for all contents of the cell, including plasma membrane, but not including the nucleus.
Deoxyribonucleic acid (DNA)	Found in the nucleus; contains all genetic information of an organism.
Diffusion	Passive movement of molecules or ions from a region of high concentration to one of low concentration until a state of equilibrium is achieved.
Endocytosis	General name for various processes by which cells ingest foodstuffs and infectious microorganisms.
Enzyme	A protein speeding up chemical reactions.
Exocytosis	The system of transporting material out of cells.
Extracellular fluid	Fluid outside the cell, bathing the body's cells.
Fibre	Any long, thin structures, including nerve fibres and muscle fibres.
Gene	The smallest physical and biological unit of heredity that encodes for a molecular cell product.
Genetic material	Mainly DNA that contains genetic information.

Glucose	Also known as dextrose, the principal sugar found in the blood; essential for life.
Glycoprotein	A protein linked to carbohydrates.
Hormone	A chemical messenger linked to the endocrine system.
Internal respiration	Use of oxygen by cells in the enzymatic release of energy from organic compounds, also called aerobic respiration.
Lipid	An energy-rich organic compound soluble in organic substances such as alcohol.
Lysosome	Organelle within the cell, an important part of the cell's digestive system.
Meiosis	Process by which the gametes (spermatozoa and ova) are reproduced.
Mitosis	The process by which cells (other than the gametes) are reproduced by simple division of the nucleus and the cell itself.
Nuclear membrane	The outer shell of the nucleus within the cell.
Nucleolus	A small spherical body found in the cell nucleus.
Nucleoplasm	Protoplasm found within the nucleus.
Organelle	A structural and functional part of a cell.
Osmosis	Passive movement of water through a selectively permeable membrane from an area of high concentration of a chemical to an area of low concentration.
Osmotic pressure	Pressure exerted on a solution to prevent passage of water into it across a semipermeable membrane from a region of higher concentration of solute to a region of lower concentration of solute.
Passive transport	Process by which substances move on their own down a concentration gradient from high concentration to one of lower concentration.
Phagocytosis	The method by which cells ingest large particles.
Pinocytosis	The method by which cells ingest small particles and fluids.
Protoplasm	Collective name for everything within the cell.
Ribosomal ribonucleic acid (rRNA)	Highly selective method by which the cell is able to ingest large particles.
Ribosome	An organelle found in cytoplasm plays a major role in the synthesis of proteins from RNA.
Simple fission	The asexual reproduction of cells by means of division of the nucleus and the cell body.
Solute	A substance dissolved in a solution.
Transmembrane ion gradient	Gradient in the concentration of ions on either side of a plasma membrane.
Vesicle	A spherical space within the cell cytoplasm involved in the storage and transfer of substances for the cell.

Multiple Choice Questions

1. Which of the following statements regarding cells is incorrect?
    a. Cells can reproduce themselves via a process called simple fission. This is achieved when full-size cells divide into two replicating themselves. A process with is reproduced many times.
    b. Cells may be acted upon or stimulated and cease to function at optimal levels.
    c. Cells do not always use all the energy they ingest via endocytosis and release what they do not use.
    d. At the end of their lifespan all cells will die – Some have a long lifespan and other very short, but all eventually die.

2. Which of the following is incorrect regarding the cell membrane?
   a. The cell membrane has a double membranous fold which is composed of phospholipids, glycolipids, and cholesterol.
   b. The cell membrane has proteins embedded within its structure and uses proteins to create specialist channels for transport into and out of the cell.
   c. The Cell has a double membrane consisting of a hydrophobic head and hydrophilic tail.
   d. The cell uses active and passive transport to move material into and out of the cell.

3. Which of the following would be considered a passive process?
   a. Osmosis
   b. Phagocytosis
   c. Active transport pumps
   d. Exocytosis

4. Which of the following is true regarding the functions of cytoplasm?
   a. The cytoplasm contains the nucleus which is responsible for regulating cellular temperature.
   b. The cytoplasm is filled with fluid called cytoplasm which may also be called extracellular fluid.
   c. Cytoplasm is approximately 50%–80% water.
   d. There are dissolved ions of Potassium, Sodium and Calcium which regulate cell function by signalling and osmolar regulation.

5. Which of the following statements is correct?
   a. The nucleus is the smallest structure found within the cell.
   b. Prior to cell division the nuclear core shortens and coils into chromatins.
   c. The protoplasm within the nucleus is called cytoplasm.
   d. Chromosomes are composed primarily of proteins and fibrin.

6. Which of the following organelles is responsible for the digestion of material taken up by endocytosis?
   a. Golgi apparatus
   b. Mitochondria
   c. Lysosomes
   d. Endoplasmic reticulum

33

7. During the process of mitosis which of the following is incorrect?
   a. This is the process in which Somatic cells replicate from the parent cell asexually producing an exact cloned copy.
   b. The daughter cell has 23 pairs of chromosomes and are referred to as diploid cells.
   c. The Cell Cycle and occurs during 2 main stages known as *Interphase* and *Mitotic phase.*
   d. Interphase is the shortest phase of Mitosis.

8. During the mitotic phase of mitosis which of the following are incorrect?
   a. Telophase sees the reforming of the nuclear envelope and the lengthening of microtubules prior to cytokinesis.
   b. During metaphase the chromosomes attach to the mitotic spindle and line up along the equator or midline of the cell.
   c. Prophase sees chromosomes form into identical stands of chromatids which join at the centromere.
   d. Anaphase sees the chromatids joined at the same end of the cell.

9. Which of the following is the most prolific tissue in the human body?
   a. Muscle tissue
   b. Nervous tissue
   c. Epithelial tissue
   d. Connective tissue

10. Which of the following is true in relation to differentiation?
   a. Differentiation is when cells are produced to become specialised for a particular purpose.
   b. Differentiation occurs when cells are damaged and need to repair themselves.
   c. The process of differentiation occurs only when cells divide during growth periods.
   d. Differentiation rarely happens in adults and is a juvenile process as children develop.

CHAPTER 3

Homeostasis

Sadie Diamond-Fox and Alexandra Gatehouse

AIM

The aim of this chapter is to provide an introduction to the many ways in which the human body maintains a state of equilibrium via multiple homeostatic mechanisms.

LEARNING OUTCOMES

On completion of this chapter you will be able to:

- Have an understanding of how the body maintains a constate of equilibrium in health.
- Understand the definition of homeostasis.
- Appreciate the interplay between body systems in maintaining homeostasis.
- Consider the disruption to normal homeostatic processes that occurs in certain disease states.

Test Your Prior Knowledge

1. What is homeostasis?
2. What are the principal body systems involved in the maintenance of homeostasis?
3. Differentiate between normal homeostatic mechanisms and those that are altered during disease.
4. What is the importance of the maintenance of homeostasis?

Introduction

Homeostasis is the cornerstone of the maintenance of normal physiology. It refers to the body's ability to maintain a balanced and stable internal environment in which normal cellular function can occur, despite changes in the external environment or related stimuli. Cell and body tissue physiology is explored in more detail in Chapter 2, but the key mechanisms that concern homeostasis are explored within this chapter.

Cells within the body require intact homeostatic mechanisms to be able to communicate with each other, and regulate their growth and division, to coordinate their functions and to allow for development and organisation into the various tissue types that exist within the body.

Fundamentals of Applied Pathophysiology for Paramedics, First Edition. Edited by Ian Peate and Simon Sawyer.
© 2024 John Wiley & Sons Ltd. Published 2024 by John Wiley & Sons Ltd.

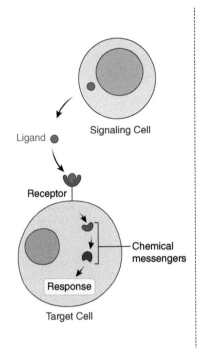

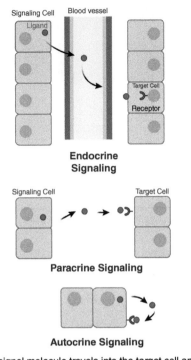

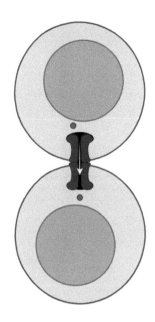

(a) Chemical messengers relay the signal from the ligand and receptor

(b) A signal molecule travels into the target cell and binds to an intracellular receptor protein within the target cells nucelus. This can occur via endocrine signalling, paracrine signalling, or autocrine signalling.

(c) A signal molecule is transferred via a junction in which adjacent cells are connected through protein channels

FIGURE 3.1 Types of cell signalling. (a) Plasma membrane-bound receptor signalling. (b) Signal molecules. (c) Gap junctions.

Cells communicate with each other via various means:

- *Receptor signalling* – cells display various plasma membrane-bound signalling molecules. There are hundreds of signalling molecules (ligands) that exist within the body. A neighbouring cell (a signalling cell) will release a signalling molecule, which will then bind to another neighbouring cell (the target cell) receptor. This type of cellular communication is known as contact signalling via plasma-membrane-bound receptors (Figure 3.1).
- *Signal molecules* – the signal molecule enters the target cell and binds to a receptor protein inside the cell itself. This type of cellular communication is known as remote signalling via secreted molecules.
- *Gap junctions* – a signalling cell and a neighbouring target cell form a gap junction (protein channel), allowing the adjacent signalling cell to coordinate activities of the target cell. This type of cellular communication is known as contact signalling via gap junctions (McCance 2019).

Cell signalling is ultimately responsible for the maintenance of homeostasis at cellular, tissue and organ-system levels.

Homeostatic Mechanisms

All human body systems are involved some way in maintaining homeostasis, but the neurological, endocrine, respiratory and renal systems play a particularly important part. The organ systems rely upon homeostatic mechanisms, which have five major components (Figure 3.2):

1. A *stimulus* – either internal or external; these stimuli cause an imbalance in the maintenance of a normal cellular environment.

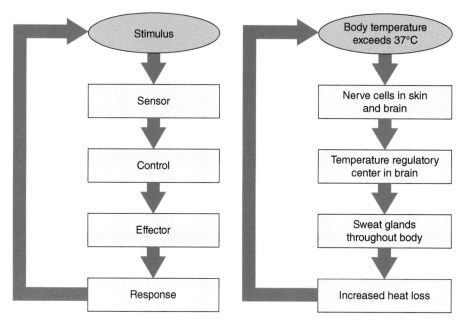

FIGURE 3.2   Five major components of homeostatic mechanisms. Source: Rice University; https://openstax.org/books/anatomy-and-physiology-2e/pages/1-5-homeostasis; CC BY 4.0.

2. *Receptor* – a cellular receptor detects the internal or external environmental change. Information from the receptor is then sent along an 'afferent' pathway to a control centre.

3. *Control centre* – the control centre determines the 'set point' at which the homeostatic variable is maintained. Information from the control centre passes via an 'efferent' pathway to an effector.

4. *Effector* – the effector responds to the commands of the control centre to either oppose or enhance the stimulus.

5. *Response* – the net effect is either opposition of an effect (negative feedback), or enhancement of an effect (positive feedback).

Each body system uses the five homeostatic control points in Figure 3.2 to regulate the internal environment. Some of the common examples of how the hemostatic mechanisms that occur via each body system are explored further within this chapter.

Reflective Learning Activity

Reflect upon the homeostatic changes you have observed within your own practice for patients who are suffering from severe sepsis.

Thermoregulation

Thermoregulation (Figure 3.3) is the body's ability to maintain a constant state of internal temperature, despite changes in the external environment. The maintenance of normal body temperature (average 37°C) is vital for cellular function, extreme deviations from this norm can result in denaturing of vital enzymes and proteins. Hyperthermia (body temperature > 38.5°C) induces thermoregulatory processes to promote heat loss, including vasodilation, sweating and increased respiratory rate. Hypothermia (body temperature < 35°C) induces thermoregulatory process such as vasoconstriction and shivering for heat gain.

The main organ involved in thermoregulation is the hypothalamus. The anterior hypothalamus responds to increased environmental temperatures, whereas the posterior hypothalamus responds to decreased environmental temperatures. Thermoreceptors present within the skin also aid in the control of body temperature and directly relay information to the hypothalamus. The thyroid gland is also involved in thermoregulation by conversion of thermogenic hormones, thyroxine (T_4) to tri-iodothyronine (T_3).

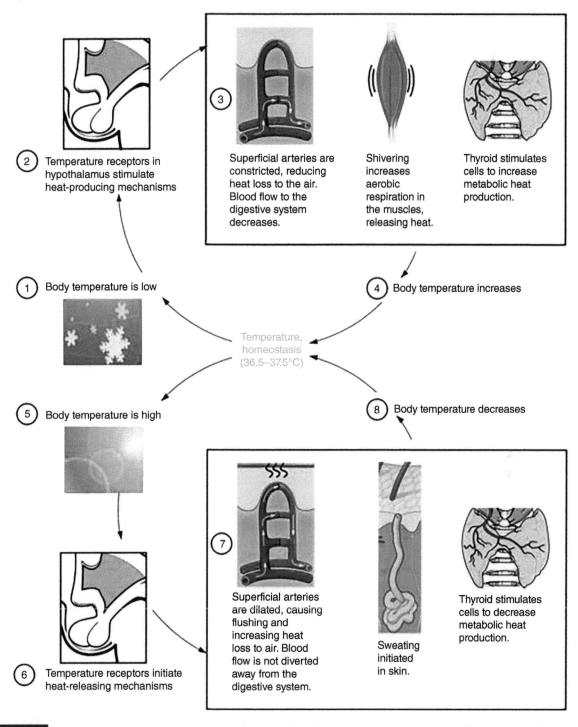

② Temperature receptors in hypothalamus stimulate heat-producing mechanisms

③ Superficial arteries are constricted, reducing heat loss to the air. Blood flow to the digestive system decreases.

Shivering increases aerobic respiration in the muscles, releasing heat.

Thyroid stimulates cells to increase metabolic heat production.

① Body temperature is low

④ Body temperature increases

Temperature, homeostasis (36.5–37.5°C)

⑤ Body temperature is high

⑧ Body temperature decreases

⑥ Temperature receptors initiate heat-releasing mechanisms

⑦ Superficial arteries are dilated, causing flushing and increasing heat loss to air. Blood flow is not diverted away from the digestive system.

Sweating initiated in skin.

Thyroid stimulates cells to decrease metabolic heat production.

FIGURE 3.3 Thermoregulatory behaviours of humans. Source: Karri Haen Whitmer, Body temperature homeostasis: cold pressor test; CC BY-SA 4.0.

Body temperature control is a major component of normal homeostatic control. Paracetamol is a common agent used for control of pyrexia (high temperature). Paracetamol's antipyretic properties have remained obscure for centuries; however, it is hypothesised that it may result from several mechanisms including inhibition of two specific enzymes implicated in temperature homeostasis; cyclooxygenase and transient receptor potential ankyrin 1 (Mirrasekhian et al. 2018).

Blood Glucose Homeostasis

Blood glucose levels are controlled by both the liver and the pancreas (Figure 3.4). When blood glucose levels begin to rise, such as after a meal, beta cells within the pancreas are stimulated top release insulin into the bloodstream. The presence of insulin causes the liver to take up glucose and store it as glycogen. Cells within other parts of the body also take up more glucose in the presence of insulin. Both uptake within the liver and other cells causes blood glucose to return to the original set point, whereby the stimulus for insulin diminishes. Conversely, when blood Glucose levels begin to drop below the homeostatic set point, alpha cells within the pancreas are stimulated to release glucagon into the blood. Glucagon breaks down glycogen stores within the liver and results in the release of glucose into the bloodstream. Blood glucose levels then rise back up to the set point and alpha cells stop releasing glucagon.

Clinical Investigations: Blood Glucose Monitoring

The body closely regulates blood glucose levels as part of metabolic homeostasis, which is crucial for cellular function. Blood glucose monitoring is one of multiple methods healthcare professionals can use to monitor the body's ability to regulate glucose homeostasis.

Preprocedure

Action:

1. Turn the machine on and ensure that the correct date and time are presented on the screen, and that there is adequate battery life. Where applicable, enter or scan operator number and/or password.
2. Ensure that the device is reading in mmol/l prior to each use.
3. Before taking the device to the patient, calibrate the monitor and test strips (where applicable) using the relevant steps below (always follow the manufacturer's instructions in case of any difference):
   a. Ensure that the testing strips are in date and have not been left exposed to air.
   b. Calibrate the monitor and test strips together.
   c. Carry out a quality control test using both high and low or level 1 and 2 solutions (in accordance with trust and manufacturer's guidelines). Ensure that the LOT number is recorded, either manually or via a bar code scanning system.
   d. Record the result (pass or fail) in the equipment log book and sign it.
   e. Where an automated device is used, ensure that the device is docked in its base unit to enable the centrally held electronic records to be updated.
   f. Ensure the meter has been decontaminated per local guidelines and is fit for use.
   g. Ensure that the meter service record is in date according to local policy.
   h. Ensure that the screen or display is intact and the 'screen safety check' has been completed in accordance with the manufacturer's guidelines (Roche Diagnostics).
4. Identify the patient, introduce yourself, explain and discuss the procedure with them, and gain their consent to proceed.
5. Select a site that is warm, well perfused and free of any skin damage. The ideal site for lancing is the palmar surface of the distal segment of the third or fourth finger (Figure 3a) of the non-dominant hand, avoiding the thumb and the index finger. Avoid sites that have recently been punctured.

Procedure

6. Ask the patient to wash their hands with soap and water and dry them thoroughly.
7. Ask the patient to sit or lie down.
8. Wash and dry hands and/ or use an alcohol-based handrub and apply personal protective equipment.
9. Turn on the device (where applicable and if not automated) and insert a testing strip.
10. Take a single-use lancet and set the appropriate depth (if applicable).
11. Using the lancet, puncture the chosen site (see step 5). If necessary, 'milk' the fingertip from the palm of the hand towards the finger to gain a large enough droplet of blood.
12. Dispose of the lancet in a sharps container.
13. Apply the drop of blood to the testing strip (some strips are hydrophilic and are dosed/filled from the side, whereas others require a drop of blood to be placed directly onto the strip). Ensure that the window on the test strip is entirely covered with blood (Figure 3b).
14. Immediately read and make note of the result on the display screen (Figure 3c). Document the result.
15. Dispose of the testing strip in a sharps container.
16. Place gauze over the puncture site, apply firm pressure and monitor for excess bleeding.
17. Once the bleeding has subsided, the site can be left exposed. It is not necessary to dress the site unless bleeding persists.
18. Remove gloves, place them in the clinical waste and perform hand hygiene again.

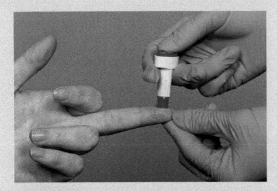

FIGURE 3a

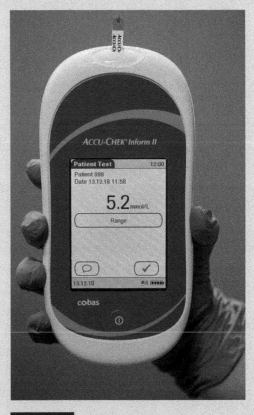

FIGURE 3c

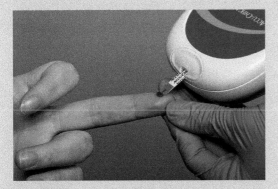

FIGURE 3b

39

Post-procedure

19. Where applicable, dock the machine.
20. Report and/or act on any unexpected results.

Source: Adapted from the *Royal Marsden Manual of Clinical Nursing Procedures* Lister et al. (2020).

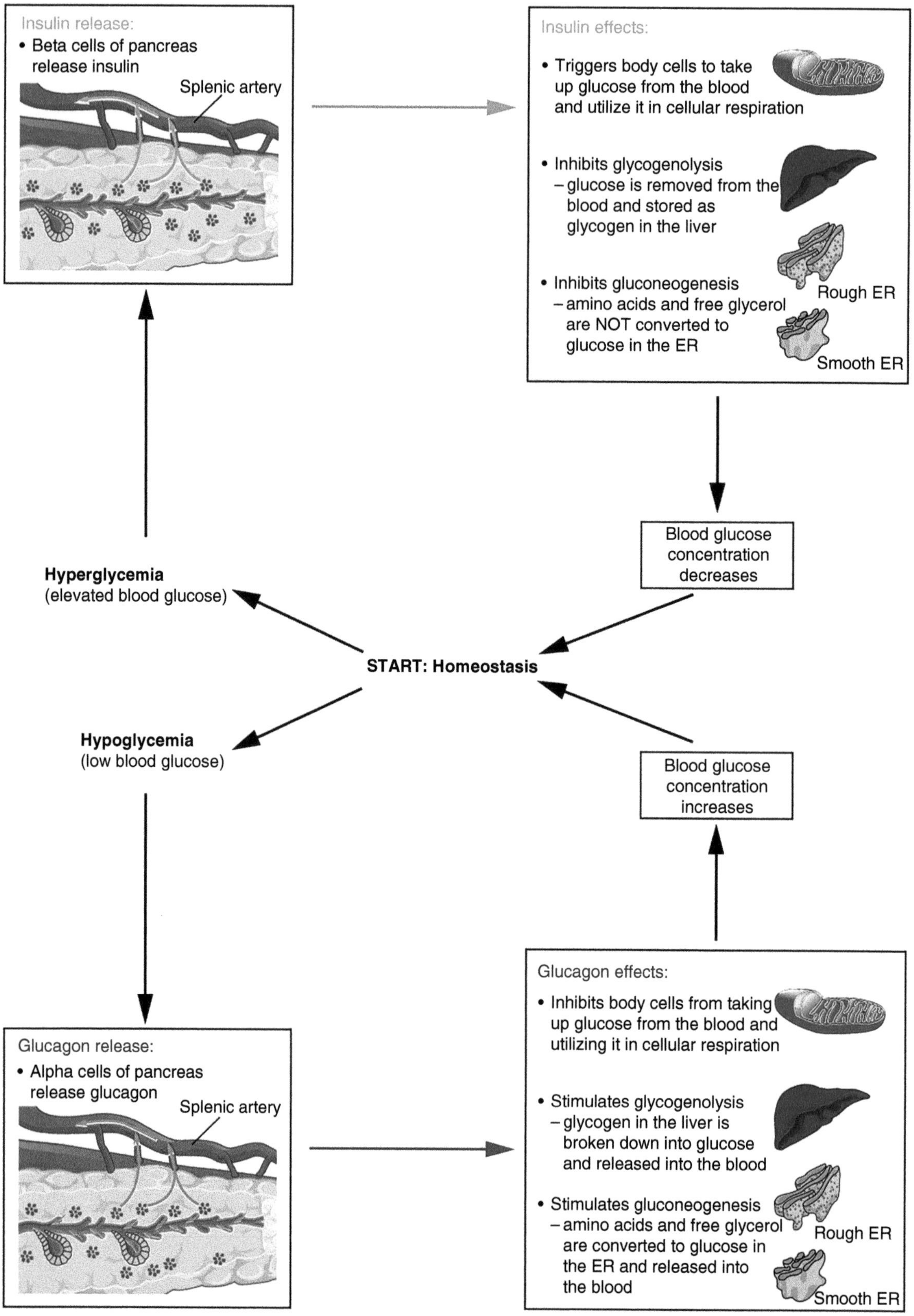

Insulin release:
- Beta cells of pancreas release insulin

Splenic artery

Insulin effects:
- Triggers body cells to take up glucose from the blood and utilize it in cellular respiration
- Inhibits glycogenolysis
  – glucose is removed from the blood and stored as glycogen in the liver
- Inhibits gluconeogenesis
  – amino acids and free glycerol are NOT converted to glucose in the ER

Rough ER

Smooth ER

Blood glucose concentration decreases

Hyperglycemia
(elevated blood glucose)

START: Homeostasis

Hypoglycemia
(low blood glucose)

Blood glucose concentration increases

Glucagon release:
- Alpha cells of pancreas release glucagon

Splenic artery

Glucagon effects:
- Inhibits body cells from taking up glucose from the blood and utilizing it in cellular respiration
- Stimulates glycogenolysis
  – glycogen in the liver is broken down into glucose and released into the blood
- Stimulates gluconeogenesis
  – amino acids and free glycerol are converted to glucose in the ER and released into the blood

Rough ER

Smooth ER

FIGURE 3.4   Glucose homeostasis. ER, endoplasmic reticulum. Source: Philschatz.com; https://philschatz.com/anatomy-book/contents/m46685.html; CC BY 4.0/public domain.

Arterial Blood Pressure Homeostasis

Under normal physiological circumstances, baroreceptors in the carotid body and aortic arch detect a fall in blood pressure, producing sympathetic stimulation and so vasoconstriction globally, as well as of the glomerular efferent arteriole. The renin–angiotensin–aldosterone system is activated and adaptations occur to compensate for changes in renal perfusion, allowing regulation of blood flow and glomerular filtration rate (GFR; Figure 3.5). A fall in renal perfusion is detected in the juxtaglomerular apparatus, as well as reduced GFR and sodium chloride concentration, which results in the release of the enzyme renin. This converts angiotensinogen, a circulating plasma protein produced by the liver, into angiotensin I. Angiotensin-converting enzyme, found in the lungs and kidneys, converts angiotensin I into angiotensin II, which has several important physiological roles, resulting in retention of salt and water and increased circulating volume.

Angiotensin II is a globally potent arteriolar vasoconstrictor and potentiates sympathetic activity, increasing blood pressure as well as causing vasoconstriction of the glomerular arterioles, the efferent more so than the afferent. GFR is maintained due to the increased pressure within the glomerulus capillaries. The sodium–hydrogen exchangers in the proximal tubule and thick ascending limb of the loop of Henle, in addition to the sodium channels in the collecting ducts, are stimulated by angiotensin II, increasing reabsorption of sodium and therefore water. The release of antidiuretic hormone from the posterior pituitary gland is stimulated by angiotensin II, causing vasoconstrictive effects, in addition to renal reabsorption of water and the sensation of thirst. Angiotensin II also causes the

41

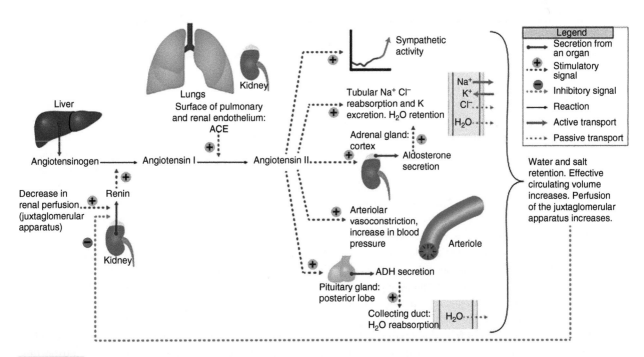

FIGURE 3.5 The renin–angiotensin–aldosterone system. Source: Soupvector; Wikimedia Commons; CC BY-SA 4.0.

release of aldosterone from the adrenal cortex, which acts upon the distal convoluted tubules and cortical collecting ducts, increasing sodium and water reabsorption.

Medications Management: Sympathomimetic Drugs

Sympathomimetic drugs such as adrenaline and noradrenaline may be required in those presenting with severe homeostatic disturbances (e.g. 'shock') resulting in severe vasodilatation and subsequent hypotension. These drugs often prescribed in micrograms per kilogramme, per minute (µg/kg/min). The following formula should be used to calculate the desired intravenous (IV) infusion rate:

$$\text{IV infusion rate (ml/hour)} = \frac{\text{Dose (µg/kg/min)} \times \text{weight (kg)} \times 60\,\text{min/hr}}{\text{Concentration (mg/ml)}\,1000\,\text{µg/mg}}$$

Red Flag Alert: Malignant Hypertension

Malignant hypertension is defined as a blood pressure 180/120 mmHg or above, with signs of progressive target organ damage (National Institute for Health and Care Excellence 2022). Signs of end-organ damage may include papilloedema, altered conscious level, seizure, chest pain and shortness of breath.

Reflective Learning Activity

Reflect upon the homeostatic changes you have observed within your own practice for patients who have experienced a cardiovascular event (e.g. myocardial infarction).

Plasma Osmolality and Electrolyte Homeostasis

Plasma osmolality concerns the solute particles sodium and potassium ions (Na^+, K^+) present within the blood (a solution) per kilogramme of solution. It is maintained within narrow limits (275–295 mOsm/kg) by several mechanisms (Figure 3.6) and determines the direction of fluid. Water will flow from a fluid compartment with low osmolality to a compartment of high osmolality if the membrane between the two compartments is permeable to water, as is the case across plasma membranes of human cells. A cell's permeability to water differs depending upon its lipid bilayer and the presence of aquaporins and other channels and carriers (see Chapter 2). Optimal osmolality is crucial for the creation of cellular homeostasis, for ion gradients between intracellular and interstitial fluid, and for subsequent generation of action potential. Changes in plasma osmolality are detected by sensory osmoreceptors in the anterior pituitary gland, which detect osmotic pressure changes and in turn trigger neuronal signals to be sent to the hypothalamus to regulate the release of antidiuretic hormone (vasopressin). Antidiuretic hormone stimulates the sensation of thirst, the formation of aquaporins within the collecting duct and, in higher concentrations, vasoconstriction. These mechanisms together serve to increase tissue perfusion via the increase in arterial blood volume and to increase blood pressure.

The renal system plays an essential role in the maintenance of homeostasis, controlling fluid, electrolyte and acid–base balance (Table 3.1). Renal disease, either acute or chronic, may affect all these processes. Fluid balance refers to the distribution of body fluid within the intracellular and extracellular (interstitial and intravascular) compartments. Total body volume, and thus total body water, is regulated within a narrow range through alteration of sodium and water content. Sodium excretion is controlled via the kidneys and is regulated by neural and endocrine responses. The sodium–potassium ion (Na^+–K^+) pumps drive sodium from the tubular cells into the blood, and this creates a lower concentration gradient within the cell. Sodium and water then move from the tubular infiltrate into the cell via various channels or co-transporters, according to the permeability of the cell membrane and the concentration gradient.

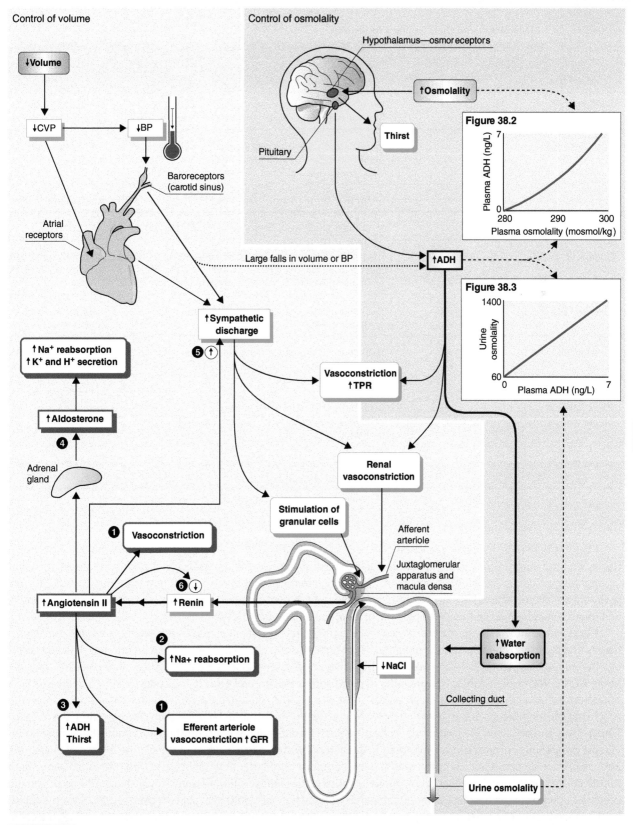

FIGURE 3.6 Control of plasma volume and osmolality. Source: Ward and Linden (2017)/John Wiley & Sons.

TABLE 3.1   Electrolytes and their primary functions.

Electrolytes	Normal values in extracellular fluid (mmol/l)	Function	Main distribution
Sodium (Na⁺)	135–145	Important cation in generation of action potentials. Plays an important role in fluid and electrolyte balance	Main cation of the extracellular fluid
Potassium (K⁺)	3.5–5	Important cation in establishing resting membrane potential. Regulates pH balance. Maintains intracellular fluid volume	Main cation of the intracellular fluid
Calcium (Ca2⁺)	2.1–2.6	Important clotting factor. Plays a part in neurotransmitter release in neurons. Maintains muscle tone and excitability of nervous and muscle tissue	Mainly found in the extracellular fluid
Magnesium (Mg2⁺)	0.5–1.0	Helps to maintain normal nerve and muscle function; maintains regular heart rate, regulates bold glucose and blood pressure. Essential for protein synthesis	Mainly distributed in the intracellular fluid
Chloride (Cl⁻)	98–117	Maintains a balance of anions in different fluid compartments	Main anion of the extracellular fluid
Bicarbonate ions (HCO³⁻)	24–31	Main buffer of hydrogen ions in plasma. Maintains a balance between cations and anions of intracellular and extracellular fluids	Mainly distributed in the extracellular fluid
Phosphate – organic (HPO₄²⁻)	0.8–1.1	Essential for the digestion of proteins, carbohydrates and fats and absorption of calcium. Essential for bone formation	Mainly found in the intracellular fluid
Sulphate (SO₄²⁻)	0.5	Involved in detoxification of phenols, alcohols and amines	Mainly found in the intracellular fluid

Source: Peate (2017) p. 511/John Wiley & Sons.

Inappropriate renal handling of sodium may occur due to a primary renal problem or an abnormality in the volume regulation mechanism. Renal tubulointerstitial disease and Addison's disease (deficiency of the hormone aldosterone) both cause excessive sodium excretion, while primary hyperaldosteronism, renal failure or oedema syndromes (liver disease, congestive heart failure, nephrotic syndrome) result in inadequate sodium excretion. The underlying cause should be identified and treated, but pharmacotherapy manipulation of renal sodium through the use of diuretics may be useful (see Chapter 9).

Potassium is integral to the maintenance of an electrochemical gradient across the cell membrane, and the ability of nerves and muscle to create an action potential. Hypokalaemia and hyperkalaemia are life threatening, causing cardiac dysrhythmias and potential cardiac arrest, and the kidneys and adrenal glands are vital in the maintenance of potassium homeostasis. Within the nephron, the majority of potassium is reabsorbed prior to the collecting duct, and excretion of potassium occurs in this segment through several mechanisms. The sodium–potassium pumps and the potassium channels in the cell membranes of the collecting duct are affected by the extracellular potassium concentration, the release of aldosterone, the pH, flow rates within the collecting duct, filtrate sodium concentration and intracellular magnesium. Plasma potassium concentration is monitored in the adrenal cortex, a rise in which results in the release of aldosterone and, as previously discussed, contributes to the maintenance of potassium homeostasis. Within the distal convoluted tubule and cortical collecting duct, aldosterone stimulates the reabsorption of sodium via the synthesis of sodium–potassium pumps in the basolateral membrane and sodium channels (epithelial sodium channel, ENaC) in the tubular luminal membrane. This creates a negative gradient within the lumen and, as potassium has been driven into the cell via the sodium–potassium pumps, it moves out into the tubular lumen via potassium channels or is co-transported with chloride. Higher flow rates also cause big potassium channels to open, increasing the secretion of potassium.

Calcium and phosphate are inextricably linked and are essential to the maintenance of bone density. They are regulated by one of several mechanisms including gut reabsorption, bone reabsorption and renal handling. Calcium is regulated by the thyroid gland and, when levels fall, parathyroid hormone stimulates bone reabsorption (release of calcium and phosphate from bone), increases vitamin D synthesis, increases renal phosphate excretion and increases renal calcium reabsorption. Vitamin D is synthesised within the kidney, increasing phosphate and calcium levels via reabsorption through the gut, bones and renal tubules. In renal failure, bone disease can be caused by vitamin D deficiency and renal phosphate retention. Because of a lack of gut reabsorption and the formation of calcium phosphate deposits (due to hyperphosphataemia), the fall in calcium stimulates parathyroid hormone, triggering further bone reabsorption and eventually hyperparathyroidism. Pharmacotherapy aims to maintain normal calcium and phosphate levels to prevent hyperparathyroidism, bone pain, poorly mineralised bone and soft tissue deposits, as typically seen in chronic kidney disease.

Medications Management

Pharmacological agents are designed to treat disease. However, pharmacological agents are used to adjust one homeostatic process by disrupting another. This disruption can lead to adverse effects. For instance, codeine phosphate may be used as an adjunct to other agents to treat pain, but it can impede intestinal motility, resulting in vomiting and constipation.

Acid–Base Homeostasis

Acid–base balance, and so pH, is controlled by the respiratory and renal systems. By regulating carbon dioxide (respiratory) and bicarbonate (renal), the pH may be normalised when acidosis or alkalosis occurs. Under normal circumstances, the kidneys excrete excess hydrogen ions (H^+) or acid through increased synthesis of the Na^+–H^+ exchangers or H^+ ATPase pump, reabsorb bicarbonate (HCO_3^-) via the Na^+–HCO_3^- co-transporters, and produce more ammonium salts (NH_4^+) for excretion. Metabolic acidosis occurs due to the loss of bicarbonate or the gain of hydrogen ions. Under normal circumstances, sodium bicarbonate is reabsorbed via the sodium gradient and hydrogen ions are secreted in the proximal tubule. In the distal tubule, hydrogen ions either contribute to reabsorption of the remaining bicarbonate or are buffered by phosphate.

Bicarbonate is lost through gut losses, increased sodium chloride administration and renal bicarbonate loss. Renal tubular acidosis results in the kidneys being unable to:

- excrete hydrogen ions and reabsorb bicarbonate ions due to disorders of the proximal tubule (rare)
- excrete hydrogen ions or absorb sodium ions due to secretory, permeability and voltage defects in the distal tubule, as seen in hypoaldosteronism.

The gain of hydrogen ions occurs in lactic acidosis, ketoacidosis, poisoning and renal failure. In renal diseases, the kidneys are unable to perform these processes effectively, so metabolic acidosis occurs, which causes hyperkalaemia due to hydrogen ions moving into cells and driving out potassium ions. Metabolic acidosis becomes more common with advancing chronic kidney disease. Damage to both the glomerulus and renal tubules significantly reduces the number of functioning nephrons and as the disease progresses, ammonia excretion is impaired (fewer hydrogen ions are excreted), bicarbonate absorption is reduced and there is insufficient production of renal bicarbonate. Patients with underlying chronic kidney disease who go on to develop an acute kidney infection are at high risk of developing metabolic acidosis.

Blood Partial Pressure of Carbon Dioxide Homeostasis

One of the main homeostatic functions of the respiratory system is the exchange of oxygen and carbon dioxide. The neurological, renal and skeletal systems also have a part to play when it comes to carbon dioxide homeostasis. Chemical control of ventilation is mediated by both central chemoreceptors and peripheral chemoreceptors. Central chemoreceptors detect both changes in pH and carbon dioxide and are made of a diffuse collection of neurons located within the medulla oblongata of the brainstem. The levels of carbon dioxide dissolved within the blood have a direct impact upon respiratory rate. High carbon dioxide levels (hypercapnia) cause a drop in blood pH. This drop is detected by central chemoreceptors located in the medulla oblongata of the brainstem. It leads to stimulation of increased rate and depth of breathing and a resulting increased rate of removal of carbon dioxide from the body. Blood carbon dioxide levels then fall, and blood pH is returned to within normal limits. Peripheral chemoreceptors detect changes in carbon dioxide and are located within the carotid and aortic bodies. When blood carbon dioxide levels increase, the firing rate of the carotid sinus nerve is increased, which results in increased ventilation and eventual restoration of normal carbon dioxide levels.

Clinical Investigations: Arterial Blood Gas

An arterial blood gas test measures the balance of multiple mechanisms of respiratory and metabolic homeostasis. Acid–base balance, and so pH, is controlled by the respiratory and renal systems. Arterial blood gas balance is a direct measure of the body's ability to maintain acid–base homeostasis.

Medications Management

Oxygen

Oxygen is one the most commonly administered drugs for patients who present with complications as a result of altered homeostatic processes. Oxygen is a drug and must be prescribed according to a targeted oxygen saturation range either on a paper or electronic drug chart such as the oxygen alert card from the British Thoracic Society 2023 (O'Driscoll et al. 2017). Normal oxygen saturation levels on room air are 94–98%, however this can be affected by pre-existing comorbidities and age (Hiley et al. 2019; O'Driscoll et al. 2017). Administration and titration of oxygen should be performed by clinical staff who are appropriately trained to detect and manage complications (World Health Organization 2016).

Oxygen saturation levels should be observed for 5–15 minutes after commencing therapy or increasing concentration and should be rechecked after one hour, then four-hourly (O'Driscoll et al. 2017; World Health Organization 2016). Monitoring of oxygen therapy is an element of the physiological track and trigger system, the National Early Warning Score (NEWS). Aany acute deterioration warrants a prompt medical review (O'Driscoll et al. 2017; Preston and Kelly 2016).

Pulse Oximetry

Pulse oximetry measures the percentage of oxygenated haemoglobin in the blood (SpO_2; Preston and Kelly 2016; World Health Organization 2016). It can be used alongside clinical examination and assessment to identify hypoxic patients (low tissue oxygenation), allowing implementation and monitoring of oxygen therapy (Preston and Kelly 2016). British Thoracic Society guidelines state that pulse oximetry should be available in all clinical settings where oxygen therapy is used, and should be documented alongside the oxygen delivery device and inspired oxygen level (FiO_2); O'Driscoll et al. 2017. Clinical staff must be trained in the use of the equipment and have awareness of its limitations to minimise inaccuracies (Preston and Kelly 2016). The Medicine and Healthcare products Regulatory Authority (2021) has issued warnings for clinicians to be aware of incidences of occult hypoxaemia in individuals with darker skin pigmentation when using pulse oximetry.

Reflective Learning Activity

Reflect upon the homeostatic changes you have observed for patients who are suffering from severe sepsis within your own practice.

Red Flag Alert: Malignant Hyperthermia

Malignant hyperthermia is a potentially fatal syndrome that results in a dramatic increase in temperature and multiple disruptions to other homeostatic processes. It results in hyperkalaemia, disseminated intravascular coagulation and acute kidney injury. Patients have a genetic susceptibility (*RYR1* gene mutation) that is often not appreciated until a triggering agent is administered. Suxamethonium, serotonergic drugs, phosphodiesterase type III inhibitors, statins, ondansetron and tetracaine are potential triggering agents.

Snapshot 3.1

Pre-arrival Information

You are dispatched to a 25-year-old man who presents feeling generally unwell with malaise, diarrhoea and vomiting, shortness of breath and myalgia. The patient is conscious and breathing.

Windscreen Report

On approaching the front door of the house, there are no signs of danger and it is safe to enter.

Entering the Location

You announce your arrival and the patient shouts to you that he is on the floor in the kitchen.

On Arrival with the Patient

As you enter, you see the patient sitting on the floor, sweating and short of breath. When you question them further, you find that there have been a few months of general malaise. They have no past medical history and do not take any regular medications.

Patient Assessment

Presenting complaint: malaise, vomiting and diarrhoea, shortness of breath and myalgia.
History of presenting complaint: He has felt generally unwell for a few days with worsening symptoms over the last 24 hours.
Past medical history: type 1 diabetes, poorly controlled.
Drug history: no known drug allergies. Insulin detemir twice daily.
Social history: full-time teacher, non-smoker, occasional alcohol, lives alone.

Primary Survey

Danger: There is no danger and the scene is safe.
Response: The patient has called out therefore they are alert on the ACVPU (alert, confusion, voice, pain, unresponsive) scale.
Catastrophic haemorrhage: No signs of major haemorrhage.
Airway: the patient spoke to you so the airway is patent; there are no added noises.
Breathing: the patient is breathing; respiratory rate 35 breaths/minute (NEWS2 = 3), saturations 94% on room air (NEWS2 = 0), auscultation – good air entry with no added sounds.
Circulation: the patient is sweating, appears well perfused and pink, heart rate is 107 beats/min (NEWS2 = 1), regular, bounding, blood pressure 115/65 mmHg (NEWS2 = 0), capillary refill time < 2 seconds.
Disability: the patient is alert (NEWS2 = 0) and moving all four limbs; pupil size 3 equal and reactive to light; blood glucose 20.1 mmol/l; ketones 4.2 mmol/l; last insulin dose over 12 hours ago.
Exposure: there is no indication to expose the patient; temperature 38.3°C (NEWS2 = 2); pear drop scented breath.
Total NEWS2 score prior to interventions = 6

Secondary Survey

Systems Examination:

- Respiratory – Nil further concerns of note.
- Cardiac – 12-lead ECG – sinus tachycardia.
- Neurological – nil further concerns of note.
- Gastrointestinal – abdomen soft, non-tender.
- Musculoskeletal – nil further concerns of note.

Last input and output: last ate over 24 hours ago; drinking small amounts of water. Bowels open today – diarrhoea, vomited prior to your arrival; passed urine this morning but very dark in colour.
Events leading up: as above.
Physical examination head to toe: no abnormal diagnosis – head, neck, upper limbs, chest, abdomen, pelvis, lower limbs

47

Paramedic Actions

- Primary survey with interventions as required, time critical transfer not indicated.
- Secondary survey with monitoring of <C>ABCD (catastrophic haemorrhage, airway, breathing, circulation, disability) throughout the clinical assessment
- Transfer to local hospital emergency department.
- Provide ATMIST handover to emergency department staff: age, time of onset, mechanisms of injury, injuries suspected, signs, treatments given.

Diagnosis

Patient presentation is that of a diabetic emergency, probably diabetic ketoacidosis due to lack of exogenous insulin administration and an infectious precipitant (gastroenteritis). A resulting metabolic acidosis is likely to be evident on arterial blood gas monitoring.

Take Home Points

- Homeostasis is the activity of cells throughout the body to maintain the physiological state within a narrow range that is compatible with life.
- Homeostatic feedback relies of five components: stimulus, receptor, control centre, effector and response.
- The maintenance of homeostasis is central to all body processes.
- Imbalances in homeostatic mechanisms can result in multiple different presentations.

Summary

As a healthcare practitioner, you will undoubtedly be involved in the care of a number of patients with one or multiple disorders resulting in altered homeostatic processes. These disorders can be very complex and have the potential to have detrimental effects on a patient's activities of daily living. As such, it is crucial that the healthcare professionals involved in supporting these patient groups have a sound understanding of the physiological and pathophysiological processes that underpins the promotion of safe and effective care.

References

Hiley, E., Rickards, E., and Kelly, C.A. (2019). Ensuring the safe use of emergency oxygen in acutely ill patients. *Nurs Times* 155: 18–21.

Lister, S., Hofland, J., and Grafton, H. (ed.) (2020). Blood Glucose Monitoring. Procedure guideline 14.8. In: *Royal Marsden Manual of Clinical Nursing Procedures*, 10e. Chichester: Wiley.

McCance, K. (2019). The cell. In: *Pathophysiology: The Biologic Basis for Disease in Adults and Children*, 8e (ed. K. McCance and S. Huether), 1–132. Philadelphia, PA: Elsevier.

Medicines and Healthcare products Regulatory Agency. (2021). The use and regulation of pulse oximeters (information for healthcare professionals). https://www.gov.uk/guidance/the-use-and-regulation-of-pulse-oximeters-information-for-healthcare-professionals (accessed 28 September 2023).

Mirrasekhian, E., Nilsson, J.L.Å., Shionoya, K. et al. (2018). The antipyretic effect of paracetamol occurs independent of transient receptor potential ankyrin 1-mediated hypothermia and is associated with prostaglandin inhibition in the brain. *The FASEB Journal* 32 (10): 5751–5759. https://doi.org/10.0.4.72/fj.201800272R. Epub 2018 May 8. PMID: 29738273.

National Institute for Health and Care Excellence. (2022). *Hypertension in Adults: Diagnosis and Management*. NICE Guideline NG136. London: National Institute for Health and Care Excellence.

O'Driscoll, B.R., Howard, L.S., Earis, J., and Mak, V. (2017). BTS guideline for oxygen use in adults in healthcare and emergency settings. *Thorax* 72 (Suppl 1): ii1–ii90.

Peate, I. (ed.) (2017). *Fundamentals of Applied Pathophysiology: An essential guide for nursing and healthcare students*. Chichester: Wiley.

Preston, W. and Kelly, C. (2016). *Respiratory Nursing at a Glance*. Chichester: Wiley.

Ward, J.P.T and Linden, R.W.A (2017). Physiology at a Glance. 4th ed. Wiley-Blackwell.

World Health Organization (2016). *Oxygen Therapy for Children*. Geneva: World Health Organization.

Further Reading

Billman, G.E. (2020). Homeostasis: the underappreciated and far too often ignored central organizing principle of physiology. *Frontiers in Physiology* 10 (11): 200. https://doi.org/10.3389/fphys.2020.00200. PMID: 32210840; PMCID: PMC7076167.

Online Resources

British Thoracic Society. Oxygen. https://www.brit-thoracic.org.uk/quality-improvement/clinical-resources/oxygen (accessed 28 September 2023).

Oxygen alert card template, policy template, guidelines and standards.

Khan Academy. Homeostasis. AP/College Biology, Unit 4 Lesson 4. https://www.khanacademy.org/science/ap-biology/cell-communication-and-cell-cycle/feedback/v/homeostasis (accessed 28 September 2023).

Osmosis.org. Acid–base disturbances: pathology review. Osmosis.org. https://www.youtube.com/watch?v=stgY1QgpGxU

Osmosis.org. Common cell signaling pathway. https://www.youtube.com/watch?v=9sF_h-bAnIE (accessed 28 September 2023).

49

Glossary

Acidosis A condition in which the body's fluids are more acidic than normal: acidosis may be either respiratory, when the lungs fail to adequately expire carbon dioxide, or metabolic, when the kidneys fail to maintain a normal balance of acid and base.

Alkalosis A condition of the blood and other body fluids in which the bicarbonate concentration is above normal, tending towards alkalaemia.

Cell membrane The semipermeable membrane enclosing the cytoplasm of a cell.

Cell receptor Any of various specific protein molecules in surface membranes of cells and organelles to which complementary molecules, as hormones, neurotransmitters, antigens or antibodies, may become bound.

Cytoplasm The cell substance between the cell membrane and the nucleus, containing the cytosol, organelles, cytoskeleton and various particles.

Effector An organ or cell that carries out a response to a nerve impulse.

Enzyme Any of various proteins, as pepsin, originating from living cells and capable of producing certain chemical changes in organic substances by catalytic action, as in digestion.

Homeostasis The tendency of a system, especially the physiological system of higher animals, to maintain internal stability, owing to the coordinated response of its parts to any situation or stimulus that would tend to disturb its normal condition or function.

Hormone Any of various internally secreted compounds, as insulin or thyroxine, formed in endocrine glands, that affect the functions of specifically receptive organs or tissues when transported to them by the body fluids.

Osmolality The concentration of an osmotic solution, usually expressed in terms of osmoles.

Multiple Choice Questions

1. Which of the following statements about feedback loops is most accurate?
   a. Positive feedback loops amplify changes to the set point of a system.
   b. Negative feedback loops amplify changes to the set point of a system.
   c. Positive feedback loops reverse changes to the set point of a system.
   d. Negative feedback loops maintain changes to the set point of a system.

2. Which of the following correctly describes how positive and negative feedback mechanisms are similar?
   a. Both feedback mechanisms move a system further from its starting point.
   b. Both feedback mechanisms amplify changes to the set point of a system.
   c. Both feedback mechanisms occur in response to stimuli.
   d. Both feedback mechanisms act to reverse changes in a system.

3. How does the body remove excess carbon dioxide from the body?
   a. By gas exchange in the lungs
   b. By gas exchange in the kidneys
   c. By gas exchange in the liver
   d. By gas exchange via the thyroid gland

4. What is the approximate normal core temperature for the body?
   a. 35°C
   b. 37°C
   c. 39°c
   d. 31°c

5. Where is the body's thermoregulatory centre?
   a. In the brain
   b. In the skin
   c. In the liver
   d. In the lungs

6. What is vasodilation?
   a. Arterioles become wider, increasing the flow of blood in the skin capillaries
   b. Arterioles become narrower, decreasing the flow of blood in the skin capillaries
   c. Arterioles become narrower, increasing the flow of blood in the skin capillaries
   d. Arterioles become wider, decreasing the flow to the capillaries

7. What effect does insulin have on blood glucose concentration?
   a. It increases the concentration of glucose
   b. It increases the concentration of glucagon
   c. It decreases the concentration of glucose
   d. It increases the concentration of glucagon AND glucose

8. What happens when blood Glucose levels become too high?
   a. Insulin is secreted, causing the conversion of glucose to glycogen
   b. Glucagon is secreted, causing the conversion of glucose to glycogen
   c. Insulin is secreted, causing the conversion of glycogen to glucose
   d. Glucagon is excreted, causing the conversion of glucose to glycogen

9. How does insulin travel around the body?
   a. In nerve cells
   b. In the bloodstream
   c. In a gland such as the pancreas

10. What type of feedback is involved in thermoregulation?
    a. Neither
    b. Positive
    c. Neutral
    d. Negative

CHAPTER 4

Trauma and Inflammation

Kylie Kendrick and Scott Stewart

AIM

This chapter aims to provide an understanding of inflammation in the setting of major trauma with a key focus on the triad of death.

LEARNING OUTCOMES

- On completion of this section, you will be able to:
- Describe inflammation in the setting of major trauma.
- Understand the mechanism of coagulopathy, metabolic acidosis and hypothermia.
- Explain the pathophysiology of the triad of death.
- Recognise a patient at risk.
- Explain how clinical management impacts on the triad.

Test Your Prior Knowledge
1. What does haemostasis mean?
2. What is your understanding of the term 'trauma'?
3. What is the coagulation cascade?
4. Describe inflammation.

Introduction

Physical trauma refers to any physical injury that is the result of external forces acting on the body. Trauma is often simply divided into blunt and penetrating, but this dichotomy ignores other causes, such as barotrauma and burns. Major trauma, which refers to injuries that have the potential to cause prolonged disability or death, is estimated to account for 10% of deaths worldwide (Haagsma et al. 2016). Trauma is considered a disease rather than an accident, as it has predictable patterns of occurrence and outcomes that can be modified by factors such as gender, age or alcohol and other drug use (Alberdi et al. 2014).

The burden of trauma falls disproportionately on the young, who suffer a significantly higher loss of disability-adjusted life years (often abbreviated to DALYs). Males are more likely to be affected by trauma as they tend to engage in higher risk activities (Nguyen et al. 2016). Low socioeconomic and low- and middle income-countries (LMICs) generally have higher rates of trauma, death and disability (Shanthakumar et al. 2021). This is due to the fewer preventative measures causing a higher incidence, as well as less effective post-trauma care, producing a higher mortality rate (Reynolds et al. 2017; Wesson et al. 2014). Trauma also has an economic burden, accounting for up to 15% of gross domestic product in LMICs (Wesson et al. 2014).

Trauma is a public health problem that requires preventative efforts at primary, secondary and tertiary levels. Survival from major trauma is often time sensitive (Gauss et al. 2019). The term 'golden hour' has been used to describe the time just after a traumatic event where medical treatment within this time frame maximises survival rates (Lerner and Moscati 2001). However, the actual time frame that differentiates survival from death for any given patient is impacted by individual factors (Rogers et al. 2015).

Immediate death at the scene of injury primarily occurs due to severe physiological derangement, such as obstructed airways, brain lacerations or massive haemorrhage. Early deaths are often attributed to a moderate haemorrhage that is not controlled in a timely manner, while late deaths are often due to organ failure and sepsis (Trunkey 1985).

Improvements in out-of-hospital care have led to sustained improvements in morbidity and mortality post trauma (Kotwal et al. 2016). For example, early deaths due to uncontrolled haemorrhage can be reduced through prehospital medical interventions such as pressure bandages (Cannon 2018), tourniquets (Epstein et al. 2023), intravenous drugs such as tranexamic acid (Roberts and Ageron 2022), topical haemostatic agents (Peng 2020) and surgical interventions such as resuscitative endovascular balloon occlusion of the aorta (Castellini et al. 2021). Later deaths due to trauma-induced coagulopathy (usually occurring in hospital) have also been studied, with changes in prehospital management suggested, such as maintaining patient temperature and reducing fluid administration (Moore et al. 2021).

Out-of-hospital trauma deaths more commonly occur in younger patients, with older patients more likely to die in hospital. Cause of injury also effects the frequency of out-of-hospital deaths, with transport accidents, penetrating injury, hanging and drowning more likely to lead to death, while falls from low heights are more likely to succumb later in hospital (Beck et al. 2019). While the paramedic responding to a trauma patient is iconic, such work often only makes up a small percentage of the case mix (Brown et al. 2018).

Major trauma, also known as polytrauma, can be defined as a patient with an injury severity score (ISS) greater than 15 (Palmer 2007). The ISS is a standardised method of measuring the severity of traumatic injury in patients with multiple injuries. Each patient receives a score between 1 for minor and 6 for unsurvivable injuries, based on injured body regions (e.g. head, face, neck, chest, abdomen, extremities or other). The three most severely injured region scores are squared and summed to generate a total ISS. With an overall range from 1 to 75 (if any region has a score of 6, the ISS is automatically set at 75), a score less than 9 reflects mild severity, 9–15 moderate, 16–24 severe injury and over 25 profound injury.

The ISS is one of the only anatomical scoring systems that directly correlates with morbidity, mortality and length of hospital stay (Javali et al. 2019). For example, a moderate pelvic fracture with an associated blood loss 20% or less by volume scores 4 for the region, which translates to an ISS of 16, designating the patient in the major trauma category (Wu et al. 2020).

Snapshot 4.1

Pre-arrival Information

A 55-year-old man, motorcycle rider vs car on rural highway. Patient unconscious and breathing. Fire and police also responding.

Windscreen Report

Motorbike deeply imbedded into the front passenger's door of an SUV. Patient supine wearing helmet and leathers, lying motionless 20 metres further up highway. Fire and police in attendance. Fire truck protecting scene from traffic.

History (From Bystanders)

Motorbike rider on rural highway has collided at approximately 100 km/h (60 mph) with an SUV pulling out from a side street. Rider travelled over the handlebars and slid along the road before ending up 20 metres further on.

On Arrival with the Patient

55-year-old man wearing a full-face helmet, full motorbike leathers and boots.

Patient Assessment: Primary Survey

Danger: controlled.
Airway: noisy respirations, tolerates oropharyngeal airway, which results in patent airway. Possible cervical spine injury due to mechanism of accident – cervical collar fitted.
Breathing: 28 breaths/minute with adequate tidal volume, L = R normal breath sounds.
Circulation: 138 beats/minute and thready. Significant haemorrhage from R thigh – controlled with pressure bandage.
Disability: AVPU = U. PEARL, bilateral periorbital ecchymosis, open fracture to right femur; pelvis is unstable with a potential fracture and abdomen is rigid.
Exposure and environment: 14°C day with light wind. Patient is warmly dressed but will have clothing removed to examine and blankets added.
Injury scores: head and neck = 5; abdomen = 3; extremities (pelvis) = 5
ISS = 59 (meeting major trauma criteria)

Pathophysiology of Trauma and Inflammation

Physical traumatic insults to the body initiate autonomic, immunological and metabolic responses, which attempt to restore homeostasis (Huber-Lang et al. 2018). The disruption of the cell walls (micro barriers) and compromise to the integrity of the skin (macro barrier) activates the innate immunity – a early, non-specific defence against pathogens (Iwasaki and Medzhitov 2015). This triggers a complex response, including initiating the clotting cascade (Satyam et al. 2019), which is aimed at limiting additional damage and promoting healing. However, this response can also be a significant factor in complications, and even fatal outcomes, following an injury (Huber-Lang et al. 2018). Appropriate and timely out-of-hospital care thus has a major role in improving the outcomes of major trauma (Bedard et al. 2020).

Homeostasis of the Trauma Patient

Homeostasis a dynamic process which describes the body's ability to self-regulate and maintain its internal stability while adjusting to external factors. In the setting of major trauma, homeostasis is most commonly impacted by hypovolaemia. As such, haemostasis is the key focus for treatment. Haemostasis occurs through three distinct processes: the vascular, the platelet and coagulation phases. These components are interlinked and compound each other, thus leading to a significant deterioration in the trauma patient (Moore et al. 2021).

Vascular Phase

When a blood vessel is damaged (cut or ruptured), there is contraction of the smooth muscle fibres within the vessel wall, which is also known as vascular spasm. These spasms are caused by the injury; they cause the smooth muscle to release thromboxane, which helps blood to clot, as well as stimulating the pain receptors (Moffatt 2013). Subsequently, the endothelium becomes sticky, with smaller blood vessels lumina stick together to occlude the vessel damage (Gando and Otomo 2015). Additionally, the spasms reduce the overall lumen size of the vessel, which slows blood loss for approximately 30 minutes from the time of injury (Moffatt 2013).

Platelet Phase

In a normal blood vessel that has not undergone injury, platelets are repelled by the endothelium. However, when a blood vessel is damaged, the platelets adhere to exposed collagen fibres. The platelets then release adenosine diphosphate (ADP), thromboxane and serotonin, which causes further vascular spasm (Moore et al. 2021). The vascular spasm attracts further platelets to the site of injury, which then release their chemical response, adding to the previously adhered platelets. This 'pile' of platelets is referred to as a platelet plug, which increases in size as the platelets aggregate (Kornblith et al. 2019).

Coagulation Phase

The activation of clotting factors is referred to as the coagulation cascade, which is what leads to haemostasis and is responsible for rapid healing (Austin 2017). Coagulation can be initiated via either the intrinsic pathway or the extrinsic pathway, leading to the activation of a fibrin mesh (Chaudhry et al. 2023). Following these pathways is the common pathway, which is the final stage of the cascade.

- The intrinsic pathway is initiated by a combination of factors that occur when protease reactions within the blood encounter the damaged blood vessel lining (endothelium; Moffatt 2013). The intrinsic pathway is slower than the extrinsic pathway and shown to take between three and six minutes.
- The extrinsic pathway is the more rapid pathway and is activated by transmembrane receptor tissue factor and plasma factor, resulting in the activation of factor X (Satyam et al. 2019). Although shorter in time, it is more complex and beyond the scope of this chapter.
- Both the intrinsic and extrinsic pathways lead to the common pathway, which is the final stage that activates fibrinogen into fibrin. Fibrin binds the platelets together, stabilising the platelet plug (Kruger-Genge et al. 2019).

Chapter 8 of this text discusses blood and associated disorders. Figure 4.1 provides a summary of these pathways.

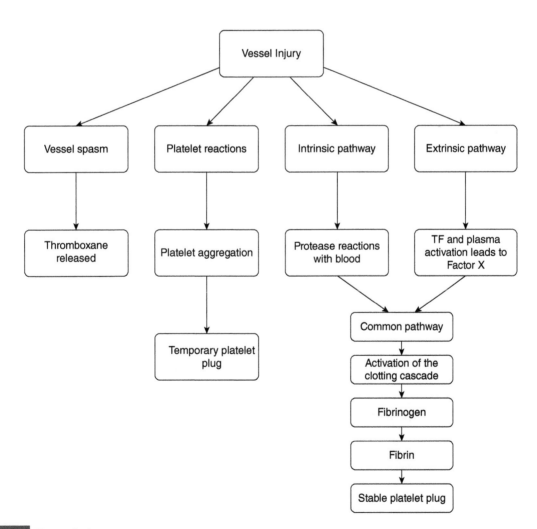

FIGURE 4.1 Haemostasis.

The Inflammatory Process

Further to the creation of the platelet plug, the inflammatory response (inflammation) is initiated when body tissues are injured by major trauma. Upon injury, the damaged cells release a range of chemical mediators such as histamine, prostaglandins and bradykinins (Chen et al. 2018). These chemicals result in leaky blood vessels, which causes fluid to be lost to the tissues, resulting in oedema (swelling), redness and pain (Abdulkhaleq et al. 2018). This can further reduce blood pressure. Additionally, these chemicals attract white blood cells and plasma proteins to the area, which attempt to destroy bacteria and engulf any dead or damaged cells.

The 'Triad of Death'

The process of homeostasis can be significantly impaired by the triad of death, also known as the lethal triad (Figure 4.2). This triad consists of coagulopathy, hypothermia and metabolic acidosis. The interconnectedness of the three physiological derangements can result in a 90% death rate among those experiencing severe trauma (Moffatt 2013).

When a patient experiences a haemorrhage, whether internal or external, it leads to a reduction in the circulating blood volume, which subsequently leads to a reduction in core body temperature and hypoperfusion (Moffatt 2013). This hypoperfusion causes the tissues to become hypoxic and uses anaerobic respiration to create lactic acid, which leads to acidosis of the blood (Mitra et al. 2012). Acidosis of the blood, in conjunction with the hypothermia, slows down the coagulation cascade, which reduces clotting ability and is referred to a *coagulopathy*. Coagulopathy prevents the body from maintaining haemostasis, which causes the haemorrhage to continue (Dobson et al. 2020). The continuing haemorrhage leads to further heat loss and hypoxia, with the acidosis also impairing myocardial performance (Dockrell and Gantner 2023). As the hypoxia and acidosis worsen, this becomes a vicious cycle leading to rapid patient deterioration (Moffatt 2013).

In the setting of major trauma, therefore, stopping the bleed, keeping the patient warm and maintaining blood pressure while minimising dilution of the blood with fluids are critical. Table 4.1 outlines important clinical assessments of the major trauma patient, together with the recognition of the triad of death.

56

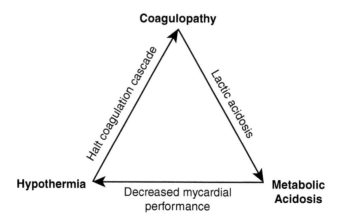

FIGURE 4.2   The triad of death. Source: Burnett 2009/Wikimedia Commons; CC BY 3.00.

TABLE 4.1 Key clinical assessments of the patient with major trauma and the recognition of the triad of death.

Out of hospital	In-hospital
Respiratory rate/pattern	pH testing
Heart rate	Clotting factors (INR testing)
Blood pressure	Ultrasound – determine source of bleeding
Glasgow Coma Scale	MRI
Environment/exposure (tympanic temp)	
pH testing if available	
Ultrasound assessment of free fluid – FAST scan	
ETCO$_2$ as required	

ETCO$_2$, end-tidal carbon dioxide; FAST, focused assessment with sonography for trauma; INR, international normalised ratio; MRI, magnetic resonance imaging.

Management

Hypothermia

To reduce the risk of hypothermia in the prehospital setting, it is important to understand how and why hypothermia occurs in the trauma patient, the associated risk factors and implications in the triad of death.

The normal core body temperature is 35.6–37.8°C, with a mean rectal temperature of 37.0°C, tympanic 36.6°C and oral 36.6°C (Geneva et al. 2019). Hypothermia is defined as a core temperature of less than 35.0°C, and up to two-thirds of all patients with major trauma are hypothermic on arrival at an emergency department (Weuster et al. 2016). The presence of hypothermia on arrival leads to an overall higher mortality, longer length of hospital stay and higher infusion rates in this cohort (van Veelen and Brodmann Maeder 2021).

Temperature that drops below normal limits causes the activation of heat-generating mechanisms to return the body to within normal limits. In someone who has a reduced body temperature, the hypothalamus causes the body to shiver, which requires an increased cellular respiration to meet the energy demand (i.e. generation of ADP; Duong and Patel 2019). Blood has a significant role in the regulation of body temperature, as it absorbs the heat generated by the skeletal muscle and redistributes this heat to other tissues (Rauch et al. 2021). When the core body temperature is below normal, warm blood flow is restricted to the vital organs (Paal et al. 2022). As heat is produced by cellular respiration, it can also be decreased by hypoperfusion or hypovolemia, as seen in the trauma patient (Liu 2023). Decreased heat production, together with the role of blood in heat distribution, means that haemorrhage can result in a rapid decrease in body temperature. In addition, hypothermia can lead to a left shift on the oxygen disassociation curve (which is where oxygen is prevented from unloading into the tissues), reduced cardiac output, dysrhythmias and coagulation (Jo 2022).

Temperature has a direct connection with clotting factors, which are optimum around 36.6°C (Hensley et al. 2021). Hypothermia delays the enzymes within the coagulation cascade and results in the prolongation of the coagulation time. Hypothermia has been shown to have a significant impact on the trauma patient (Balvers et al. 2016), with a temperature of less than 32.0°C on hospital admission associated with a survival rate approaching 0% (Moffatt 2013). Several risk factors for hypothermia in trauma are influenced by paramedic care. These include the seriousness of the injury, out-of-hospital intubation, wet clothing, environmental temperature and the administration of cold fluids (Balmer et al. 2022).

Best practice management includes actions that prevent heat loss such as removing the patient from any cold or wet environments, providing blankets (thermal if necessary) and including the provision of heat, which may include using the heater in the ambulance, or the use of warm fluids or heat packs (Haverkamp et al. 2018). Gentle handling of the patient is also imperative, as cardiac dysrhythmias are also a risk in the patient with hypothermia (Brown et al. 2012).

Coagulopathy

Coagulopathy is described as a problem with blood clotting and can happen for a number of reasons. It is common in approximately 25% of patients presenting with trauma (Kornblith et al. 2019). Coagulopathy occurs from a combination of haemorrhage, haemodilution, clotting factors, hypothermia and acidotic conditions (Moffatt 2013). Extensive injuries can lead to disseminated intravascular coagulation (DIC), which is a form of coagulopathy. DIC leads to the formation of small blood clots within the blood vessels, which can obstruct blood flow to vital organs. DIC also results in a deficiency of clotting factors that are needed to maintain haemostasis allowing the haemorrhage to continue.

Best practice management in the out-of-hospital setting includes preventing hypothermia, which increases risk of metabolic acidosis, preventing further blood loss and restoring circulating volume. Although large volumes of crystalloids such as physiological (0.9%) saline can increase blood pressure, they may exacerbate coagulopathy and dislodge clots (Moore et al. 2021).

The addition of coagulation factor concentrates and rapid transport to an emergency department with trauma management capabilities are imperative in this patient cohort. Vitamin K is commonly used in the hospital setting, as it plays an important role in coagulation (Nascimento et al. 2012).

Metabolic Acidosis

Under normal conditions, aerobic respiration provides energy in the form of adenosine triphosphate (ATP), which is demonstrated in Figure 4.3.

Hypovolaemia leads to a decrease in oxygen delivery, which means that the body is unable to meet the overall oxygen demand. Due to the hypoxic conditions, tissues start to respire anaerobically, which creates lactic acid. The continuing production of lactic acid leads to metabolic acidosis (Burša and Pleva 2014). The various clotting factors that become active during haemostasis and the associated coagulation cascade are affected by pH. Normal body pH is 7.35–7.45. A pH outside

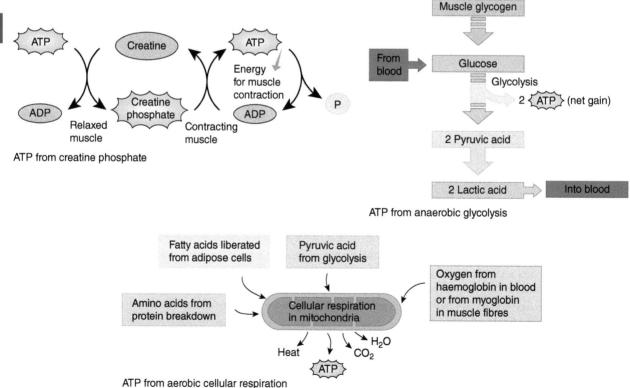

FIGURE 4.3   Aerobic respiration.

this range can result in the denaturing of the clotting enzymes, which has a negative effect on coagulation. The ability of thrombin to generate is altered at a pH below 7.3 and acidosis also slow both the intrinsic and extrinsic coagulation pathways. In addition, acidosis decreases myocardial contractility and cardiac output and causes vasodilation, hypotension, reduced blood flow to organs such as the kidney and liver, and can cause ventricular dysrhythmias (Lier et al. 2008).

Best practice management of metabolic acidosis in the out-of-hospital setting includes the management of hypoxia and hypoperfusion, as these are the two key factors that lead to metabolic acidosis. High-flow oxygen and rapid fluid administration are essential (Spahn et al. 2019). Where available, both tranexamic acid and prothrombin have been demonstrated to reverse severe acidosis effectively (Porta et al. 2013).

Red/Orange Flag Alerts

Red and orange flags are used to identify clinical assessments that are known to be an indicator of deterioration/severity. Red flags identify significant derangement and are a clear warning sign, whereas orange flags identify increasing risk and/or deterioration.

Red flags	Orange flags
Respiration rate < 10 or > 30 breaths/min	GCS < 15
Heart rate < 60 or > 120 beats/min	Respiration rate gradually increasing or at the higher end of normal post trauma
Blood pressure < 90 mmHg systolic	Shivering
Oxygen saturation (SpO$_2$) < 90	Significant comorbidities
GCS < 13	
Temperature < 35.6°C or > 37.8°C	

GCS, Glasgow Coma Scale score.

59

Out-of-Hospital Medications

A variety of medications are given in the prehospital environment. A summary is given in Table 4.2.

TABLE 4.2 Out of hospital medications.

Medication	Use
0.9% NaCl physiological (normal) saline	Isotonic fluid that expands blood volume to increase blood pressure but carries little oxygen and dilutes clotting factors (Curran et al. 2021). It has a short intravascular half-life of 30 minutes, which may be increased in shocked individuals (Hahn and Lyons 2016). Beware of haemodilution and disrupting clots
Oxygen therapy	Provided in efforts to relieve hypoxaemia. It does not improve ventilation or resolve the underling issue
Fentanyl	Powerful synthetic opioid that has a faster onset than morphine and less histamine is released, hence it causes less vasodilation and is therefore better for a patient following hypotensive trauma (Huang et al. 2022; Watso et al. 2022). Can be administered intravenously, intraosseously, intranasally, subcutaneously, orally, transmucosally
Sodium bicarbonate	Hypertonic crystalloid solution which can be used to normalise the acid–base imbalance associated with metabolic acidosis; It does not resolve the underlying cause
Tranexamic acid	Used in efforts to prevent excessive blood loss; it works by slowing the breakdown of blood clots

Snapshot 4.2

Pre-arrival Information

36-year-old woman trapped under tractor at rural location. Fire and police also responding.

Windscreen Report

Adult female trapped under tractor that has rolled over on a farm in a rural location. Fire and police in attendance.

History

A 36-year-old woman is working on her hobby farm. The tractor she is driving flipped over and she was trapped with the roll bar across her abdomen and mid-thigh region. Unable to reach her phone or two-way radio to call for help, she was found four hours later when her partner returned from work.

Patient Assessment: Primary Survey

Danger: controlled – fire brigade has stabilised the tractor and can lift off when directed.
Airway: patient is maintaining patent airway. Glasgow Coma Scale score: 14 (E3, V5, M6).
Breathing: 20 breaths/minute with adequate tidal volume, L = R normal breath sounds. Speaking in sentences.
Circulation: 66 beats/minute; blood pressure: 98/60 mmHg, no significant external haemorrhage.
Skin: pale and cool, dry with delayed capillary refill above the mid-thigh crush point while dusky below it, with no capillary refill or pedal pulses.
Disability: AVPU = A. PEARL: patient has some minor cuts and grazes to her face. She has 4/10 pain at the crush site and numbness distally. Her pelvis appears intact.
Exposure and environment: 8°C day with light wind. Patient is warmly dressed but is in contact with the ground and will have clothing removed to examine and blankets added. Tympanic temperature: 34.0°C.
Injury scores: head and neck = 0; face = 1; chest = 0; abdomen = 4; extremities 5; external = 1
ISS = 42 (meeting major trauma criteria)

Pathophysiology of Injury

This patient has been exposed to a cold environment and is hypothermic. She has also suffered blood loss, resulting in hypotension. The injury itself includes a crush injury. Skeletal muscle can tolerate ischaemia for two hours before irreversible changes occur, with necrosis beginning at six hours (Cote et al. 2020). The patient has a localised injury to her thighs, including crush syndrome. Crush syndrome is a condition characterised by traumatic rhabdomyolysis, which occurs when pressure is released after an extended period of muscle compression (Kodadek et al. 2022). This leads to the systemic release of muscle cell contents, including potassium and myoglobin. The damage to the muscle sarcolemma, the protective covering of muscle fibres, results in increased membrane permeability and the leakage of cellular contents. The compression of the muscle reduces tissue perfusion, leading to ischaemia and a switch from aerobic to anaerobic metabolism (Bjertnæs et al. 2022). This metabolic shift causes the accumulation of lactic acid, resulting in metabolic acidosis. The cellular membrane damage allows sodium, water and calcium to enter the cell, causing swelling, while potassium, myoglobin, purines and other toxins leak out into the surrounding tissue (Chavez et al. 2016). When the pressure is released, these cell contents are released into the systemic circulation. This can cause profound hypotension due to the permeable membranes in the injured tissues (Bjertnæs et al. 2022).

Management

The patient is cold, acidotic and hypovolemic, meaning she is time critical given the triad of death. Bilateral large-bore intravenous access is gained, and she is given 20 ml/kg of warmed 0.9% NaCl before release of the compression by the tractor (Bolt 2006). Analgesia is via fentanyl 50 µg. She is handled gently to reduce stimulating arrhythmias (Vardon et al. 2016). Her wet clothing is removed and she is wrapped in layers of cotton and mylar 'space' blankets to reduce further heat loss (Forristal et al. 2020). Inside the ambulance, the heater is tuned up and further warmed fluids are titrated to a blood pressure of 90 mmHg systolic (Lott et al. 2021). Fluid demands can be significant as each injured limb can sequester 10 l in odema due to increased permeability. (Cote et al. 2020).

Take Home Points

- Trauma is a public health problem that requires efforts at primary, secondary and tertiary prevention.
- Major trauma accounts for 10% of deaths worldwide and requires rapid identification and management to reduce mortality and length of stay in hospital.
- One of the most significant findings in major trauma is the triad of death, which includes hypothermia, metabolic acidosis and coagulopathy.
- The management of each of these components is imperative and requires both pharmacological and non-pharmacological actions to be undertaken.
- Rapid transport to an emergency department with trauma capabilities should also be considered early in the management of these patients.

Summary

Major trauma is a common cause of death in the out-of-hospital care environment. The unique pathophysiology of the body's response to trauma provides three key outcomes which must be assessed and managed by paramedics – the triad of death, which includes hypothermia, coagulopathy and metabolic acidosis. Best practice management includes stopping the bleed and providing fluids to prevent hypotension and preventing heat loss and actively warming the patient to avoid hypothermia. Acidosis management may also be initiated prehospitally. Rapid transport to an emergency department with major trauma capabilities is essential to reduce morbidity and mortality.

References

Abdulkhaleq, L., Assi, M., Abdullah, R. et al. (2018). The crucial roles of inflammatory mediators in inflammation: a review. *Veterinary World* 11 (5): 627. https://www.ncbi.nlm.nih.gov/pmc/articles/PMC5993766/pdf/VetWorld-11-627.pdf.

Alberdi, F., Garcia, I., Atutxa, L. et al. (2014). Epidemiology of severe trauma. *Medicina Intensiva* 38 (9): 580–588. https://doi.org/10.1016/j.medin.2014.06.012.

Austin, S.K. (2017). Haemostasis. *Medicine* 45 (4): 204–208.

Balmer, J.C., Hieb, N., Daley, B.J. et al. (2022). Continued relevance of initial temperature measurement in trauma patients. *The American Surgeon* 88 (3): 424–428. https://doi.org/10.1177/00031348211048833.

Balvers, K., Van der Horst, M., Graumans, M. et al. (2016). Hypothermia as a predictor for mortality in trauma patients at admittance to the intensive care unit. *Journal of Emergencies, Trauma, and Shock* 9 (3): 97–102. https://doi.org/10.4103/0974-2700.185276.

Beck, B., Smith, K., Mercier, E. et al. (2019). Differences in the epidemiology of out-of-hospital and in-hospital trauma deaths. *PLoS One* 14 (6): e0217158. https://doi.org/10.1371/journal.pone.0217158.

Bedard, A.F., Mata, L.V., Dymond, C. et al. (2020). A scoping review of worldwide studies evaluating the effects of prehospital time on trauma outcomes. *The International Journal of Emergency Medicine* 13 (1): 64. https://doi.org/10.1186/s12245-020-00324-7.

Bjertnæs, L.J., Næsheim, T.O., Reierth, E. et al. (2022). Physiological changes in subjects exposed to accidental hypothermia: an update. *Frontiers in Medicine* 9: 824395.

Bolt, B. (2006). *Earthquakes: 2006 Centennial Update*. Macmillan.

Brown, D.J., Brugger, H., Boyd, J., and Paal, P. (2012). Accidental hypothermia. *New England Journal of Medicine* 367 (20): 1930–1938.

Brown, E., Williams, T.A., Tohira, H. et al. (2018). Epidemiology of trauma patients attended by ambulance paramedics in Perth, Western Australia. *Emergency Medicine Australasia* 30 (6): 827–833. https://doi.org/10.1111/1742-6723.13148.

Burnett, C. (2009). *Trauma triad of death.svg*. Retrieved 23 May from https://commons.wikimedia.org/wiki/File:Trauma_triad_of_death.svg

Burša, F. and Pleva, L. (2014). Anaerobic metabolism associated with traumatic hemorrhagic shock monitored by microdialysis of muscle tissue is dependent on the levels of hemoglobin and central venous oxygen saturation: a prospective, observational study. *Scandinavian Journal of Trauma, Resuscitation and Emergency Medicine* 22 (1): 1–9.

Cannon, J.W. (2018). Hemorrhagic shock. *New England Journal of Medicine* 378 (4): 370–379. https://doi.org/10.1056/NEJMra1705649.

61

Castellini, G., Gianola, S., Biffi, A. et al. (2021). Resuscitative endovascular balloon occlusion of the aorta (REBOA) in patients with major trauma and uncontrolled haemorrhagic shock: a systematic review with meta-analysis. *World Journal of Emergency Surgery: WJES* 16 (1): 41. https://doi.org/10.1186/s13017-021-00386-9.

Chaudhry, R., Usama, S.M., and Babiker, H.M. (2023). *Physiology, Coagulation Pathways*. Treasure Island, FL: StatPearls Publishing.

Chavez, L.O., Leon, M., Einav, S., and Varon, J. (2016). Beyond muscle destruction: a systematic review of rhabdomyolysis for clinical practice. *Critical Care* 20 (1): 1–11.

Chen, L., Deng, H., Cui, H. et al. (2018). Inflammatory responses and inflammation-associated diseases in organs. *Oncotarget* 9 (6): 7204–7218. https://doi.org/10.18632/oncotarget.23208.

Cote, D.R., Fuentes, E., Elsayes, A.H. et al. (2020). A "crush" course on rhabdomyolysis: risk stratification and clinical management update for the perioperative clinician. *Journal of Anesthesia* 34 (4): 585–598. https://doi.org/10.1007/s00540-020-02792-w.

Curran, J.D., Major, P., Tang, K. et al. (2021). Comparison of balanced crystalloid solutions: a systematic review and meta-analysis of randomized controlled trials. *Critical Care Exploration* 3 (5): e0398. https://doi.org/10.1097/cce.0000000000000398.

Dobson, G.P., Morris, J.L., Davenport, L.M., and Letson, H.L. (2020). Traumatic-induced coagulopathy as a systems failure: a new window into hemostasis. *Seminars in Thrombosis and Hemostasis* 46: 199–214.

Dockrell, L. and Gantner, D. (2023). Shock: causes, assessment and investigation. *Anaesthesia and Intensive Care Medicine* 24 (2): 99–107. <Go to ISI>://WOS:000964960400001.

Duong, H. and Patel, G. (2019). *Hypothermia*. Treasure Island, FL: StatPearls Publishing.

Epstein, A., Lim, R., Johannigman, J. et al. (2023). Putting medical boots on the ground: lessons from the war in Ukraine and applications for future conflict with near peer adversaries. *Journal of the American College of Surgeons* https://doi.org/10.1097/XCS.0000000000000707.

Forristal, C., Van Aarsen, K., Columbus, M. et al. (2020). Predictors of hypothermia upon trauma center arrival in severe trauma patients transported to hospital via EMS. *Prehospital Emergency Care* 24 (1): 15–22.

Gando, S. and Otomo, Y. (2015). Local hemostasis, immunothrombosis, and systemic disseminated intravascular coagulation in trauma and traumatic shock. *Critical Care* 19: 1–11.

Gauss, T., Ageron, F.X., Devaud, M.L. et al. (2019). Association of prehospital time to in-hospital trauma mortality in a physician-staffed emergency medicine system. *JAMA Surgery* 154 (12): 1117–1124. https://doi.org/10.1001/jamasurg.2019.3475.

Geneva, I.I., Cuzzo, B., Fazili, T., Javaid, W. (2019). Normal body temperature: a systematic review. Open Forum Infectious Diseases 6: ofz032.

Haagsma, J.A., Graetz, N., Bolliger, I. et al. (2016). The global burden of injury: incidence, mortality, disability-adjusted life years and time trends from the global burden of disease study 2013. *Injury Prevention* 22 (1): 3–18. https://doi.org/10.1136/injuryprev-2015-041616.

Hahn, R.G. and Lyons, G. (2016). The half-life of infusion fluids: an educational review. *European Journal of Anaesthesiology* 33 (7): 475–482. https://doi.org/10.1097/eja.0000000000000436.

Haverkamp, F.J., Giesbrecht, G.G., and Tan, E.C. (2018). The prehospital management of hypothermia – an up-to-date overview. *Injury* 49 (2): 149–164. https://www.injuryjournal.com/article/S0020-1383(17)30777-5/fulltext https://www.sciencedirect.com/science/article/pii/S0020138317307775?via%3Dihub.

Hensley, N.B., Kostibas, M.P., Koch, C.G., and Frank, S.M. (2021). Perioperative blood management in cardiac surgery. In: *Evidence-Based Practice in Perioperative Cardiac Anesthesia and Surgery* (ed. D.C.H. Cheng, J. Martin, and T. David), 273–286. Cham: Springer.

Huang, M., Watso, J.C., Belval, L.N. et al. (2022). Low-dose fentanyl does not alter muscle sympathetic nerve activity, blood pressure, or tolerance during progressive central hypovolemia. *American Journal of Physiology. Regulatory, Integrative and Comparative Physiology* 322 (1): R55–r63. https://doi.org/10.1152/ajpregu.00217.2021.

Huber-Lang, M., Lambris, J.D., and Ward, P.A. (2018). Innate immune responses to trauma. *Nature Immunology* 19 (4): 327–341. https://doi.org/10.1038/s41590-018-0064-8.

Iwasaki, A. and Medzhitov, R. (2015). Control of adaptive immunity by the innate immune system. *Nature Immunology* 16 (4): 343–353. https://doi.org/10.1038/ni.3123.

Javali, R.H., Krishnamoorthy, P.,.A., Srinivasarangan, M. et al. (2019). Comparison of injury severity score, new injury severity score, revised trauma score and trauma and injury severity score for mortality prediction in elderly trauma patients. *Indian Journal of Critical Care Medicine* 23 (2): 73–77. https://doi.org/10.5005/jp-journals-10071-23120.

Jo, K.W. (2022). Target temperature management in traumatic brain injury with a focus on adverse events, recognition, and prevention. *Acute and Critical Care* 37 (4): 483–490. https://doi.org/10.4266/acc.2022.01291.

Kodadek, L., Carmichael, S.P., Seshadri, A. et al. (2022). Rhabdomyolysis: an American association for the surgery of trauma critical care committee clinical consensus document. *Trauma Surgery & Acute Care Open* 7 (1): e000836.

Kornblith, L.Z., Moore, H.B., and Cohen, M.J. (2019). Trauma-induced coagulopathy: the past, present, and future. *Journal of Thrombosis and Haemostasis* 17 (6): 852–862. https://www.ncbi.nlm.nih.gov/pmc/articles/PMC6545123/pdf/nihms-1023740.pdf.

Kotwal, R.S., Howard, J.T., Orman, J.A. et al. (2016). The effect of a golden hour policy on the morbidity and mortality of combat casualties. *JAMA Surgery* 151 (1): 15–24. https://doi.org/10.1001/jamasurg.2015.3104.

Kruger-Genge, A., Blocki, A., Franke, R.P., and Jung, F. (2019). Vascular endothelial cell biology: an update. *International Journal of Molecular Sciences* 20 (18): 4411. https://doi.org/10.3390/ijms20184411.

Lerner, E.B. and Moscati, R.M. (2001). The golden hour: scientific fact or medical "urban legend"? *Academic Emergency Medicine* 8 (7): 758–760. https://doi.org/10.1111/j.1553-2712.2001.tb00201.x.

Lier, H., Krep, H., Schroeder, S., and Stuber, F. (2008). Preconditions of hemostasis in trauma: a review. The influence of acidosis, hypocalcemia, anemia, and hypothermia on functional hemostasis in trauma. *Journal of Trauma and Acute Care Surgery* 65 (4): 951–960.

Liu, L. (2023). Hemorrhagic shock. In: *Explosive Blast Injuries: Principles and Practices*, 211–226. Springer.

Lott, C., Truhlář, A., Alfonzo, A. et al. (2021). European resuscitation council guidelines 2021: cardiac arrest in special circumstances. *Resuscitation* 161: 152–219.

Mitra, B., Tullio, F., Cameron, P.A., and Fitzgerald, M. (2012). Trauma patients with the 'triad of death'. *Emergency Medicine Journal* 29 (8): 622–625. https://emj.bmj.com/content/29/8/622.long https://emj.bmj.com/content/emermed/29/8/622.full.pdf.

Moffatt, S.E. (2013). Hypothermia in trauma. *Emergency Medicine Journal: EMJ* 30 (12): 989–996. https://doi.org/10.1136/emermed-2012-201883.

Moore, E.E., Moore, H.B., Kornblith, L.Z. et al. (2021). Trauma-induced coagulopathy. *Nature Reviews Disease Primers* 7 (1): 30. https://doi.org/10.1038/s41572-021-00264-3.

Nascimento, B., Al Mahoos, M., Callum, J. et al. (2012). Vitamin K-dependent coagulation factor deficiency in trauma: a comparative analysis between international normalized ratio and thromboelastography (CME). *Transfusion* 52 (1): 7–13. https://onlinelibrary.wiley.com/doi/pdfdirect/10.1111/j.1537-2995.2011.03237.x?download=true.

Nguyen, R., Fiest, K.M., McChesney, J. et al. (2016). The international incidence of traumatic brain injury: a systematic review and meta-analysis. *Canadian Journal of Neurological Sciences* 43 (6): 774–785.

Paal, P., Pasquier, M., Darocha, T. et al. (2022). Accidental hypothermia: 2021 update. *International Journal of Environmental Research and Public Health* 19 (1): 501. https://doi.org/10.3390/ijerph19010501.

Palmer, C. (2007). Major trauma and the injury severity score--where should we set the bar? *Annual Proceedings. Association for the Advancement of Automotive Medicine* 51: 13–29. https://www.ncbi.nlm.nih.gov/pubmed/18184482 https://www.ncbi.nlm.nih.gov/pmc/articles/PMC3217501/pdf/aam51_p013.pdf.

Peng, H.T. (2020). Hemostatic agents for prehospital hemorrhage control: a narrative review. *Military Medical Research* 7 (1): 13. https://doi.org/10.1186/s40779-020-00241-z.

Porta, C.R., Nelson, D., McVay, D. et al. (2013). The effects of tranexamic acid and prothrombin complex concentrate on the coagulopathy of trauma: an in vitro analysis of the impact of severe acidosis. *Journal of Trauma and Acute Care Surgery* 75 (6): 954–960. https://doi.org/10.1097/TA.0b013e31829e20bf.

Rauch, S., Miller, C., Brauer, A. et al. (2021). Perioperative hypothermia-a narrative review. *International Journal of Environmental Research and Public Health* 18 (16): 8749. https://doi.org/10.3390/ijerph18168749.

Reynolds, T.A., Stewart, B., Drewett, I. et al. (2017). The impact of trauma care systems in low- and middle-income countries. *Annual Review of Public Health* 38: 507–532. https://doi.org/10.1146/annurev-publhealth-032315-021412.

Roberts, I. and Ageron, F.X. (2022). The role of tranexamic acid in trauma – a life-saving drug with proven benefit. *Nature Reviews. Disease Primers* 8 (1): 34. https://doi.org/10.1038/s41572-022-00367-5.

Rogers, F.B., Rittenhouse, K.J., and Gross, B.W. (2015). The golden hour in trauma: dogma or medical folklore? *Injury* 46 (4): 525–527. https://doi.org/10.1016/j.injury.2014.08.043.

Satyam, A., Graef, E.R., Lapchak, P.H. et al. (2019). Complement and coagulation cascades in trauma. *Acute Medicine & Surgery* 6 (4): 329–335. https://doi.org/10.1002/ams2.426.

Shanthakumar, D., Payne, A., Leitch, T., and Alfa-Wali, M. (2021). Trauma care in low-and middle-income countries. *The Surgery Journal* 7 (04), e281–e285.

Spahn, D.R., Bouillon, B., Cerny, V. et al. (2019). The European guideline on management of major bleeding and coagulopathy following trauma. *Critical Care* 23: 1–74.

Trunkey, D. (1985). Towards optimal trauma care. *Archives of Emergency Medicine* 2 (4): 181–195. https://doi.org/10.1136/emj.2.4.181.

Vardon, F., Mrozek, S., Geeraerts, T., and Fourcade, O. (2016). Accidental hypothermia in severe trauma. *Anaesthesia Critical Care & Pain Medicine* 35 (5): 355–361.

van Veelen, M.J. and Brodmann Maeder, M. (2021). Hypothermia in trauma. *International Journal of Environmental Research and Public Health* 18 (16): https://doi.org/10.3390/ijerph18168719.

Watso, J.C., Belval, L.N., Cimino, F.A. 3rd et al. (2022). Low-dose morphine reduces tolerance to central hypovolemia in healthy adults without affecting muscle sympathetic outflow. *American Journal of Physiology. Heart and Circulatory Physiology* 323 (1): H89–h99. https://doi.org/10.1152/ajpheart.00091.2022.

Wesson, H.K., Boikhutso, N., Bachani, A.M. et al. (2014). The cost of injury and trauma care in low- and middle-income countries: a review of economic evidence. *Health Policy and Planning* 29 (6): 795–808. https://doi.org/10.1093/heapol/czt064.

Weuster, M., Bruck, A., Lippross, S. et al. (2016). Epidemiology of accidental hypothermia in polytrauma patients: an analysis of 15,230 patients of the TraumaRegister DGU. *Journal of Trauma and Acute Care Surgery* 81 (5): 905–912. https://doi.org/10.1097/TA.0000000000001220.

Wu, Y.T., Cheng, C.T., Tee, Y.S. et al. (2020). Pelvic injury prognosis is more closely related to vascular injury severity than anatomical fracture complexity: the WSES classification for pelvic trauma makes sense. *World Journal of Emergency Surgery* 15 (1): 1–9. https://doi.org/10.1186/s13017-020-00328-x.

Further Reading

Friedman, M.J., Resick, P.A., Bryant, R.A. et al. (2011). Classification of trauma and stressor-related disorders in DSM-5. *Depression and Anxiety* 28 (9): 737–749. https://doi.org/10.1002/da.20845.

Gallaher, J., An, S.J., Kayange, L. et al. (2023). Tri-modal distribution of trauma deaths in a resource-limited setting: perception versus reality. *World Journal of Surgery* https://doi.org/10.1007/s00268-023-06971-0.

Galvagno, S.M. Jr., Sikorski, R., Hirshon, J.M. et al. (2015). Helicopter emergency medical services for adults with major trauma. *Cochrane Database of Systematic Reviews* 2015 (12): CD009228. https://doi.org/10.1002/14651858.CD009228.pub3.

Gando, S. and Otomo, Y. (2015). Local hemostasis, immunothrombosis, and systemic disseminated intravascular coagulation in trauma and traumatic shock. *Critical Care* 19 (1): 72. https://doi.org/10.1186/s13054-015-0735-x.

Nellist, E. and Lethbridge, K. (2013). Rhabdomyolysis: an overview for pre-hospital clinicians. *Journal of Paramedic Practice* 5 (8): 442–446.

Paniker, J., Graham, S. M., and Harrison, J. W. (2015). Global trauma: the great divide. *SICOT-J,* 1: 19.

Online Resources

Evidencio. Injury Severity Score: https://www.evidencio.com/models/show/369 – this online resource supports clinical decision making and calculates the ISS based on data entry and can be used for either training or clinical purposes.

Gerecht, R. (2014). Trauma's lethal triad of hypothermia, acidosis and coagulopathy create a deadly cycle for trauma patients. *JEMS Journal of Emergency Medical Services* 4 February: https://www.jems.com/patient-care/trauma-s-lethal-triad-hypothermia-acidos.

NHS England. (2020). Clinical guidelines for major incidents and mass casualty events: https://www.england.nhs.uk/publication/clinical-guidelines-for-major-incidents-and-mass-casualty-events.

Glossary

Adenosine diphosphate (ADP)	Molecule responsible for the transfer and provision of energy within the cell
Adenosine triphosphate (ATP)	An organic compound providing energy to drive and support many processes in living cells
Aggregation	Binding together
Anaerobic respiration	The process of energy use (ATP) without adequate oxygen supply to the tissues
Bradykinin	Compound in the blood that causes contraction of smooth muscle and dilation of blood vessels
Coagulation	Usually associated with the cessation of blood loss from a damaged blood vessel by converting a liquid to a semisolid state or gel, forming a blood clot
Coagulopathy	Alteration of haemostasis resulting in excessive bleeding or clotting
Crystalloids	A aqueous solution of minerals that are water soluble and able to pass through a semipermeable membrane
Disability adjusted life years (DALYs)	1 DALY = loss of the equivalent of one year of health
Disseminated intravascular coagulation (DIC)	Condition which causes abnormal clotting of the blood, leading to micro thrombi

Factor X	An enzyme in the coagulation cascade
Fibrin	A protein formed from fibrinogen during the process of blood clotting
Golden hour	Used to suggest that an individual requires urgent medical care; it is also suggested that if care is not received in the first hour following injury, there is an increase in both morbidity and mortality
Haemorrhage	The loss of blood from a damaged blood vessel
Haemodilution	Increase in fluid concentration in the blood, leading to a lower amount of red blood cells
Haemostasis	The body's natural reaction to cease bleeding and repair damage
Histamine	Compound released by the cells in response to injury or allergic or inflammatory reactions, leading to contraction of the smooth muscles and dilation of the capillaries
Homeostasis	The ability of an organism to self-regulate and maintain internal stability irrespective of the external environment
Hypoperfusion	Decreased blood flow to the vital organs
Hypothermia	Core body temperature of less than 35°C
Hypoxia	Deficiency of oxygen reaching the tissues
Hypotension	Decrease in systemic blood pressure below accepted values (accepted values are variable but typically considered to be >100 mmHg systolic in the 'standard' adult)
Injury severity score (ISS)	A medical score used to establish trauma severity
Inflammation	Normal part of the body's response to injury and infection where the body releases chemicals to trigger an immune response to fight off infection or heal damaged tissue
Lactic acid	A chemical that the body makes when using carbohydrates for energy; lactic acid increases when oxygen decreases
Metabolic acidosis	The build-up of too many acids within the blood
Oxygen dissociation curve	A graph which shows how oxygen binds to haemoglobin
Phagocytosis	The process of engulfing and eliminating particles such as microorganisms or apoptotic cells
pH	Scale representing the acidity or alkalinity of a solution; normal body pH is 7.35–7.45
Platelet	Cells within the blood that bind together when they recognise a damaged vessel
Prostaglandins	Lipids made at the site of tissue damage or infection, directly involved in the healing process
Prothrombin	Protein in the blood which converts to thrombin during coagulation
Serotonin	Naturally occurring hormone which has implications for mood; it also acts as neurotransmitter that has the ability to constrict blood vessels
Thromboxane	Vasoconstricting agent, which is also facilitates platelet aggregation
Tranexamic acid	Synthetic compound that inhibits the breakdown of fibrin within blood clots
Vitamin K	Vitamin essential for clotting processes

Multiple Choice Questions

1. Major trauma accounts for what percentage of deaths worldwide?
   a. 5%
   b. 10%
   c. 15%
   d. 20%

2. The time just after a traumatic event where treatment maximises the survival rate is:
   a. 60 minutes
   b. Immediately
   c. 24 hours
   d. Varies with the extent of trauma and the patient

3. Which of the following phases is NOT part of haemostasis?
   a. Coagulation phase
   b. Haemorrhage phase
   c. Platelet phase
   d. Vascular phase

4. Vascular spasm post traumatic injury causes the smooth muscle to release which chemical mediator?
   a. Prostaglandins
   b. Thromboxane
   c. Adenosine diphosphate
   d. Bradykinins

5. Which of the following is correct?
   a. The intrinsic pathway is faster than the extrinsic pathway
   b. The extrinsic pathway is superior to the intrinsic pathway
   c. The common pathway activates fibrinogen into fibrin
   d. The primary pathway is initiated by vessel injury

6. The presence of which physiological derangement post major trauma leads to higher mortality and longer length of stay at hospital?
   a. Hypertension
   b. An ISS < 15
   c. Shivering
   d. Hypothermia

7. What is the cornerstone management of metabolic acidosis?
   a. High-flow oxygen and rapid fluid administration
   b. Rapid fluid administration and blood products
   c. High-flow oxygen and thromboxane
   d. Rapid fluid administration and rapid warming

8. Anaerobic respiration creates which concern in the trauma patient?
   a. Acidosis
   b. Coagulopathy
   c. Hypothermia
   d. Hyperoxia

9. Hypothermia is defined as a temperature lower than:
   a. 37.2°C
   b. 36.6°C
   c. 35.0°C
   d. 34.5°C

10. A limb that has been crushed can sequester up to what volume of fluid?
    a. 500 ml
    b. 1 l
    c. 5 l
    d. 10 l

CHAPTER 5

Shock

Matt Wilkinson-Stokes

AIM

This chapter provides an overview of physiological shock, including pathophysiology, identification and paramedic management.

LEARNING OUTCOMES

On completion of this chapter you will be able to:

- Define shock and summarise its pathophysiology.
- List the types of shock and their major causes.
- Identify shock and determine its stage.
- List common treatments and their mechanisms of action.

Test Your Prior Knowledge

1. What is shock?
2. What is the most common cause of shock?
3. What are the four main types of shock?
4. What are the three stages of shock, and how can you identify them?

Introduction

A functioning circulatory system is necessary to deliver the nutrients that tissues need to survive (in particular oxygen and glucose) and to remove waste products (including carbon dioxide and water). Having adequate circulation to maintain normal function in the tissues is referred to as *perfusion*. Any disruption is often described as either inadequate perfusion, hypoperfusion or malperfusion These three terms all mean the same thing and can be used interchangeably.

Fundamentals of Applied Pathophysiology for Paramedics, First Edition. Edited by Ian Peate and Simon Sawyer.
© 2024 John Wiley & Sons Ltd. Published 2024 by John Wiley & Sons Ltd.

This circulatory system can be thought of as having three core components:

1. A pump – the heart.
2. Pipes – the arteries, capillaries, and veins.
3. Liquid – mainly referring to blood, but also affected by the volume of interstitial fluid, intracellular fluid, and lymph.

Problems can occur in any part or a combination of these three components that can then lead to malperfusion.

With the heart, malperfusion can occur when it is unable to pump enough blood to meet tissue demands. The main causes of heart dysfunction are due to:

- Tissue death (myocardial infarction).
- Tissue changes or weakness (congestive cardiac failure, ventricular hypertrophy or dilated cardiomyopathy).
- Infection (myocarditis).
- Electrical system malfunctions causing the heart rate to speed up, slow down, or become irregular (dysrhythmia).
- Valvular disorders (stenosis, regurgitation, prolapse or rupture).

If the heart is not able to pump adequately, the amount of blood being pushed into circulation reduces – leading to insufficient blood flow to the tissues.

Malperfusion can also occur due to the vessels becoming flaccid, wider (due to vasodilation) or leaky (due to infection causing a fluid shift), or by becoming blocked or constricted (such as pulmonary embolism). These conditions can lead to liquid pooling rather than flowing freely (causing hypotension), or lead to fluid leaving the vessels completely and entering the interstitial fluid (reducing circulating volume).

With blood, malperfusion is usually caused by a lack of circulating volume, which is called hypovolaemia. Hypovolaemia occurs when the blood leaves the vessels and cannot get back in. The most obvious example of this is external bleeding; however, it also includes internal bleeding, which can be harder to detect. Rarely, it can be caused by severe dehydration.

Failure of any of these three components to function that leads to a widespread lack of circulation of the tissues is shock.

Shock

Shock is defined as a state of systemic inadequate perfusion. Shock does not refer to an interruption to blood flow to any single area of the body – as happens with a heart attack or stroke – but it occurs instead when there is inadequate blood flow to the entire body (or multiple major systems).

Blood flow is difficult to measure, so we largely use blood pressure as a proxy. However, blood pressure does not directly correlate with shock, and patients may be in shock with a normal or high blood pressure.

Medical shock is not a state of surprise, and should not be confused with psychological conditions such as acute stress disorder. Nor is shock disease in itself, but instead a state of malperfusion that can occur as a result of many different disease processes. Because of this, there is no single cause or treatment for shock.

Shock is a medical emergency in all cases and is fatal in nearly 40% of cases (De Backer et al. 2010).

Shock is usually categorised into four broad types: cardiogenic, distributive, obstructive and hypovolaemic. We discuss each in turn, and a summary is provided in Table 5.1.

A Note on Terminology

In this area of medicine, clinicians tend to use varied terminology. A person in shock from a severe bleed is equally likely to be referred to as being in haemorrhagic shock, hypovolaemic shock, having irreversible blood loss, having absolute

TABLE 5.1   An overview of the types of shock and their subtypes and major causes.

Hypovolaemic shock (absolute hypovolaemia)	Cardiogenic shock	Obstructive shock	Distributive shock (relative hypovolaemia)	Combined shock

• Haemorrhagic shock:
  • External traumatic
  • Internal traumatic
  • Non-traumatic
 	
• Non-haemorrhagic shock
  • Dehydration
	• Reduced cardiac output:
	  • Acute myocardial infarction
	  • Dysrhythmia
	  • Overdose
	  • Congestive heart failure
	  • Valvular disease
	  • Cardiomyopathy
		• Physical obstruction:
		  • Pulmonary embolism
		  • Tension pneumothorax
		  • Cardiac tamponade
			• Loss of vascular tone and fluid shift:
			  • Sepsis
			  • Neurogenic shock
			  • Anaphylaxis
				• Burn shock

blood loss, or even being described in looser terms such as having traumatic shock. Therefore, while the following definitions and examples are all accurate, you may hear alternative terms in practice.

Pathophysiology of Shock

Hypovolaemic Shock

Hypovolaemic shock refers to inadequate perfusion due to low circulating fluid volume. While the fluid here refers mainly to blood, it is important to remember that normal fluid *homeostasis* is a balance between blood, interstitial fluid, intracellular fluid and lymphatic fluid. Remember to differentiate between whole blood loss and plasma loss, each of which presents in different causes of hypovolaemic shock (the former in haemorrhage, the latter in dehydration), and has a different treatment (discussed below).

   All forms of hypovolaemic shock are referred to as irreversible loss of fluid, shown in Figure 5.1. Hypovolaemic shock is divided into two main types: haemorrhagic shock and non-haemorrhagic shock.

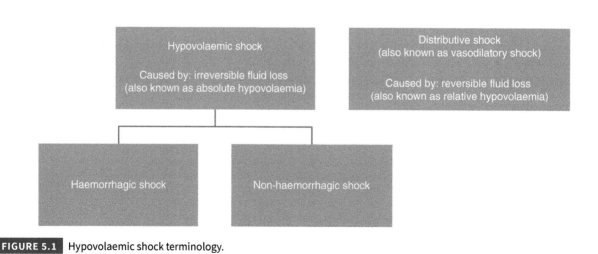

FIGURE 5.1   Hypovolaemic shock terminology.

Haemorrhagic Shock

Haemorrhagic shock includes external and internal haemorrhage. While this can be due to blunt or penetrating trauma (consider the orange flag alert), it can also occur in any medical condition that leads to severe bleeding, such as the rupture of a dissecting thoracic or abdominal aortic aneurysm or rupture of an ectopic pregnancy. The most common cause of haemorrhagic shock is gastrointestinal haemorrhage (De Backer et al. 2010).

Orange Flag Alert: Psychological Harm

Witnessing a major trauma, such as a significant external haemorrhage, can be psychologically harmful, particularly for bystanders who are neither trained nor prepared for it. A key part of the paramedic's role is ensuring the safety of everyone, including the psychological safety of both bystanders and the paramedics themselves. Consider both offering and seeking support.

Haemorrhagic shock is traditionally divided into four classes, depending on the amount of blood loss and the body's ability to compensate (Table 5.2). While they remain standard currently, it is good to know that these classes have been criticised for difficulty in practical application (see Clinical Investigations: Estimating blood loss). The most severe progression of this absolute blood loss is called *exsanguination*, where the patient effectively loses all circulating volume.

Clinical Investigations: Estimating Blood Loss

The amount of blood lost is useful information for determining hospital treatment. Doctors will almost always want a best guess – however unreliable – from paramedics. However, there is strong evidence that everyone, from university students to senior consultant physicians, cannot accurately judge the amount of blood lost even in relaxed, well-lit classroom simulations (Ashburn et al. 2012; Patton et al. 2001; Tall et al. 2003; Williams and Boyle 2007). Accurate estimation becomes exponentially harder in cramped environments, at night or when on any surface that may mask blood loss (such as carpet or car footwell) or dilute blood (such as in a toilet), all of which are the paramedic's usual workplaces. Transport all blood-soaked pads, clothing, bedding or similar to hospital if possible. The hospital can weigh the items to get a more accurate estimation of blood loss. Be sure to put all items in a sterile bag and to use good personal protective equipment.

TABLE 5.2 Haemorrhagic shock classes for adults

Class	Percent of blood lost	Actual blood flost (70 kg adult)			Basic vital signs to expect		
		Female	Pregnant (near term)	Male	Blood pressure	Heart rate	Mental status
I	<15%	<700 mL	<1000 mL	<750 mL	Normal	Normal or minor increase	Normal or anxious
II	15-30%	700-1400 mL	1000 – 2000 mL	750 – 1500 mL			Anxious
III	30-40%	1400-1800 mL	2000 – 2800 mL	1500 – 2000 mL	Decreased	Increased	Altered
IV	>40%	>1800 mL	>2800 mL	>2000 mL			

* Rounded using approximate values of 65 mL/kg in birth females, 100 mL/kg in term pregnant females, 70 mL/kg in birth males; these values vary significantly across populations and should not be relied on.

Non-haemorrhagic Shock

A less common cause of hypovolaemic shock is dehydration. Dehydration occurs where natural fluid loss (via urine, faeces, vomiting, evaporation and exhalation) is excessive or not replaced, eventually leading to a reduction in blood volume. In dehydration, there is loss of plasma alone, rather than whole blood.

In both haemorrhagic and non-haemorrhagic shock, there is a reduced venous return to the heart. The body can compensate for minor blood loss by vasoconstriction and temporarily maintain cardiac output by increasing heart rate or force of contraction. However, if the blood loss is severe, no amount of squeezing empty vessels or pumping an empty heart chamber will make any difference. The shock then becomes decompensatory, and rapid intervention is required to prevent death.

Cardiogenic Shock

Cardiogenic shock occurs when cardiac output drops below the body's minimum requirements to maintain perfusion, due to a primary cardiac cause. Cardiac output is a function of stroke volume and heart rate. Stroke volume depends on *preload* (amount of blood in the heart before contraction), *afterload* (force the heart has to push against to eject blood) and *inotropy* (force of contraction). Heart rate depends on chronotropy (rate of impulse generation), dromotropy (rate of conduction), bathmotropy (excitability of tissues to impulses; how reactive the tissues are) and lusitropy (rate of relaxation prior to the next contraction).

Clinical Investigations: Cardiac Output

$$CO = SV \times HR$$

$$\text{Cardiac output}\,(\text{mL}/\text{min}) = \text{stroke volume}\,(\text{mL}/\text{stroke}) \times \text{heart rate}\,(\text{strokes}/\text{min})$$

Stroke volume factors: preload, afterload, inotropy
Heart rate factors: chronotropy, dromotropy, bathmotropy, lusitropy

---

Cardiac output is always measured over one minute. For a healthy adult, a normal stroke volume ranges from 50 to 100 mL, with a normal heart rate ranging from 60 to 100 beats/min (lower rates may be normal for some people, such as athletes). Normal cardiac output could range from $50 \times 60 = 3\,l$ to as high as $100 \times 100 = 10\,l$ of blood/min, with the normal amount being 5–6 l/min. When cardiac output drops below this level, there is a potential for cardiogenic shock.

Cardiogenic shock is formally defined as signs of hypoperfusion combined with a systolic blood pressure less than 90 mmHg for over 30 minutes or a requirement for *vasopressors* (medications that squeeze the vessels, discussed below) to maintain perfusion.

There are many causes for cardiogenic shock, including:

- Acute myocardial infarction.
- Dysrhythmias.
- Overdose (particularly on beta or calcium channel blockers).
- Congestive cardiac failure.
- Valvular diseases.
- Myocarditis.
- Cardiomyopathy.

These conditions cause a reduction in either stroke volume or heart rate, in turn leading to a reduction in cardiac output. Initially, there is often an attempt to counterbalance the reduced cardiac output with a compensatory tachycardia. However, this increases myocardial demand, potentially worsening any myocardial injury.

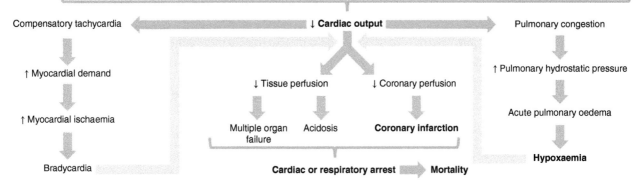

FIGURE 5.2 A summary of cardiogenic shock pathology.

A reduction in cardiac output can also lead to congestion in the pulmonary circuit. As the hydrostatic pressure increases and eventually overwhelms oncotic pressure, fluid moves into the interstitial space and then the alveoli, leading to acute pulmonary oedema. The fluid in the alveoli reduces the surface area available for gas exchange, in turn reducing the amount of oxygen able to bind to haemoglobin and leading to hypoxaemia. This can also wash out surfactant in the alveoli, leading to atelectasis. The main pathological pathways of cardiogenic shock are summarised in Figure 5.2.

Reduced cardiac output and hypoxaemia lead to inadequate perfusion of the tissues throughout the body. The tissues will initially compensate with anaerobic metabolism; however, this leads to acidosis. As anaerobic metabolism fails, the inadequate perfusion, hypoxaemia and acidosis all cause multiple organ distress. Uncorrected, this will lead to cardiac arrest and death.

Obstructive Shock

Obstructive shock occurs when a physical blockage disrupts systemic circulation. Any blockage can cause the tissues to infarct distally, such as in an acute myocardial infarction or cerebrovascular accident; however, we reserve the term shock for when the entire body is malperfused. This can occur when the obstruction is in a large enough vessel to stop the entire circulatory system from working properly. There are three major causes: pulmonary embolism, tension pneumothorax and cardiac tamponade. Pulmonary embolisms may be large enough to block the pulmonary circuit, leading to reduced blood flow and also to the alveoli with ventilation but no perfusion (referred to as V/Q mismatch or dead space), causing both hypotension and hypoxaemia.

Tension pneumothoraces or haemothoraces increase intrathoracic pressure, leading to compression of the lungs (reducing pulmonary blood flow and gas exchange) and occlusion of the major veins (especially the vena cava, which reduces venous return to the heart).

Cardiac tamponade is caused by an effusion or inflammation in the pericardium that compresses the heart, limiting expansion and reducing preload and output.

Less common causes for obstructive shock include an arterial gas embolus from SCUBA diving, a fat embolus released post long-bone fracture, tumours that grow near a vessel, and aortic diseases such as coarctation.

In all cases, obstructive shock shares the same aetiology – a physical blockage that reduces circulation throughout the body.

Distributive Shock

Distributive shock occurs when the vessels fail to maintain adequate blood flow. This can occur for two reasons, which often occur together. The first is that the vessels relax and become flaccid and large, reducing peripheral vascular resistance. This is called a reduction in vasomotor tone, and distributive shock is therefore also often known as vasodilatory shock. As pressure is inversely related to volume, the increase in vessel volume leads to a decrease in blood pressure.

The second reason is that the vessel walls can become leaky, a normal part of healing in inflammation (as the leaky vessels allow leukocytes and other cells to reach a site of injury), sometimes known as third spacing. However, if it occurs at too great a scale, it can reduce circulating volume to a level that impacts perfusion.

Distributive shock can be differentiated from hypovolaemic shock as there is a normal volume of fluid within the body. However, although the amount of fluid is normal, there is a change in the distribution of fluid among the body's compartments.

Distributive shock itself has four main subtypes: septic, anaphylactic, neurogenic and other.

Septic Shock

Sepsis – an exaggerated immune response to infection mediated by cytokines and the complement cascade – leads to vasodilation, endothelial permeability, third-space fluid shift, cytopathic injury and apoptosis. When this process leads to reduced perfusion to the tissues, septic shock occurs. The pathology of sepsis is summarised in Figure 5.3.

Septic shock is the single most common cause of shock, making up over 60% of all shock cases and with a mortality rate nearing 40% (De Backer et al. 2010; Bauer et al. 2020; Hotchkiss et al. 2016; Vincent et al. 2019). Cold sepsis is a more deadly subset of sepsis.

Red Flag Alert: Cold Sepsis

As compensatory mechanisms fail and normal thermoregulatory responses become deranged, sepsis may present with hypothermia rather than hyperthermia. This is known as 'cold sepsis'. It occurs in up to 20% of sepsis cases and has more than double the rate of mortality (Fullerton 2015; Young and Bellomo 2014).

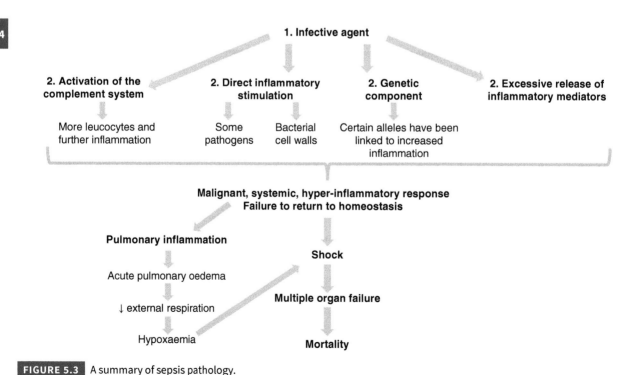

FIGURE 5.3 A summary of sepsis pathology.

Anaphylactic Shock

In anaphylactic shock, a fundamentally similar inflammatory response as septic shock occurs; however, here it is triggered by an acute response from re-exposure to an antigen, activating immunoglobulin E (IgE) and causing degranulation of granulocytes. There is a second rarer type of anaphylaxis where degranulation is not triggered by IgE activation, but instead by direct causes from chemicals within the cell, usually opioids or radiocontrast dye.

The epidemiology of anaphylaxis triggers is shown in Figure 5.4, with the pathology summarised in Figure 5.5. In anaphylactic shock, up to 35% of the circulating volume can be lost to the extravascular space within just 10 minutes (Fisher 1986).

Anaphylaxis can present in many different ways, with common signs including cutaneous rash (90%), respiratory distress (85%), gastrointestinal symptoms such as nausea or vomiting (45%), and hypotension (45%) (Campbell et al. 2023; Cardona et al. 2020).

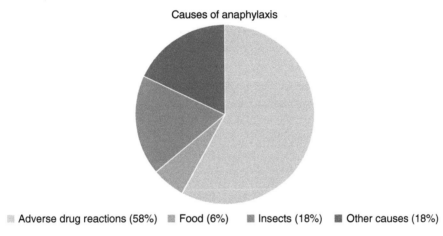

Causes of anaphylaxis

■ Adverse drug reactions (58%) ■ Food (6%) ■ Insects (18%) ■ Other causes (18%)

FIGURE 5.4 Causes of anaphylaxis.

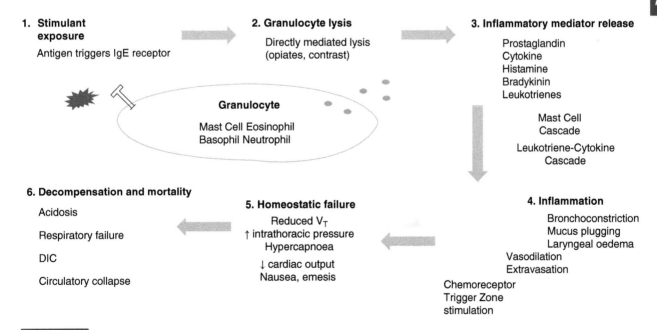

1. Stimulant exposure
Antigen triggers IgE receptor

2. Granulocyte lysis
Directly mediated lysis (opiates, contrast)

Granulocyte
Mast Cell Eosinophil
Basophil Neutrophil

3. Inflammatory mediator release
Prostaglandin
Cytokine
Histamine
Bradykinin
Leukotrienes

Mast Cell
Cascade

Leukotriene-Cytokine
Cascade

6. Decompensation and mortality
Acidosis
Respiratory failure
DIC
Circulatory collapse

5. Homeostatic failure
Reduced V_T
↑ intrathoracic pressure
Hypercapnoea
↓ cardiac output
Nausea, emesis

4. Inflammation
Bronchoconstriction
Mucus plugging
Laryngeal oedema
Vasodilation
Extravasation

Chemoreceptor
Trigger Zone
stimulation

FIGURE 5.5 A simple summary of anaphylaxis pathology.

Neurogenic Shock

Neurogenic shock occurs when there is damage to the high spinal column, usually the cervical vertebrae, although it can occur as low as the tenth thoracic vertebra (well below the level of the axillae).

The injury physically interrupts neuronal signalling via the spinal column. As sympathetic regulation occurs from nerves originating in the spinal column while parasympathetic regulation is mediated directly by the vagus nerve (cranial nerve X), this means that there is an unopposed parasympathetic response. This parasympathetic drive causes both bradycardia and vasodilation, especially peripherally, leading to malperfusion.

It is important not to confuse neurogenic shock with spinal shock, which refers to a temporary stunning of the spinal column from trauma that eventually resolves and which is not a form of physiological shock.

Other Causes of Distributive Shock

Other causes of distributive shock include endocrine shock (including adrenal insufficiency, hypothyroidism, hyperthyroidism, hyperglycaemia, or from electrolyte imbalance causing severe acidosis or alkalosis), pancreatitis, and overdose of vasodilatory drugs. After a heart attack and/or cardiac arrest, there is a massive release of inflammatory mediators, which may lead to a post-arrest distributive shock.

Burn Shock

Burn shock is a unique combination of distributive, hypovolaemic and cardiogenic shock. Damage to cells releases inflammatory mediators, leading to vasodilation and third-space shift (distributive shock). The loss of skin integrity causes evaporative fluid loss (hypovolaemic shock) and disrupts thermoregulation, contributing to coagulopathy. Many inflammatory mediators released have cardiodepressive effects (cardiogenic shock). Airway burns may cause oedema, reducing tidal volume, causing hypoxaemia.

The loss of skin integrity and release of immunosuppressants can increase the risk of a subsequent infection; sepsis accounts for up to 90% of deaths after burns (Belba et al. 2017; Tripathee and Basnet 2017). Over a longer period (several hours through to three years), a hypermetabolic response occurs, where the body becomes stuck in a destructive loop. Burn pathology is summarised in Figure 5.6.

Undifferentiated Shock

The term undifferentiated shock is used when shock is identified but the cause is unknown.

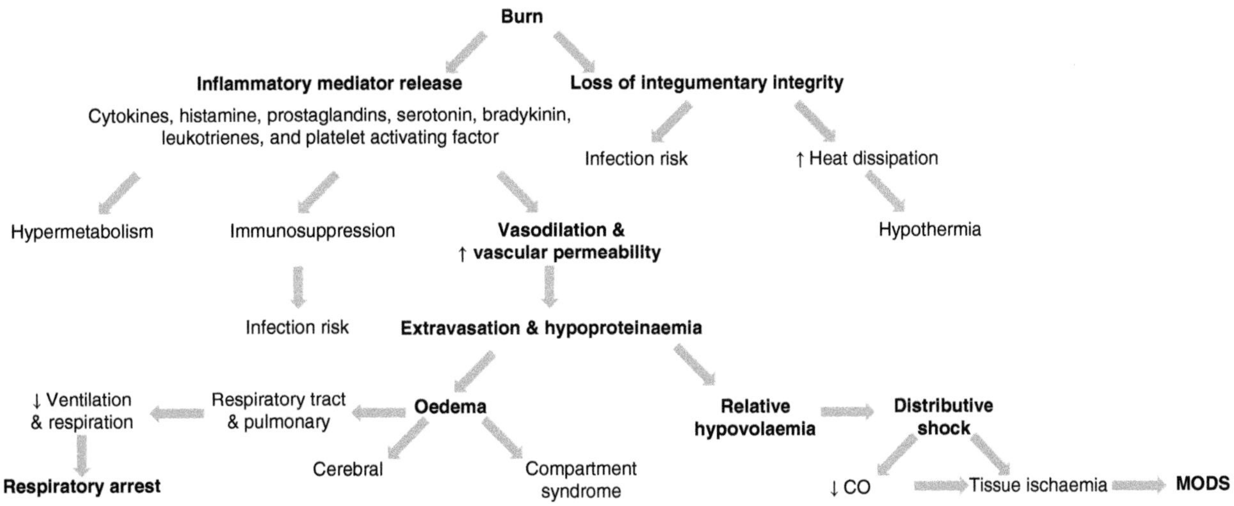

FIGURE 5.6 A summary of burn pathology.

Reflective Learning Activity

How can you 'rule in' or 'rule out' different causes of shock?
What investigations and tools are available where you work?

Snapshot 5.1

It is 3 a.m. and dark. You attend an elderly man in a solo highway car accident.
Scene: Airbags deployed, all windows broken, columns intact, not entrapped. Safe scene.
Immediate impression: Semi-conscious, self-ventilating with difficulty.

Primary Survey

Skin: Cold
Pulse: Weak and rapid
Respiration rate: 30 breaths/min
V_T: Shallow
$EtCO_2$: 30
Heart rate: 125 beats/min
SpO_2: 88%
Blood pressure: 85 mmHg palpated
Capillary refill: unable to see
Glasgow Coma Scale score: E2 V4 M6
Temperature: 34.8°C
Blood glucose level: not yet taken
Auscultation: Left laminar, right diminished
ECG: sinus tachycardia
Head to toe: airbag abrasion to forehead, cervical tenderness, major seatbelt contusion, probable right rib fractures, compound femur fracture, blood lost in footwell, no paresis or paraesthesia

Questions to Ask

- Does this patient have shock?
- If so, what stage is it at?
- What are your next actions?

Responses

- Does this patient have shock? Yes.
- If so, what stage is it at? Decompensation.
- What are possible causes of shock? Haemorrhagic hypovolaemic shock either external from the femur, or internal in the abdomen (seatbelt contusion) or pelvis (mechanism alone makes this plausible). Obstructive shock from a right tension pneumothorax.
- What are your next actions? Rapid extrication, right thoracostomy, stop bleeding (femoral and pelvic splints, haemostatic dressing, possible femoral torniquet, tranexamic acid), bilateral large-bore cannulation, maintain blood pressure (blood products, vasopressors, fluids), oxygenate, warm aggressively, prepare for traumatic cardiac arrest, and transport with pre-notification. Ultrasonography if available.

Stages of Shock

While the pathophysiology of the different root causes of shock may differ between patients, the physiological symptoms tend to follow a predictable pattern that can be summarised in three broad stages: compensatory, decompensatory and refractory.

Compensatory Stage

Compensation refers to the early stage of shock, when the body is able to adjust to the interruption in perfusion using a series of mechanisms to avoid tissue injury. As this stage of shock often does not present with abnormal vital signs, it is also referred to as pre-shock or cryptic shock.

Reflective Learning Activity

What are considered 'vital signs' where you work?
(Consider capillary refill, SpO_2, blood glucose, pulse rate, blood pressure, ECG, auscultation, respiratory rate, $EtCO_2$, pupillary reflexes, temperature, skin assessment and a head-to-toe assessment.)
What are the parameters used within the various populations and specific contexts?

Maintenance of Blood Pressure

When the initial interruption to perfusion occurs, changes in blood pressure are sensed by the baroreceptors, mechanical stretch receptors that sense physical tugging on the artery wall. These have two effects: nervous and endocrine.

The main nervous baroreceptors are located in the carotid sinus and the aortic arch. There are also low pressure baroreceptors throughout the body. Changes in blood pressure are transferred via cranial nerves IX (glossopharyngeal) and X (vagus) to the medulla, which causes vasoconstriction and increases chronotropy and inotropy.

The endocrine baroreceptors are located in the juxtaglomerular apparatus in the kidney and are able to directly stimulate the release of renin by the juxtaglomerular cells, initiating the renin–angiotensin–aldosterone system (RAAS). This system ultimately leads to the release of multiple hormones, including angiotensin II (a strong vasoconstrictor that also increases renal reabsorption), antidiuretic hormone (also known as vasopressin, another strong vasoconstrictor that also increases renal reabsorption, and a medication that some paramedics provide) and aldosterone (that increases renal reabsorption).

Maintenance of Blood Chemistry

Simultaneously, changes in carbon dioxide levels are sensed by chemoreceptors, thermochemical receptors that sense the amount of oxygen, carbon dioxide, pH and temperature. There are three main locations of chemoreceptors. The medulla contains the central chemoreceptors. The other two locations are, similar to the baroreceptors, just next to the carotid sinus and in the aortic arch. They are called the carotid body and aortic bodies, and together are referred to as the peripheral chemoreceptors.

As with the baroreceptors, changes in blood chemical composition sensed by the carotid and aortic chemoreceptors are transferred via cranial nerves IX (glossopharyngeal) and X (vagus) to the medulla, that in turn increases ventilation rate and tidal volume (increasing gas exchange) and increases excretion of bicarbonate (neutralising hydrogen and raising pH).

Compensation Generally

In combination, all of these mechanisms – vasoconstriction, increased stroke volume and heart rate, increased tidal volume, increased respiratory rate, activation of the RAAS and bicarbonate excretion – allow for normal perfusion to be temporarily maintained, despite the increased strain on the body. This compensation can mean that vital signs appear normal initially or present with only small variations from normal.

Medications Management: Cardioactive Drugs

Patients taking cardioactive medications, such as beta blockers, may be unable to increase their heart rate despite being in shock.

Mitochondria are extremely sensitive even to minor lapses in perfusion, resulting in small amounts of anaerobic metabolism occurring. This produces lactic acid as a by-product (detectable via lactate blood test). Acidaemia is one of the first signs to occur in shock – often preceding changes in heart rate or blood pressure. Initial stages of acidosis may be masked by the release of bicarbonate from the kidneys. The amount of bicarbonate, usually taken as base excess (bases being chemicals that react with acids by donating electrons), can be measured by blood tests.

When these mechanisms are working adequately and the patient appears well perfused despite causes of shock, paramedics may refer to them as compensating well or maintaining their perfusion. Some populations may compensate differently from others.

Red Flag Alert: Compensation in Special Populations

Certain populations compensate particularly well until a late stage of shock, including paediatric and obstetric populations. Children and pregnant women may appear well for a longer period of time before a rapid deterioration into death, and it is therefore particularly important to treat them as a high-risk group.

Decompensatory Stage

When the initial mechanisms used to maintain perfusion begin to fail, the body initiates further mechanisms that aim to preserve life even if they cause harm. These mechanisms are a last-ditch attempt at saving life. This is called the *decompensatory* stage, also sometimes known as progressive shock. Significant injury usually precedes decompensation (see Red Flag Alert: Hypovolaemic Blood Pressure).

Initially, patients will experience hypotension, extreme peripheral vasoconstriction and central vasodilation as the body seeks to shunt all remaining circulating blood to the central organs (especially the brain, heart and kidneys), even if this causes ischaemia to other parts of the body.

Red Flag Alert: Hypovolaemic Blood Pressure

Humans can maintain a normal blood pressure until one-third of their total blood volume is lost (Bonanno 2020). It is therefore critical not to wait until a patient is hypotensive before commencing treatment.

Widespread anaerobic metabolism will occur, which in turn depletes base excess, meaning that the body can no longer repress acidosis. The body may temporarily try to correct acidosis further via more pronounced hyperpnoea or tachypnoea (to off-gas carbon dioxide and reduce acidosis). Where hyperpnoea and tachypnoea occur together, this is referred to as Kussmaul respirations, and is a common sign in decompensatory shock.

The reduction in adenosine triphosphate (ATP) leads to failure of the sodium–potassium pump, calcium pump, and consequently (with the loss of ion gradients) to failure of the sodium–calcium exchanger and calcium–hydrogen exchanger. Without normal repolarisation, the increase in intracellular calcium leads to myocardial irritability, and in turn can cause dysrhythmias.

Once anaerobic metabolism fails, heat generation reduces and patients become hypothermic. This hypothermia also contributes to worsening coagulopathy.

The affected tissues will begin to dysfunction and then ultimately necrotise. Cell necrosis has three key negative consequences. First, the cell walls lyse and the contents of the cell are released. This includes numerous inflammatory mediators (potentially leading to distributive shock), dysrhythmics (impacting cardiac function, and risking cardiac arrest), and may cause rhabdomyolysis (impacting renal function). Second, nearby cells also die because the cell contents include cytotoxic chemicals. Third, the organ containing the dysfunctioning cells can cease to function correctly, leading to specific organ system problems; for example, in the kidney, this may include acute kidney injury and accumulation of waste products, while for the heart it may lead to a reduced cardiac output. When this occurs across multiple organs, it is known as multiple organ dysfunction syndrome.

The resultant inadequate perfusion to the brain can lead to altered levels of consciousness. At this stage, patients often have a reduced response to stimulus, and you may see a reduced Glasgow Coma Scale or AVPU (alert, voice, pain, unresponsive) score.

Patients who are in decompensatory shock may also develop multiple specific conditions, including acute respiratory distress syndrome, multiple organ dysfunction syndrome and disseminated intravascular coagulopathy (hypercoagulation followed by depletion of coagulation factors and unopposed haemorrhage).

Refractory Stage

The *refractory* stage of shock is when the patient remains malperfused despite vasopressors, fluids and oxygenation. If the shock occurs rapidly (such as via a major trauma), the patient may only be in shock for a few minutes before cardiac arrest. If the shock is prolonged (such as multiple days in intensive care with sepsis), multiple organ dysfunction syndrome usually occurs first.

In this stage, you will probably see vital signs inconsistent with recovery, such as unresponsive bradycardia, hypotension, hypopnoea, hypothermia, and altered conscious state or unconsciousness.

Refractory shock is not necessarily fatal, although mortality rates exceed 50% (Jenkins et al. 2009; Jentzer et al. 2018; Reyentovich et al. 2016).

The three stages of shock are summarised in Table 5.3.

TABLE 5.3   The stages of shock.

Stage of shock	Signs and symptoms
Compensatory	Normal blood pressure
	Normocardia or tachycardia
	Eupnoea or tachypnoea
	Oliguria or anuria
	Normal consciousness
Decompensatory	Hypotension
	Tachycardia (or, later, bradycardia)
	Kussmaul respirations
	Slightly altered consciousness
	Cool peripheral skin
Refractory	Periarrest
	Hypotension, or unrecordable blood pressure
	Bradycardia
	Kussmaul respirations (or, later, hypopnoea)
	Severely altered consciousness or comatose
	Cold skin

Identification of Shock

As discussed, shock is not a specific pathology but a state of malperfusion occurring for any of many reasons. Consequently, there is no single test used to identify shock; instead, holistic assessment of the patient is necessary.

Clinical Investigations: Blood Pressure

Is the current blood pressure sufficient to perfuse the vital organs? There is no consensus on what blood pressure achieves perfusion, although most evidence suggests a mean arterial pressure (MAP) around 65 mmHg (Kato and Pinsky 2015). Targeting the minimum pressure to perfuse vital organs is referred to as permissive hypotension and is a common strategy in some types of shock.

- Remember that a traumatic brain injury is a unique scenario requiring a close to normal blood pressure to be targeted. In this instance, preserving neurological function is considered the priority.
- Remember that blood pressure does not directly correlate with blood flow and shock. Avoid over-reliance on blood pressure and evaluate the patient holistically.

There are three key considerations when assessing vital signs:

1. Assess the patient in context. People become tachycardic and diaphoretic when exercising, have altered consciousness when sleepy, and have cold hands on a cold day. However, these are not pathological and do not suggest shock.

2. Consider population variations. Neonates and young children have a heart muscle that is not fully developed, with little ability to vary the stroke volume. They are dependent on heart rate to maintain cardiac output, so you would have a higher suspicion index and lower tolerance for variations of vital signs in such populations.

3. Monitor for trends. This is more important than any single set of vital signs and can additionally be used to determine whether treatment is effective.

Shock Index

One indicator for shock is the shock index, calculated by dividing heart rate by systolic blood pressure. An index below 0.8 is considered normal, and shock should be considered any time this is exceeded. A useful memory aid for those who struggle with fractions is to consider shock any time that heart rate exceeds systolic blood pressure.

$$\text{Shock index} = \frac{\text{heart rate}}{\text{systolic blood pressure}}$$

Clinical Investigations: A Palpable Carotid Pulse

Many paramedics have historically been taught that a palpable pulse suggests adequate blood pressure, but this is not true (Deakin 2000; Paxton and O'Neil 2019; Poulton 1988). Patients may retain a palpable carotid pulse with a systolic blood pressure below 40 mmHg (inadequate to perfuse the brain) and may have no palpable pulses with a systolic blood pressure of 75 mmHg (adequate to perfuse the vital organs).

Management of Shock

Treatments for shock can be either definitive or supportive and are summarised in Table 5.4. Definitive treatments for shock fix the underlying problem and are only occasionally provided by paramedics (such as thrombolysis, thoracostomy or blood products).

TABLE 5.4   Treatments by cause of shock.

Shock type	Subtype or cause	Primary treatments
Hypovolaemic	Haemorrhagic	Stop the bleed (direct pressure, splinting, torniquet, tranexamic acid, surgery; Figure 5.7)
		Restore circulation (blood products or fluids)
	Non-haemorrhagic	Restore circulation (blood products or fluids)

TABLE 5.4 *(Continued)*

Shock type	Subtype or cause	Primary treatments
Cardiogenic	Multiple causes (see Cardiogenic Shock section)	Varies with cause. May include medications (anti-dysrhythmics, vasopressors, thrombolytics) or interventions (pacing, cardioversion, percutaneous coronary intervention, open surgery)
Obstructive	Pulmonary embolism	Remove emboli (thrombolysis or percutaneous embolectomy)
	Tension haemo/pneumothorax	Decompress pleura (thoracostomy)
	Cardiac tamponade	Decompress pericardium (pericardiocentesis or surgery)
Distributive	Septic	Destroy pathogen (antibiotics/antiviral/antifungal)
		Restore circulation (fluids, vasopressors, inotropes)
	Anaphylactic	Remove antigen
		Restore circulation (fluids, vasopressors, inotropes)
	Neurogenic	Restore circulation (fluids, vasopressors, inotropes)
Combined	Burn	Prevent infection
		Restore circulation (fluids, vasopressors, inotropes)

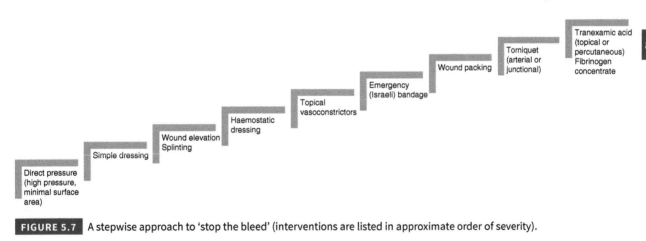

FIGURE 5.7 A stepwise approach to 'stop the bleed' (interventions are listed in approximate order of severity).

Supportive treatments provided by paramedics mainly focus on improving circulation to keep the patient alive until definitive treatment, and is achieved mainly through volume replacement, vasopressors, inotropes and oxygenation. A common mantra for managing shock is 'defend the MAP'; this refers to maintaining a perfusing blood pressure. The rationale behind treatments is summarised in Table 5.5.

TABLE 5.5   Common treatments for shock.

Treatment		Purpose
Pharmacology		
Fluids	Sodium chloride 0.9% (normal saline)	Replaces intravascular volume, increasing blood pressure
	Balanced salts (sodium lactate, Hartmann's solution, Plasma-Lyte® (Baxter Healthcare), lactated Ringer's)	
	Colloid fluids	
Blood products	Whole blood	Replaces blood
	Extended life plasma (thawed fresh frozen plasma)	Replaces volume and coagulation factors
	Packed red blood cells	Replaces erythrocytes
Vasopressors and inotropes	Adrenaline	Agonises all adrenergic receptors and stabilises mast cells
	Noradrenaline	Agonises A_1 receptors, increasing vasoconstriction
	Isoprenaline	Agonises B_1 and B_2 receptors, increasing cardiac output and ventilation
	Dobutamine	
	Dopamine	As dosage increases, progressively agonises D_1 and D_2 receptors (increasing inotropy), B_1 and B_2 receptors, and A_1 receptors
	Vasopressin (anti-diuretic hormone)	Agonises V_{1A}, V_{1B}, V_2 and oxytocin receptors, increasing vasoconstriction
	Metaraminol	Agonises A_1 receptors, increasing vasoconstriction, and indirectly increases free noradrenaline
	Phenylephrine	
Oxygen		Increases alveolar partial pressure, increasing gas exchange and minimising hypoxaemia
		Causes vasoactive effects and produces free radicals
Interventions		
Intubation: includes rapid sequence induction, delayed sequence induction, medication facilitated intubation, ketamine-only breathing intubation and unassisted intubation		Provides reliable ventilation
		Increases the fraction of inspired oxygen (FiO_2) to 100%
		Reduces the risk of aspiration
		Reduces gastric insufflation (that can lead to splinting of the diaphragm and inability to inhale)
		Reduces the work of breathing
		Reduces spikes in intracranial pressure
CPAP, BiPAP, PEEP		Increases expiratory resistance, reducing dynamic airway collapse and alveolar collapse from atelectasis. This recruits surface area for external respiration, reducing hypoxaemia

TABLE 5.5 (*Continued*)

Treatment	Purpose
Maintain normothermia	Reduces mortality, coagulopathy, and minimises left shift in the oxygen-disassociation curve
Consult	Patients with complex needs often benefit from a team approach, and discussion with on-call colleagues is entirely appropriate. The saying 'more brains are better than one' is apt. Some paramedics have historically been resistant to consultation, viewing it as a sign of personal incompetence. However, this is not only untrue, but also not what occurs in hospital (where multiple senior doctors routinely have team discussions during critical care) or in the best interests of the patient. A cultural change increasing acceptance of consultation is underway and this solitary mentality is increasingly rare
Pre-notification of hospital	Provides time for a multidisciplinary team to be assembled to minimise impacts on continuity of care

BiPAP, biphasic positive airway pressure; CPAP, continuous positive airway pressure; PEEP, positive end expiratory pressure.

Medications Managements: Risks of Fluids

Fluids are a mainstay of treatment for all types of shock, even cardiogenic shock, and a targeted fluid challenge will benefit most patients. However, fluids carry significant risks. Depending on the formulation, they are acidotic (sodium chloride has a pH of 5.5), isotonic (worsening oedema and, most dangerously, exacerbating acute respiratory distress syndrome), cold (most fluids are routinely stored at room temperature, below core body temperature), reduce haematocrit (they do not carry erythrocytes, and cannot transport oxygen) causing dilutional anaemia, and for haemorrhagic hypovolaemia can exacerbate bleeding and dislodge clots. Finally, fluids tend to be a temporising measure – they only provide short-term benefit and buy time to fix the underlying disease. Fluids must therefore be administered cautiously and with constant monitoring. When providing fluids, monitor continuously for the development of acute pulmonary oedema or cerebral oedema.

Take Home Points

- Shock is a state of systemic inadequate perfusion.
- Shock results from a problem with one or more of the heart, vessels, or blood causing a failure of the tissues to receive nutrients and remove waste.
- Shock can be caused by many disease processes; the most common is sepsis at 60%.
- Shock is usually classified in one of four ways, depending on where the main circulatory problem is: cardiogenic, distributive, obstructive or hypovolaemic.
- There are also some special cases that overlap with several categories and may sometimes be described under one of them or listed separately: septic, burn, anaphylactic, neurogenic and endocrine shock.
- There is no single way to diagnose shock or to exclude it. Patients may be in shock with normal GCS and normal blood pressure.
- Shock is always a medical emergency and has a mortality of nearly 40%.

Summary

- Identify and resolve the underlying pathology.
- If the cause is haemorrhagic, stop the bleeding (Figure 5.7).
- Consider sepsis early.
- Defend the MAP. For haemorrhagic hypovolaemia, this may include permissive hypotension; for traumatic brain injury, a higher MAP will be appropriate. Be careful when giving fluids.
- Consult colleagues, work as a team, and pre-notify the receiving hospital.

Acknowledgement

All Figures are original creations by Matt Wilkinson-Stokes, first published in The Shift Extension (Wilkinson-Stokes, 2023). Reproduced with permission of the publisher.

References

Ashburn, J., Harrison, T., Ham, J., and Strote, J. (2012). Emergency physician estimation of blood loss. *Western Journal of Emergency Medicine* 13 (4): 376–379. http://dx.doi.org/10.5811/westjem.2011.9.6669.

Bauer, M., Gerlach, H., Vogelmann, T. et al. (2020). Mortality in sepsis and septic shock in Europe, North America and Australia between 2009 and 2019 – results from a systematic review and meta-analysis. *Critical Care* 24 (1): 239. http://dx.doi.org/10.1186/s13054-020-02950-2.

Belba, M.K., Petrela, E.Y., and Belba, A.G. (2017). Epidemiology and outcome analysis of sepsis and organ dysfunction/failure after burns. *Burns* 43 (6): 1335–1347. http://dx.doi.org/10.1016/j.burns.2017.02.017.

Bonanno, F. (2020). The need for a physiological classification of hemorrhagic shock. *Journal of Emergencies, Trauma, and Shock* 13(3): 177. https://doi.org/10.4103/JETS.JETS_153_19

Campbell, R., Kelso, J., Walls, R., and Feldweg, A. (2023). *Anaphylaxis: Acute diagnosis.* UpToDate.

Cardona, V., Ansotegui, I.J., Ebisawa, M. et al. (2020). World allergy organization anaphylaxis guidance 2020. *World Allergy Organization Journal* 13 (10): 100472. http://dx.doi.org/10.1016/j.waojou.2020.100472.

Deakin, C. D. (2000). Accuracy of the advanced trauma life support guidelines for predicting systolic blood pressure using carotid, femoral, and radial pulses: observational study. *BMJ,* 321 (7262), 673–674. https://doi.org/10.1136/bmj.321.7262.673

De Backer, D., Biston, P., Devriendt, J. et al. (2010). Comparison of dopamine and norepinephrine in the treatment of shock. *New England Journal of Medicine* 362 (9): 779–789. http://dx.doi.org/10.1056/NEJMoa0907118.

Fisher, M.M.D. (1986). Clinical observations on the pathophysiology and treatment of anaphylactic cardiovascular collapse. *Anaesthesia and Intensive Care* 14 (1): 17–21. http://dx.doi.org/10.1177/0310057X8601400105.

Fullerton, J. N. (2015). Increased Mortality in "Cold Sepsis." *Critical Care Medicine,* 43(6), 1327–1329. https://doi.org/10.1097/CCM.0000000000000987

Hotchkiss, R.S., Moldawer, L.L., Opal, S.M. et al. (2016). Sepsis and septic shock. *Nature Reviews Disease Primers* 2 (1): 16045. http://dx.doi.org/10.1038/nrdp.2016.45.

Jenkins, C.R., Gomersall, C.D., Leung, P., and Joynt, G.M. (2009). Outcome of patients receiving high dose vasopressor therapy: a retrospective cohort study. *Anaesthesia and Intensive Care* 37 (2): 286–289. http://dx.doi.org/10.1177/0310057X0903700212.

Jentzer, J.C., Vallabhajosyula, S., Khanna, A.K. et al. (2018). Management of refractory vasodilatory shock. *Chest* 154 (2): 416–426. http://dx.doi.org/10.1016/j.chest.2017.12.021.

Kato, R., & Pinsky, M. R. (2015). Personalizing blood pressure management in septic shock. *Annals of Intensive Care,* 5(1), 41. https://doi.org/10.1186/s13613-015-0085-5

Patton, K., Funk, D., McErlean, M., and Bartfield, J. (2001). Accuracy of estimation of external blood loss by EMS personnel. *The Journal of Trauma: Injury, Infection, and Critical Care* 50 (5): 914–916.

Paxton, J. H., & O'Neil, B. J. (2019). When is PEA really ROSC? *Resuscitation,* 142, 182–183. https://doi.org/10.1016/j.resuscitation.2019.06.012.

Poulton, T. J. (1988). ATLS paradigm fails. *Annals of Emergency Medicine,* 17(1), 107. https://doi.org/10.1016/S0196-0644(88)80538-9

Reyentovich, A., Barghash, M.H., and Hochman, J.S. (2016). Management of refractory cardiogenic shock. *Nature Reviews Cardiology* 13 (8): 481–492. http://dx.doi.org/10.1038/nrcardio.2016.96.

Tall, G., Wise, D., Grove, P., and Wilkinson, C. (2003). The accuracy of external blood loss estimation by ambulance and hospital personnel. *Emergency Medicine Australasia* 15 (4): 318–321. http://dx.doi.org/10.1046/j.1442-2026.2003.00469.x.

Tripathee, S. and Basnet, S.J. (2017). Epidemiology and outcome of hospitalized burns patients in tertiary care center in Nepal: two year retrospective study. *Burns Open* 1 (1): 16–19. http://dx.doi.org/10.1016/j.burnso.2017.03.001.

Vincent, J.-L., Jones, G., David, S. et al. (2019). Frequency and mortality of septic shock in Europe and North America: a systematic review and meta-analysis. *Critical Care* 23 (1): 196. http://dx.doi.org/10.1186/s13054-019-2478-6.

Wilkinson-Stokes, M. (2023). *Clinical Guideline Posters.* The Shift Extension.

Williams, B. and Boyle, M. (2007). Estimation of external blood loss by paramedics: is there any point? *Prehospital and Disaster Medicine* 22 (6): 502–506. https://doi.org/10.0.3.249/S1049023X0000532X.

Young, P. J., & Bellomo, R. (2014). Fever in sepsis: is it cool to be hot? *Critical Care,* 18(1), 109. https://doi.org/10.1186/cc13726

Online Resources

Farkas, J. (2021). Approach to shock. *Internet Book of Critical Care.* https://emcrit.org/ibcc/shock (accessed 29 September 2023).

Gaieski, D.F. and Mikkelson, M.E. (2023). Definition, classification, aetiology, and pathophysiology of shock in adults. *UpToDate* 16 June. https://www.uptodate.com/contents/definition-classification-etiology-and-pathophysiology-of-shock-in-adults (accessed 29 September 2023).

Nickson, C. and Pearlman, J. (2023). Shock. *Life In The Fast Lane* 25 February. https://litfl.com/shock (accessed 29 September 2023).

Shock [podcast] *The Resus Room* (14 January). www.theresusroom.co.uk/shock (accessed 29 September 2023).

The Calgary Guide to Understanding Disease. Shock. https://calgaryguide.ucalgary.ca/category/cardiology (accessed 29 September 2023).

Glossary

Afterload	The pressure the ventricles have to push against (in the aortic and pulmonary arteries) to eject blood; higher afterload reduces cardiac output.
Compensation	The ability of the body to adjust to a disruption in normal homeostasis, such as by vasoconstriction or increased heart rate.
Decompensation	The loss of ability to adjust to a disruption in normal homeostasis, such as ongoing hypotension despite compensatory mechanisms.
Exsanguination	The effective loss of all circulating volume; commonly called bleeding out.
Homeostasis	The maintenance of a stable, normal physiological state.
Inotropes	Medications that increase the force of cardiac contraction, increasing cardiac output but also myocardial demand.
Perfusion	Delivery of adequate nutrients and removal of waste from the tissues. When this is not occurring, it is referred to as inadequate perfusion, malperfusion or hypoperfusion.
Preload	The amount of blood in the heart before contraction; lower preload decreases cardiac output.
Refractory	When current treatments become ineffective.
Vasopressors	Medications that vasoconstrict, increasing perfusion. While research is continuing, there is currently no strong evidence favouring any one vasopressor.

Multiple Choice Questions

1. Which of these is not a type or subtype of shock?
   a. Spinal shock
   b. Distributive shock
   c. Non-haemorrhagic shock
   d. Neurogenic shock

2. The term 'relative hypovolaemia' refers to what type of shock?
   a. Distributive shock
   b. Obstructive shock
   c. Hypovolaemic shock
   d. Haemorrhagic shock

3. Which of these is not a cause of obstructive shock?
   a. Arterial gas embolism from scuba diving
   b. Aortic coarctation
   c. Fat embolism from a long bone fracture
   d. Coronary thrombus

4. Can a patient with a normal GCS have shock?
   a. No
   b. Yes
   c. Only if moderate-severe (GCS < 12)
   d. Only if severe (GCS < 9)

5. Neurogenic shock has unopposed stimulation from which system?
   a. Ganglionic
   b. Parasympathetic
   c. Spinal reflex arcs
   d. Sympathetic

6. What is the most common cause of shock?
   a. Major traumatic haemorrhage
   b. Gastrointestinal haemorrhage
   c. Sepsis
   d. Acute myocardial infarction

7. Approximately what percentage of patients with shock will ultimately die?
   a. 10%
   b. 20%
   c. 30%
   d. 40%

8. The combination of hyperpnoea and tachypnoea is known as what?
   a. Biot's
   b. Apneustic
   c. Kussmaul's
   d. Cheyne–Stokes

9. Which of these terms refers to the second stage of shock rather than the first?
   a. Pre-shock
   b. Progressive shock
   c. Cryptic shock
   d. Compensatory shock

10. Acidosis, dilutional anaemia, hypothermia, exacerbating oedema and exacerbating haemorrhage are potential adverse effects of which treatment?
    a. Inotropes
    b. Vasopressors
    c. Fluids
    d. Blood products

CHAPTER 6

The Nervous System and Its Associated Disorders

Tom E. Mallinson

AIM

This chapter aims to provide an introduction to diseases that affect the human nervous system, including their assessment and management.

LEARNING OUTCOMES

On completion of this chapter you will be able to:

- Describe the anatomical regions of the brain and how nerves transmit information around the body.
- Understand the roles of the central and the peripheral nervous systems.
- Understand the assessment of neurological function.
- Gain an insight into the care required by patients with neurological disorders.

Test Your Prior Knowledge

1. List the components of the central and peripheral nervous systems.
2. What are the differences between the sympathetic and parasympathetic division of the autonomic nervous system?
3. Explain the function of the blood–brain barrier.
4. What is the difference between a primary and secondary brain injury?

Introduction

The nervous system is both the *computer* and *wiring* of the human body. The brain is responsible for controlling both voluntary and involutory action, while nerves transmit electrical signals throughout the body, both sensing and causing actions to be undertaken by various organ systems. The nervous system is the lynchpin in both our interaction with the wider world and our ability to maintain homeostasis. This chapter discusses the structure and function of the central

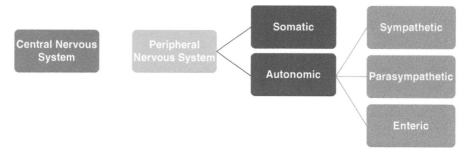

FIGURE 6.1   Divisions of the nervous system.

(CNS) and peripheral (PNS) nervous systems, and also some of the common disorders of the nervous system. Snapshot scenarios explore the clinical presentations caused by various pathologies.

Anatomy of the Nervous System

The nervous system can be considered in two main parts: the CNS and the PNS:

1. The CNS consists of the brain, the spinal cord, the retina and two cranial nerves (CNI and CNII).

2. The PNS consists of the other cranial and spinal nerves and all other peripheral neurons. These nerves, or neurons, carry impulses towards and away from the spinal cord. The PNS includes most of the cranial nerves that emanate from the brain and the spinal nerves arising from the spinal cord. The PNS can also be divided into the somatic (voluntary) and the autonomic (involuntary or homeostatic) nervous systems. The autonomic nervous system (ANS) is then further divided into the parasympathetic and sympathetic divisions and the enteric nervous system (Figure 6.1).

Central Nervous System

Brain

The brain or encephalon (*en* – within and *cephalon* – head), which is encased in the cranial vault (or skull), is the body's control system. It can be divided anatomically into four distinct but interconnected sections (Figure 6.2):

1. Cerebrum.
2. Cerebellum.
3. Diencephalon.
4. Brainstem.

Cerebrum

The cerebrum is made up of the outer cerebral cortex, the internal cerebral white matter containing myelinated nerve axons, and the grey matter nuclei deeper within the white matter. The cerebral cortex lies uppermost in the skull and contains billions on neurons, arranged in layers. The surface of the cerebrum appears wrinkled due to the numerous gyri (raised areas), fissures (deep grooves) and sulci (shallow grooves).

The cerebrum is divided into two distinct hemispheres or halves, each having four lobes: frontal, parietal, temporal and occipital (Table 6.1; Figure 6.3). While it can be helpful to simplify the roles of various areas of the brain, complex processes may span multiple regions of the brain.

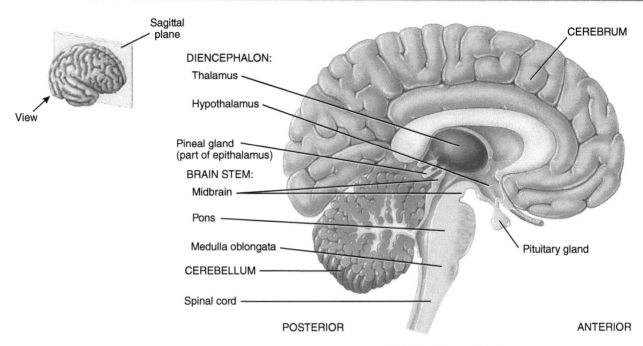

Sagittal plane

View

DIENCEPHALON:
- Thalamus
- Hypothalamus
- Pineal gland (part of epithalamus)

BRAIN STEM:
- Midbrain
- Pons
- Medulla oblongata

CEREBELLUM

Spinal cord

POSTERIOR

CEREBRUM

Pituitary gland

ANTERIOR

Sagittal section, medial view

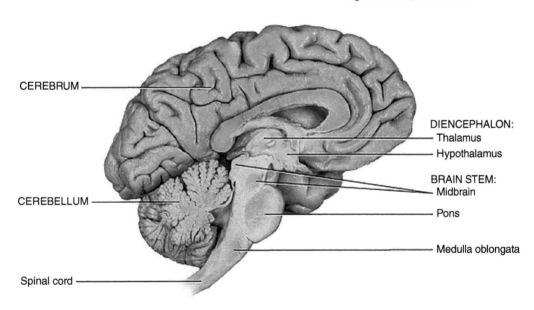

CEREBRUM

CEREBELLUM

Spinal cord

DIENCEPHALON:
- Thalamus
- Hypothalamus

BRAIN STEM:
- Midbrain
- Pons

Medulla oblongata

Sagittal section, medial view

FIGURE 6.2 The gross anatomy of the human brain.

Each hemisphere is able to communicate with the other via the corpus callosum, a thick area of axonal nerve fibres. Deep within each cerebral hemisphere lies a region historically called the basal ganglia (although 'basal nuclei' is more correct). The basal ganglia are vitally important in a number of key brain functions including the coordination of motor control, eye movements, learning and thinking, as well as modulating emotional responses. Encircling the upper brainstem and corpus callosum is the limbic system, which is important in moderating emotional responses and in processing smells and memories.

TABLE 6.1   The lobes of the cerebral hemispheres.

Anatomical region	Function
Frontal lobe	Personality and conscious thought, abstract thinking, memory and judgement, affective reactions and initiation of motor activity in the precentral gyrus (Figure 6.3)
Parietal lobe	Receiving and interpreting stimuli from sensory neurones in the postcentral gyrus (Figure 6.3) and spatial awareness
Temporal lobe	Processing of visual memories, processing sensory input and language recognition and comprehension
Occipital lobe	Visual processing

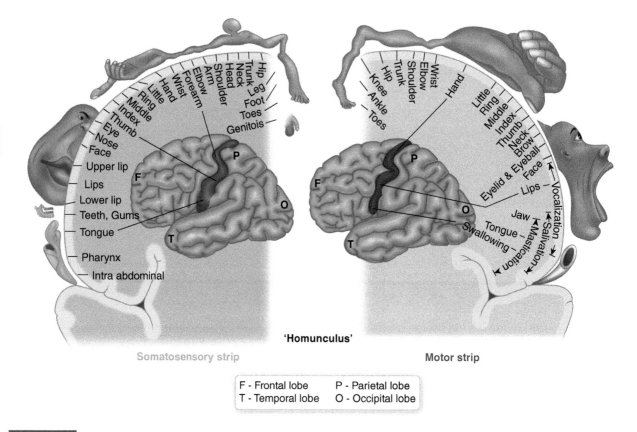

'Homunculus'

Somatosensory strip   Motor strip

F - Frontal lobe   P - Parietal lobe
T - Temporal lobe   O - Occipital lobe

FIGURE 6.3   Homunculus.

Cerebellum

The cerebellum lies under the occipital lobe of the cerebrum. It consists of an inner layer of white matter and an outer layer of grey matter, and its surface is convoluted like the surface of the cerebrum. The cerebellum is responsible for smoothing and coordinating voluntary movement. It also plays a key role in balance and movement. Cerebellar dysfunction can present in a number of ways, making identification of insults to this part of the brain difficult to detect. The area is also poorly visualised on imaging scans, further exacerbating the problem.

Diencephalon

The diencephalon consists of the thalamus, hypothalamus and the pineal gland. It lies between the brainstem and the cerebrum.

The thalamus acts as a relay centre, receiving information from the body via the spinal cord and forwarding it on to the appropriate areas of the brain. It plays a crucial role in sleep and wakefulness as well as the conscious experience of pain. Ischaemia or infarct of the thalamus can lead to thalamic pain syndrome and akinetic mutism and is implicated in Korsakoff syndrome, which occurs in alcoholism due to thiamine deficiency. The hypothalamus is located below the thalamus and is significant in the regulation of homeostasis. The hypothalamus acts to coordinate the ANS, serum electrolyte equilibrium and acid–base balance. The pineal gland is a small endocrine gland that produces the hormone melatonin.

93

Cranial Nerves

Most cranial nerves are part of the PNS, as they require an intermediate synapse between the origin nerve and the peripheral sensory or motor nerve (CNI, CNII and the retina being the exceptions; Table 6.2).

Brainstem

The brainstem connects the spinal cord to the rest of the brain. It is responsible for many essential homeostatic functions, as well as being the entry point for 10 of the 12 cranial nerves (Figure 6.2). Within the brainstem, a complex and anatomically diffuse network of nerve cells, known as the reticular formation, controls vital reflexes (Mangold and Das 2022). The reticular formation plays a vital role in coordinating cardiovascular and ventilatory actions, as well as for maintaining wakefulness and physiological arousal. Physiologically, this region is often referred to as the reticular activating system, which plays a key role in some types of coma, has been implicated in some symptoms of schizophrenia and is involved various disorders including post-traumatic stress disorder and some sleep disorders.

Anatomically, the brainstem is made up of the midbrain, the pons and the medulla oblongata. The midbrain is made up of bundles of nerve fibres forming a connection between the diencephalon and the pons. It is involved in the control of voluntary and involuntary eye movements as well as the startle reflex. The substantia nigra, part of the basal nuclei is also found within the midbrain, with other parts of the basal nuclei being more cephalad within the diencephalon. The pons, measuring approximately 2.5 cm in length, relays nerve impulses between the cerebral hemispheres, the cerebellum and the brainstem. It is also the origin of four cranial nerves (Table 6.2). The pons also plays a vital role in the control of the rate and depth of ventilation. A pontine stroke can affect ventilation, the functions of CNV–VIII and consciousness, in severe cases, leading to locked-in syndrome. The 3-cm medulla oblongata is in essence an extension of the spinal cord as it lies just inside the cranial cavity above the foramen magnum. Within the medulla are a number of reflex centres for control of

TABLE 6.2   Cranial nerves.

Cranial nerve		Types[a]	Anatomical origin	Function
I	Olfactory	S	Olfactory bulb	Olfaction (smell)
II	Optic	S	Thalamus	Vision (sight)
III	Oculomotor	M	Midbrain	Movement of eyeballs and upper eyelid, accommodation of vision and pupillary constriction
IV	Trochlear	M	Midbrain	Movement of eyeballs
V	Trigeminal	B	Pons	Sensory: light touch, pain, temperature to scalp, face and oral cavity
				Motor: muscles of mastication and the tensor tympani muscle of the ear
VI	Abducens	M	Pons	Eye movement (Lateral rectus muscle of the eye)
VII	Facial	B	Pons	Sensory: taste, external auditory canal
				Motor: muscles of facial expression, lacrimal and salivary secretion
VIII	Vestibulocochlear	S	Pons	Hearing and equilibrium
IX	Glossopharyngeal	B	Medulla oblongata	Sensory: taste, proprioception of muscle involved in swallowing
				Motor: swallowing and salivary secretion
X	Vagus	B	Medulla oblongata	Sensory: small areas of epithelial sensation around the ear and visceral sensory innervation to various organs
				Motor: swallowing, vocalisation and coughing; modulates many other organ systems
XI	Spinal accessory	M	Medulla oblongata	Pectoral and neck muscles
XII	Hypoglossal	M	Medulla oblongata	Speech and swallowing

[a] M, Motor; S, Sensory; B, Both (motor and sensory). Often remembered using the mnemonic: Some Say Marry Money But My Brother Says Big Brains Matter Most.

blood vessel diameter, heart rate, ventilation, coughing, swallowing, vomiting and sneezing. In cases of cerebellar herniation out of the foramen magnum (tonsillar herniation), both the pons and medulla oblongata can be compromised resulting in cerebellar signs (Figure 6.2) followed by a rapid deterioration of Glasgow Coma Scale (GCS) score, terminating in a deep coma and death.

Blood Supply to the Brain

The brain requires approximately 20% of the cardiac output to receive the necessary oxygen and glucose to function. This equates to around 800 ml of blood passing through the cerebral circulation every minute.

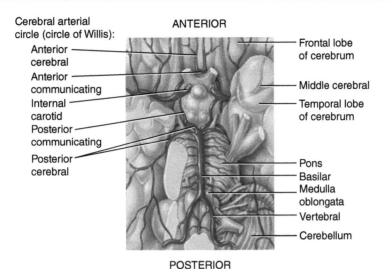

FIGURE 6.4 The circle of Willis.

TABLE 6.3 Lipid solubility of opioids.

Drug	Lipid solubility
Morphine	+
Pethidine	++
Fentanyl	++++

The blood supply to the brain is via the two vertebral, two internal carotid and the anterior spinal arteries. These vessels intersect at the circle of Willis (Figure 6.4), providing a degree of redundancy for any one vessel becoming compromised. The circle of Willis is clinically important as a site of aneurysmal bleeding in atraumatic subarachnoid haemorrhage. Cerebral blood flow is modulated by a number of factors, including in response to signals from the chemoreceptors and baroreceptors in the common carotid artery and aorta (Claassen et al. 2021). This modulation occurs through constriction and dilation of the cerebral vasculature, either decreasing or increasing flow.

Blood–Brain Barrier

The brain requires a constant supply of oxygen and nutrients, with a very limited capability to withstand changes in the supply of these or the levels of circulating electrolytes or dissolves gases (oxygen, carbon dioxide, etc). This means that the maintenance of a constant environment is crucial to allow consistent function of the brain parenchyma. This is facilitated in part through the action of the blood–brain barrier. The blood–brain barrier is a semipermeable network of endothelial cells in the capillaries adjacent to brain tissue, which act as a filter between the systemic circulation and the brain tissue to provide the brain with some protection against toxins and harmful metabolites. The blood–brain barrier is, however, permeable to dissolves gases and fat-soluble/hydrophobic molecules. Clinically, this is useful as more lipid soluble drugs will cross the blood–brain barrier more readily. Lipid solubility may vary greatly, even within a pharmacological class (Table 6.3).

Cerebrospinal Fluid

Cerebrospinal fluid (CSF) flows within the cranial vault, circulating nutrients, surrounding the brain and providing a shock-absorbing cushion. This cushioning reduces damage to the brain parenchyma and the associated nerves and vessels. CSF is clear (or straw coloured), odourless, with similar constituent parts to blood plasma (water, glucose, proteins and electrolytes). It is produced by specialised epithelial cells called the choroid plexus, found within the ventricles of the brain and is absorbed by the arachnoid granulations (Fame and Lehtinen 2020). These arachnoid granulations can easily become blocked (e.g. by blood in a subarachnoid haemorrhage) leading to accumulation of CSF, hydrocephalus and raised intracranial pressure (ICP).

Meninges

The brain and spinal cord are surrounded by three layers of protective tissue, known as the meninges (membranes). The first and most superficial of these meninges is the dura mater (or meninx fibrosa), which is a thick fibrous membrane. Within the skull, the dura mater has two layers, the most superficial being the periosteal layer. This layer is closely adherent to the inside of the cranial vault, with the inner layer referred to as the meningeal layer, which extends down the spinal cord as the dural (or thecal) sac. The dura mater has four important areas where it projects as flat protrusions into the cranial vault (Figure 6.5):

- *Falx cerebri* is the largest of these folds; it descends vertically from anterior to posterior, separating the two cerebral hemispheres.
- *Tentorium cerebelli* is a large crescent-shaped sheet of the dura that separates the occipital lobes from the cerebellum.
- *Falx cerebelli* has a similar vertical orientation to the falx cerebri but lies inferior to the tentorium cerebelli and separates the cerebellar hemispheres.
- *Diaphragma sellae* is a small sheet of dura mater which covers the pituitary gland, forming a roof over the pituitary fossa in the base of the skull.

The remaining two meningeal layers are the *arachnoid mater* and *pia mater*. The arachnoid mater, named after its spidery appearance, is a fibrous mesh adherent to the dura. There is a space between the arachnoid mater and pia mater in which CSF circulates; this is the subarachnoid space. The final meningeal layer, the pia mater, is a delicate membrane that is closely adherent to the surface of the brain and spinal cord.

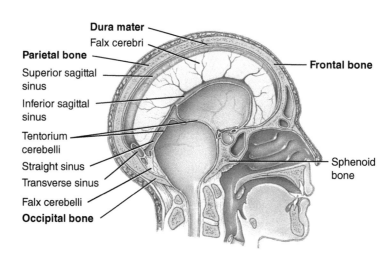

FIGURE 6.5   Folds and reflections of the dura mater.

Spinal Cord

The spinal cord lies within the protective vertebral canal of the vertebral column. It provides communication between the brain and the rest of the body. The meninges are continuous between the brain and spinal cord. This is clinically useful when considering Brudzinski's sign in suspected meningitis, and in considering the risk of inadvertent dura puncture and spinal anaesthesia when a patient receives intercostal nerve blocks for rib fractures.

Peripheral Nervous System

The spinal nerves and all the cranial nerves apart from CN1 and CN2 make up the PNS. The cranial nerves are named in relation to their function but are also numbered roughly in order of their origins from the brain; anterior to posterior.

Reflective Learning Activity

You can remember the names of the cranial nerves by using mnemonics, one of which is:

On Old Olympus's Towering Tops A Friendly Viking Grew Vines And Hops.

Full testing of the cranial nerves can be extremely helpful for eliciting subtle clinical signs and is a key skill in prehospital care (Table 6.2). There are 31 pairs of spinal nerves: 8 cervical, 12 thoracic, 5 lumbar, 5 sacral and 1 coccygeal, according to their point of origin from the spinal cord (Figure 6.6).

Spinal nerves have sensory and motor neurons and relay information to and from various peripheral structures, including the skin and skeletal muscle groups. It is useful in clinical practice to have a good understanding of which spinal nerves innervate specific areas of skin. The regions of skin innervation are described as dermatomes and are often presented as a diagrammatical dermatomal map (Figure 6.7), while the groups of muscles being innervated are described as myotomes (Table 6.4). There are also a number of groupings of spinal nerves known as plexuses, including the cervical plexus, brachial plexus and lumbosacral plexus. These have important clinical relevance, for example, understanding of the brachial plexus is important in relation to some nerve blocks, injuries occurring at birth and assessing injuries to the arm.

The PNS is also divided into the somatic and ANS. The ANS is further subdivided into the parasympathetic, sympathetic and enteric divisions.

Somatic Nervous System

The somatic nervous system consists of sensory and motor neurons which connect the CNS to the rest of the body. These control both our perception of the world (and our bodies position within it) and our interaction with the world through movement. The somatic nervous system also hosts the somatic reflex arcs, being those relating to skeletal muscle function (as opposed to autonomic reflex arcs).

Autonomic Nervous System

The ANS works to maintain homeostasis within the body through regulation of the body's involuntary functions. The ANS is also the site of a number of autonomic reflex arcs. These are reflexes which affect the internal organs. An example of their use in clinical practice is the *vagal manoeuvres* used to terminate a supraventricular tachycardia (Table 6.5).

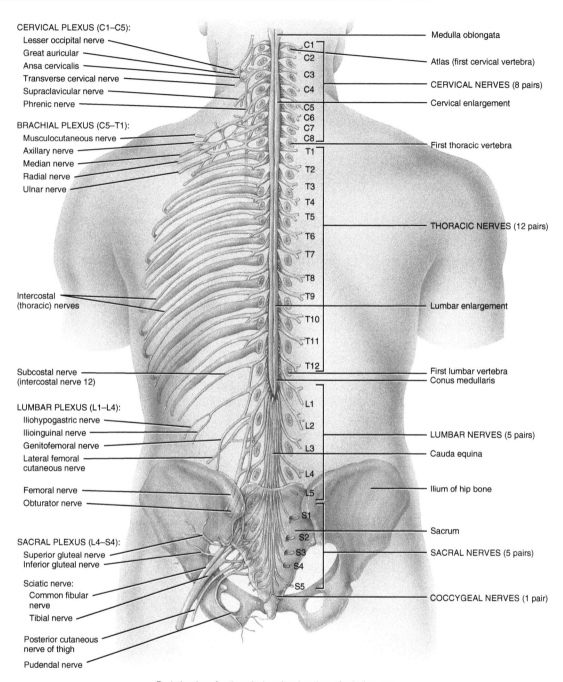

CERVICAL PLEXUS (C1–C5):
 Lesser occipital nerve
 Great auricular
 Ansa cervicalis
 Transverse cervical nerve
 Supraclavicular nerve
 Phrenic nerve

BRACHIAL PLEXUS (C5–T1):
 Musculocutaneous nerve
 Axillary nerve
 Median nerve
 Radial nerve
 Ulnar nerve

Intercostal
(thoracic) nerves

Subcostal nerve
(intercostal nerve 12)

LUMBAR PLEXUS (L1–L4):
 Iliohypogastric nerve
 Ilioinguinal nerve
 Genitofemoral nerve
 Lateral femoral
 cutaneous nerve

 Femoral nerve
 Obturator nerve

SACRAL PLEXUS (L4–S4):
 Superior gluteal nerve
 Inferior gluteal nerve

 Sciatic nerve:
  Common fibular
  nerve
  Tibial nerve

 Posterior cutaneous
 nerve of thigh
 Pudendal nerve

C1
C2
C3
C4
C5
C6
C7
C8
T1
T2
T3
T4
T5
T6
T7
T8
T9
T10
T11
T12
L1
L2
L3
L4
L5
S1
S2
S3
S4
S5

Medulla oblongata

Atlas (first cervical vertebra)

CERVICAL NERVES (8 pairs)

Cervical enlargement

First thoracic vertebra

THORACIC NERVES (12 pairs)

Lumbar enlargement

First lumbar vertebra
Conus medullaris

LUMBAR NERVES (5 pairs)

Cauda equina

Ilium of hip bone

Sacrum

SACRAL NERVES (5 pairs)

COCCYGEAL NERVES (1 pair)

Posterior view of entire spinal cord and portions of spinal nerves

FIGURE 6.6   The spinal cord and the location of the 31 pairs of spinal nerves.

98

The ANS is further divided into the sympathetic and parasympathetic divisions. The sympathetic division modulates the activity of many internal organs in response to physiological or psychological stress (Table 6.6). In cases of significant stress, this is known as the 'fight or flight' response, typified by a hormonal cascade that results in the release of catecholamines. The hormonal activity of the sympathetic division also influences the secretion of the sex hormones cortisol, serotonin and dopamine, as well as affecting multiple organ systems (Table 6.1). The parasympathetic division uses acetylcholine to control the internal responses associated with relaxation (Table 6.6).

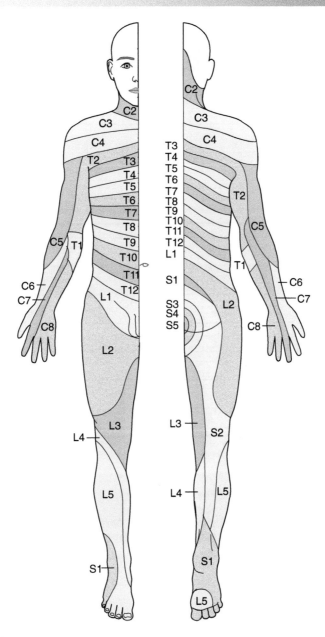

FIGURE 6.7 Dermatome map.

TABLE 6.4   Myotomes.

Innervation	Muscle group or *reflex arc*
Cervical 3, 4 and 5	Diaphragm
Cervical 5 and 6	Elbow flexion
Cervical 5 and 6	*Biceps jerk*
Cervical 7	Elbow extension
Thoracic 1	Intrinsic muscles of the hand
Thoracic 8–12	*Abdominal reflex*
Lumbar 1 and 2	Hip flexors
Lumbar 2 and 3	Hip adductors
Lumbar 3 and 4	Knee extensors
Lumbar 3 and 4	*Quadriceps knee jerk*
Lumbar 4 and 5 and Sacral 1	Knee flexors
Sacral 1 and 2	Toe flexors
Sacral 2, 3 and 4	Anal sphincter

TABLE 6.5   Vagal manoeuvres.

Vagal manoeuvre	Method	Mechanism	Contraindications	Risks
Carotid sinus massage	Fingertip massage of the patient's carotid sinus	The baroreceptors within the carotid body are stimulated, triggering bradycardia via the vagus nerve	Bruits on neck auscultation, bilateral carotid massage	Embolic stroke – perhaps as frequent in 1:1000 in elderly patients. Asystole, hypotension or other dysrhythmias
Mammalian diving reflex	Immersion of face and head into a container of ice water for 5 seconds, or application of a cold wet cloth or ice pack to the face	Stimulation of the trigeminal nerve, resulting in a reflex arc causing bradycardia via brainstem and vagus nerve	Unable to safely hold their breath; fear of drowning	Aspiration of water; asystole, hypotension or other dysrhythmias
Modified Valsalva manoeuvre	Forceful exhalation against resistance which raises intrathoracic pressure Followed by passive leg elevation and supine positioning	Stimulation of baroreceptors in the carotid body and aortic arch leading to an increase in vagal tone	Acute myocardial infarction, Aortic stenosis, glaucoma or retinopathy	Asystole, hypotension or other dysrhythmias

Enteric Nervous System

The enteric nervous system is a division of the ANS concerned with the gastrointestinal tract. It modulates the tract's motor functions, secretory functions, blood flow and endocrine activity (see Chapter 11).

TABLE 6.6 Physiological effects of the sympathetic and parasympathetic nervous systems.

Organ/system	Sympathetic effects	Parasympathetic effects
Eyes	Dilates pupils (mydriasis)	Constricts pupils (miosis)
Heart	Positive inotropic and chronotropic effects	Negatively chronotropic
Lungs	Dilation of bronchioles	Constriction of bronchioles
Renal system	Decreased urine output, contraction of urinary bladder sphincter	Relaxation of urinary bladder sphincter
Adrenal medulla	Secretion of adrenaline and noradrenaline	No effect
Liver	Increased glucose production and decreased glycogen production	Reduced glucose production with increased production of glycogen
Digestive tract	Reduced peristalsis and constriction of the digestive system sphincters	Increased peristalsis and relaxation of the digestive system sphincters
Lacrimal glands	Inhibits secretion of lacrimal fluid (tears)	Increased secretion of lacrimal fluid (tears)
Salivary glands	Reduces salivary production	Increases salivary production
Sweat glands	Stimulates perspiration and diaphoresis	No effect in normal physiology
Cellular metabolism	Increases metabolism, stimulating lipid breakdown	Homeostatic maintenance
Blood vessels	Constriction of peripheral blood vessels and dilation of some central vessels blood vessels	Vasodilation to selected vessels (e.g. genital erectile tissues, cerebral arteries)

Disorders of the Nervous System

Snapshot 6.1 Road Traffic Collision

Pre-Arrival Information

A pedestrian has been struck by a vehicle, believed to be deliberate. Police are en route. The patient is unconscious and their breathing status is unknown.

Windscreen Assessment

On arrival at the scene, you can see that a number of cars have stopped, blocking the road. There is a pedestrian lying in the carriageway on her back.

Primary Survey

DR CABCDE:
Danger: the scene is relatively safe, traffic is stopped.
Response: there is no response to painful stimuli.
Catastrophic haemorrhage: no catastrophic bleeding.

Airway: compromised
Breathing: no ventilatory effort.
Circulation: palpable radial pulse.
Disability: unresponsive to pain, pupils bilaterally dilated.
Exposure: a brief secondary survey identifies a scalp laceration with venous bleeding. Chest and abdomen appear grossly uninjured and long bones appear intact.

Analysis

Laksmi Basnyat is a 28-year-old woman who was a pedestrian struck by a car, which subsequently left the scene of the accident. On your arrival, Laksmi is lying in the road, bleeding from a laceration to her forehead. She is unresponsive and apnoeic but has a palpable pulse at her wrist. You place a supraglottic airway and ventilate her with an FiO_2 (fraction of inspired oxygen) of 0.9. En route to hospital she regains consciousness but remains confused and agitated. Her eyes are open spontaneously, and she pulls out the supraglottic airway, but she will not do as you ask of her. She seems to be very confused and keeps asking when the plane will take off. Her pupils are now equal and reactive to light, estimated at 3 mm.

Vital Signs

Her vital signs in the ambulance are as follows:

Vital sign	1000 h	1010 h	1020 h	Normal values
Temperature (°C)	Not recorded	35.7	Not repeated	36.0–37.9
Pulse (beats/min)	93	88	91	60–100
Respiration (breaths/min)	Apnoeic	Ventilated at 12	Self-ventilating at 18	12–20
Blood pressure (mmHg)	Radial pulse present	155/79	140/88	100–139 (systolic)
O_2 saturation (%)	Not obtained	99	98	94–98
AVPU	Unresponsive	Unresponsive	Alert (confused)	Alert

Reflective Learning Activity

Reflect on Snapshot 6.1 and consider the following:

- What is Laksmi's current GCS score?
- Consider what may have caused Laksmi's apnoeic episode?
- Discuss the role of the GCS score in identifying improvement or deterioration in a patient with a head injury.
- If Laksmi had remained apnoeic, what further resources would you have wanted to attend scene or rendezvous with you en route?
- In your locality, which receiving unit would be most appropriate for this patient and why?

Traumatic Brain Injury

Traumatic brain injury is a leading cause of death in the under 40s and can occur from a plethora of mechanisms of injury (road traffic collisions, falls from height, etc.) and a high index of suspicion must be held for such injuries when assessing a patient (Figure 6.8). Injuries range from very minor head injuries to concussions and on to serious and life-threatening injury (Figure 6.9).

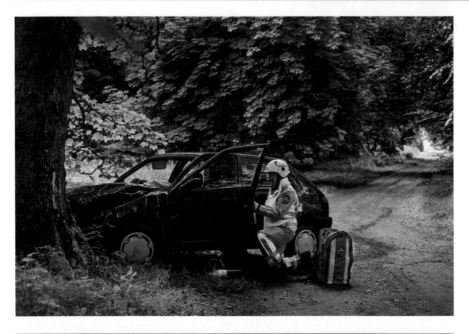

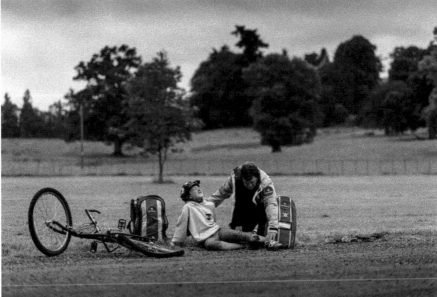

FIGURE 6.8 Head injuries can result from an array of traumatic incidents.

Minor Head Injury > Concussion > Serious Head Injury

FIGURE 6.9 Continuum of head injuries.

Primary Brain Injury

Primary brain injuries are injuries that occur from direct energy transfer at the time of injury to the brain tissue. This includes focal injuries such as penetrating trauma to the brain or bone fragments being displaced into the brain parenchyma and the more diffuse injuries seen in brains subjected to rapid acceleration or deceleration forces. Such diffuse injuries form a spectrum from a mild concussion to significant diffuse axonal injuries. These injuries are also seen in cases of non-accidental head injury (historically known as shaken baby syndrome). Direct trauma or rapid velocity change to the skull can also lead to a phenomenon called coup/contrecoup injuries. Coup injuries are those occurring to the brain under the point of impact with the skull. Contrecoup injuries occur where brain parenchyma strikes or grates against in inside of the cranial vault as a result of impact elsewhere, typically to the opposite side of the brain.

Impact Brain Apnoea

Primary brain injury also includes impact brain apnoea, which is the cessation of breathing after traumatic brain injury (Wilson et al. 2016). This condition is associated with the previous alcohol intake. The duration of apnoea appears to be linked to the degree of energy transfer occurring to the brain. Basic airway manoeuvres and artificial ventilation are essential to prevent secondary hypoxia brain injury. The clinical case presented in Snapshot 6.1 describes the initial clinical course of a patient with impact brain apnoea.

Secondary Brain Injury

Secondary brain injuries are those occurring after and as a consequence of the initial insult. These are the injuries that we have the greatest ability to limit during our prehospital care of a patient. Once damaged, the cells of the brain parenchyma become inflamed and oedematous and ICP rises (Figure 6.10). This rise in ICP leads to worsening of brain tissue ischaemia and neuronal death. Secondary brain injury is worsened by reduced cerebral perfusion, hypoxia or free radical formation due to hyperoxaemia, hypercapnia and hypotension.

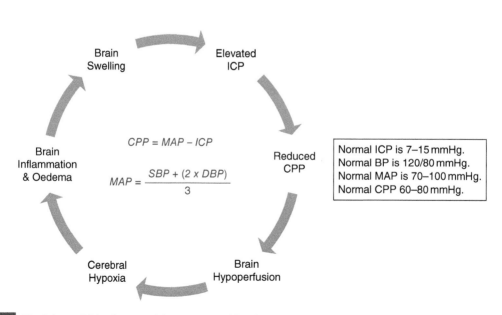

FIGURE 6.10   Physiology of rising intracranial pressure. BP, blood pressure; CPP, cerebral perfusion pressure; DBP, diastolic blood pressure; ICP, intracranial pressure; MAP, mean arterial pressure; SBP, systolic blood pressure.

Raised Intracranial Pressure

ICP is the pressure exerted by the fluids within the skull on both the skull vault and the brain tissue. ICP depends on the volume of brain tissue, CSF and blood within the fixed space of the cranium. There is a limited ability for venous blood and, to a lesser extent, CSF to be shunted out of the cranial vault to produce room for a swelling brain, but this can only provide compensation for a short time. The addition of another mass, such as a brain tumour or haematoma, into the cranial vault will raise ICP.

ICP is a key component in the ability of the body to perfuse the brain. In cases where the ICP is elevated, a greater mean arterial pressure is required to overcome the ICP and provide cerebral perfusion in the form of the cerebral perfusion pressure (Figure 6.10). Once cerebral perfusion has been interrupted or compromised, the subsequent hypoperfusion leads to reactive cerebral vasodilation and cerebral oedema which both further raise the ICP, leading to a cycle of worsening perfusion and brain injury (Figure 6.10).

While clinical indicators of raised ICP seen in the prehospital phase appear to correlate poorly to the degree of rise in ICP (ter Avest et al. 2021), it is important to be aware of such findings. Common indications of raised ICP include:

- Early indications:
  - Irritability
  - Confusion
- Late indications:
  - Progressively reduced consciousness
  - Cushing's triad
    - Bradycardia
    - Hypertension
    - Irregular breathing pattern
  - Posturing (decorticate/decerebrate; Figure 6.11)
  - Pupillary changes
    - Unequal pupils
    - Bilaterally fixed and dilated >5 mm

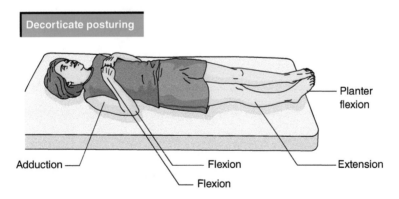

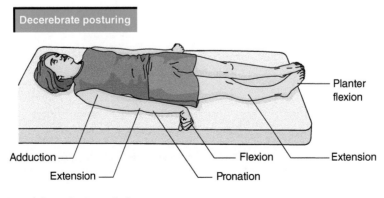

FIGURE 6.11 Decorticate and decerebrate posturing.

Red Flag: Cushing's Triad

Irregular ventilation, bradycardia and a widening pulse pressure is the Cushing's triad. This can indicate a rise in intracerebral pressure.

Brain Herniation

A significant and rapid rise in ICP can lead to herniation of brain parenchyma (Figure 6.12). There is a shift of intracranial contents from one region of the skull to another or through the foramen magnum. There are six main types of brain herniation (Table 6.7); frustratingly, the medical profession seems divided on how to classify them.

Red Flag

New-onset confusion or a drop of two or more points in the Glasgow Coma Scale score indicate significant worsening neurological function.

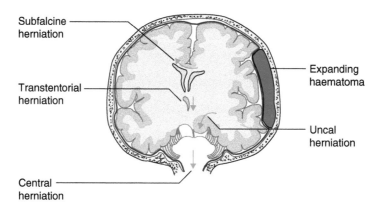

Subfalcine herniation

Transtentorial herniation

Central herniation

Expanding haematoma

Uncal herniation

FIGURE 6.12   Brain herniation.

TABLE 6.7   The main types of brain herniation.

Type	Region
Supratentorial	Uncal
	Central
	Subfalcine
	Trancalvarial
	Tectal
Infratentorial	Upward (upward cerebellar herniation)
	Tonsillar (downward cerebellar herniation), often called coning

Assessing Global Neurological Function

Glasgow Coma Scale

The Glasgow Coma Scale (Table 6.8) is the most widely accepted assessment tool for measuring level of consciousness. It should be documented for any patient with a head injury or any other cause of confusion or decreased consciousness. The GCS was developed specifically for detecting and monitoring changes in a patient's neurological status after neurosurgery but is now used more widely (Teasdale et al. 2014).

Assessment is achieved by evaluating three categories of behaviour: eye opening, best verbal response and best motor response. For each category, the best level of response achieved is allocated a numerical value. The lower the patient scores for each element, the more significant the neurological dysfunction (Teasdale et al. 2014). Scores should be presented in a standard order: eyes (E) then verbal (V) and then motor (M). A fully conscious person would therefore have a GCS score of E4 V5 M6, with a total score of 15. In patients who are intubated, the score for verbal response is replaced by a T. This means the minimum and maximum scores for an intubated patient are 2–10 T. The GCS score has been criticised for its lack of validity when used for non-neurogenic pathology and the sole use of the cumulative score is also less helpful than detailing the three components of the score separately. A GCS score, scoring as it does the 'best response', is limited in its ability to assess unilateral pathology.

TABLE 6.8   The Glasgow Coma Scale.

Behaviour	Response in adults	Score	Response in children (<5 years)
Best eye opening	Spontaneous	4	Spontaneous
	To speech	3	To speech
	To pain	2	To pain
	No response	1	No response
Best verbal response	Orientated conversation	5	Alert, babbles, coos or words/sentences to usual ability level
	Confused conversation	4	Less than usual ability level or irritable crying
	Inappropriate words	3	Cries to pain
	Incomprehensible sounds	2	Moans to pain
	No verbal response to pain	1	No verbal response to pain
	Intubated	T	Intubated
Best motor response	Obeys commands	6	Normal spontaneous movements
	Localises pain	5	Localises to pain or withdraws to touch
	Withdraws from pain	4	Withdraws from pain
	Abnormal flexion to pain (decorticate posturing)	3	Abnormal flexion to pain (decorticate posturing)
	Abnormal extension to pain (decerebrate posturing)	2	Abnormal extension to pain (decerebrate posturing)
	No motor response	1	No motor response

ACVPU

AVPU is an acronym for 'alert, voice, pain, unresponsive'. It is a quick assessment of consciousness that can be made as part of your primary survey. It is much quicker than undertaking an assessment of GCS score. In some settings, a C is added to make the score sensitive for new-onset confusion.

Vital Signs Recording

While GCS and ACVPU scores are good assessments of neurological function, the other vital signs are also important when assessing a patient with a brain injury. Assessing pupil function is also an important neurological observation; however, while the presence of a 'fixed blown pupil' is a reliable indicator of raised ICP (ter Avest et al. 2021), where it likely represents uncal herniation and compression of CNIII, more subtle changes are less helpful and clinicians perform poorly at estimating pupil size (Olson et al. 2016).

Decision Making and Management of a Head Injury

Emergent Management of Significant Head Injuries

Significant head injuries are an emergency requiring rapid evacuation to a suitable receiving unit. During the prehospital phase, all efforts should be made to avoid raising the ICP further (Table 6.9). If transfer times will be prolonged, the involvement of an enhanced care team may be beneficial. Some further management options include:

- *Maintaining perfusion and oxygenation*: maintenance of an appropriate CPP with adequate oxygenation is the mainstay of prehospital treatment.
- *Encourage venous drainage*: placing a patient in a position of a 20- to 30-degree head-up tilt and removal or loosening of a cervical collar will assist venous drainage from the cranial vault (Nathanson et al. 2020).
- *Osmotherapy*: treatment with hypertonic saline or another osmotically active drug may reduce ICP by drawing water out of the oedematous brain (Nathanson et al. 2020). The evidence for these interventions is, however, mixed (Bergmans et al. 2020; Williams 2021).
- *Anaesthesia and ventilation*: providing prehospital anaesthesia reduces the oxygen demand of the injured brain (Figure 6.13). Once anaesthetised, normocapnia and normoxia can be more easily targeted (AAGBI 2006; Nathanson et al. 2020). In extremis, hyperventilation may also be used as a temporising measure to reduce ICP by reducing $PaCO_2$ (partial pressure of carbon dioxide in arterial blood), resulting in cerebral vasoconstriction.
- *Decompressive surgery*: in austere settings, a prehospital or emergency craniotomy or burr-hole insertion may be used to reduce ICP (Wilson et al. 2012).

TABLE 6.9   Avoiding iatrogenic rises in intracranial pressure.

Interventions that can raise ICP	Mitigating these risks
Circumferential endotracheal tube ties	Tape endotracheal tube in place
Laryngoscopy	Blunt reflex sympathetic response to laryngoscopy with fentanyl and anaesthetic drugs; airway manipulation undertaken by an expert
Cervical collars	Loosen or remove collar for transport
Head down position/Trendelenburg	30-degree head-up tilt
Transfer by helicopter (Maissan et al. 2018)	Consider land transport, if unavoidable ensure head-up tilt is applied
Rapid acceleration or deceleration	Smooth and progressive driving
Physiological arousal (e.g. pain, vibration, coughing, gagging)	Reduce external stimuli (reduce light and noise), ensure adequate analgesia and consider prehospital anaesthesia and continuing sedation

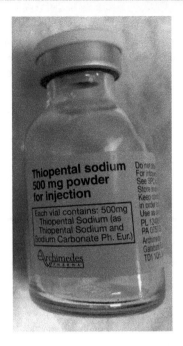

FIGURE 6.13 Thiopentone, an anaesthetic agent.

Minor Head Injuries

When considering whether trauma can be considered a minor head injury, we need to have a working knowledge of the indications for computed tomography (CT) of the head:

- More than one episode of vomiting
- Anticoagulant treatment (There is increasing evidence that patients taking antiplatelet therapy, especially dual anti-platelet therapy, are at increased risk of intracranial haemorrhage after head injury. It would be prudent to treat such patients as if they were anticoagulated.)
- Amnesia
- Dangerous mechanism
- Focal neurological deficit
- GCS score less than 13
- Post-traumatic seizure
- Suspected skull fracture.

If none of these indications and no other concerning features are present, a patient may be suitable for discharge on scene. Verbal and printed information should be provided, including appropriate safety nets, information about return to work/school and about anticipated recovery. It is also appropriate to advise that a responsible adult stays with the patient for the first 24 hours post injury.

Safety Netting
It is important to provide appropriate safety netting for patients with minor head injuries, and to the responsible adult who will be staying with your patient. Safety netting should cover a number of core areas.

Snapshot 6.2 Stroke

Mr Regan is a 66-year-old man whose wife called an ambulance for him when he started slurring his words and stumbling while they were at the playground with their grandchildren. On your arrival, you notice that Mr Regan appears muddled and is having trouble finding the right words. His mouth appears to droop slightly on the right side and, on holding his arms out in front of him, he has slight pronator drift on the right. He has a history of moderate hypertension, controlled with ramipril. He is overweight and drinks around five units of alcohol a week but has never smoked.

Physical Examination

On examination:

Cranial nerve		Assessment
I	Olfactory	Unable to test in the ambulance
II	Optic	Visual acuity appears grossly normal on a hand-held Snellen chart; visual fields appear compromised on the right side
III	Oculomotor	The patient finds it difficult to track your movements and complains of diplopia
IV	Trochlear	
VI	Abducens	
V	Trigeminal	Sensation: diminished on the right side of the face.
		Motor: muscles of mastication are noticeably weak on the right
VII	Facial	Sensory: unable to assess taste
		Motor: notable right sided facial weakness, able to 'wrinkle forehead'
VIII	Vestibulocochlear	Hearing appears grossly normal as does balance
IX	Glossopharyngeal	Swallow and cough not formally assessed
X	Vagus	
XI	Spinal accessory	Pectoral and neck muscles appear weak on the right
XII	Hypoglossal	Speech appears normal apart from the difficulty with word finding

Chest: Equal bilateral air entry with no added sounds. Heart sounds I+I+0. Jugular venous pressure unremarkable.
Abdomen: Abdomen soft and non-tender. Bowel sounds normal.
Calves: Soft and non-tender.

Vital Signs

The following vital signs were noted and recorded:

Vital sign	On scene	Normal values
Temperature (°C)	37.2	36.0–37.5
Pulse (beats/min)	110	60–100
Respiration (breaths/min)	22	12–20
Blood pressure (mmHg)	171/98	100–139 (systolic)
O_2 saturation (%)	95	95–98

- Alert on the AVPU scale.
- GCS score: E4 V4 M6.
- His NEWS (National Early Warning Score) is 4 on scene.

Reflective Learning Activity

Take some time to reflect on Snapshot 6.2 and then consider the following:

1. What type of stroke has Mr Regan experienced (Table 6.4 may help you)?
2. Discuss Mr Regan's risk factors for stroke.
3. From your reading, what are the limitations with using the GCS score for Mr. Regan?
4. What is the evidence to support the use of the NEWS in the prehospital setting?
5. Outline, with reference to relevant guidance, the immediate care that Mr Regan requires.

Stroke

A stroke occurs when the blood (and oxygen) supply to a discrete area of brain is interrupted or reduced for a prolonged amount of time. While some strokes are fairly easy to detect clinically using a scoring system such as the FAST (face, arm, speech, time) or ROSIER scores (Sibson 2017), others will be much harder to recognise (Ataullah and Naqvi 2021; Devlin 2022). There are also a large number of conditions which can present in a similar way to a stroke, considered stroke mimics (McClelland et al. 2019). During the prehospital phase, it is extremely difficult to identify all these conditions accurately, and such patients will usually require rapid transport and brain imaging.

111

Red Flag: The Anna King Rule

Any instantaneous onset of central neurological signs or symptoms is a stroke until proven otherwise.

Stroke Pathophysiology

Interruption in oxygen delivery can occur due to occlusion or compression of an artery supplying brain tissue, haemorrhage from one of these vessels, or systemic hypoperfusion. In simplistic terms, around 87% of strokes are ischaemic in nature, while the remaining 13% are haemorrhagic (Stroke Association 2018). Many of the risk factors for ischaemic stroke are common to other atherosclerotic disorders:

- Diabetes mellitus type 2
- Family history of stroke (age < 50 years)
- Hyperlipidaemia
- Hypertension
- Obesity
- Smoking.

In an ischaemic stroke, blood flow to an area of the brain is interrupted, leading to an area of brain parenchyma becoming deficient in oxygen (ischaemic), which may progress to cell death (infarction). Such interruptions from blood flow are most often caused by the rupture of an atherosclerotic plague in one of the cerebral arteries. The process of atherosclerosis is discussed more fully in Chapter 7. It can be helpful to conceptualise an area of salvageable tissue around the central area of cell death (the penumbra). This viable tissue may progress to worsening ischaemia and death or, if reperfusion therapy is provided rapidly, may be saved (Liu et al. 2010). Reperfusion can be provided by thrombolysis or clot retrieval.

A haemorrhagic stroke occurs when one of the blood vessels in or around the brain ruptures, leading to bleeding, interrupted blood supply, increased ICP and compression and ischaemia of brain parenchyma. These strokes share many of the risk factors as ischaemic events, with old age and hypertension being key features.

The Bamford classification defines a number of stroke syndromes that correlate clinical presentation with location and extent of injury (Table 6.10). Further localisation is possible with a detailed neurological examination (Devlin 2022). Some areas of the brain control very specific functions, so a loss of these particular functions will indicate localised damage. An example of this is in relation to the understanding and expression of the spoken word. An area of the brain called Broca's area in the frontal lobe is concerned with the fluent production of speech, while an interconnected area in the temporal lobe called Wernicke's area is responsible for language comprehension (Figure 6.14). You could therefore have damage only to Wernicke's area and be presenting with *fluent dysphasia*, meaning that you can fluently talk but

TABLE 6.10   Bamford classification of stroke syndromes.

Stroke syndrome		Blood vessel involvement	Clinical presentation
TACS	Total anterior stroke	Middle and anterior cerebral arteries	All three of the following: • Unilateral motor or sensory deficit to at least two of the following areas: face, arm or leg. • Homonymous visual field defect. • High cerebral dysfunction (e.g. dysphasia)
PACS	Partial anterior stroke	Middle and anterior cerebral arteries	At least two of the following: • Unilateral motor or sensory deficit to at least two of the following areas: face, arm or leg. • Homonymous visual field defect. • High cerebral dysfunction (e.g. dysphasia)
POCS	Posterior circulation stroke	Vertebral or basilar arteries, or posterior cerebral artery	Any of the following: • Cerebellar dysfunction • Homonymous visual field defect • Eye movement disorder • Bilateral motor or sensory deficit • Ipsilateral cranial nerve palsy with contralateral motor or sensory deficit
LACS	Lacunar stroke	Subcortical small vessels	Isolated motor or sensory symptoms, or ataxic hemiparesis in the absence of higher cerebral dysfunction and hemianopia

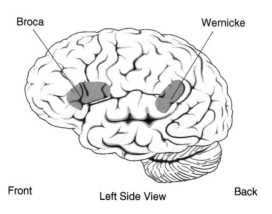

FIGURE 6.14   Broca's and Wernicke's areas.

what you are saying may lack meaning. Equally, you could have isolated damage to Broca's area and present with *non-fluent dysphasia*, where fluency is lost but meaning is still present in the words produced. Rapid CT of the brain will be essential for these patients; transporting them to an appropriate facility is a priority.

Transient Ischaemic Attack

A transient ischaemic attack (TIA) is sometimes referred to as a mini-stroke and represents a temporary interruption to cerebral blood flow (Clissold et al. 2020). These may present with paraesthesia, paralysis and impaired speech or vision. Symptoms must fully resolve within 24 hours to define an event as a TIA. As TIA is often a warning of significant underlying atherosclerotic disease, these patients require urgent assessment, by a specialist TIA clinic (Clissold et al. 2020). Assessment tools such as the ABCD2 (age, blood pressure, clinical features, duration of TIA, presence of diabetes) score should not be used, as all TIAs need urgent follow-up.

Pharmacological Management: Acute Phase

Acute pharmacological management of stroke depends on whether it is haemorrhagic or ischaemic in nature; delineating these two pathologies in prehospital care is a challenge. The mainstay of prehospital treatment is maintaining normoxia and rapid transport to an appropriate hospital. In hospital, an ischaemic stroke may be treated with thrombolysis or thrombectomy.

Non-pharmacological Management: Acute Phase

Thrombectomy is indicated within six hours of symptom onset for individuals with ischaemic strokes where there has been large occlusion of a major cerebral artery (National Institute for Health and Care Excellence 2022).

Orange Flag: Psychological Impact Following a Stroke

Many patients experience low mood after experiencing a stroke. In around 12–15% of cases, this low mood results in suicidal ideation, with the presence of comorbidities and low family income being specific risk factors for such depressive illness (Zhang et al. 2022).

Clinical Investigation: Computed Tomography of the Brain

A CT of the brain is the investigation of choice for the majority of suspected strokes. Patients in whom a cerebellar stroke is suspected are the exception to this rule, where magnetic resonance imaging (MRI) with diffusion-weighted imaging may be preferred.

Dementia

Dementia is a progressive neurological disorder typified by the progressive and irreversible loss of cerebral function. The term 'dementia' describes a constellation of symptoms including amnesia, mood changes and difficulties with communication and reasoning. There are a number of subclassifications of dementia, which have slightly different clinical presentations and causes. Some common subtypes are presented in Figure 6.15; a good working knowledge of some of these dementias is beneficial in clinical practice.

- Common
- 17% of all diagnoses of dementia
- Associated with ischaemic injury to the brain

Vascular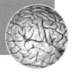

- Loss of dopaminergic neurones with typical symptomatology of:
- rigidity
- bradykinesia
- unsteadiness

Parkinson's Disease

- Most Common
- 60% of all diagnoses of dementia
- Associated with amyloid plaques and neurofibrillary tangles

Alzheimer's Disease

- Typically a gradual progression of behaviour change, loss of empathy and judgement.
- Executive dysfunction and language impairment

Fronto-temporal

- Caused by prolonged and excessive alcohol intake.
- Exacerbated by thiamine deficiency and hepatic encephalopathy.
- May coexist with Wernick'es Syndrome.

Alcohol Related Brain Damage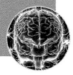

- Rare.
- Causes problems with facial recognition, reading, writing and spacial awareness.

Posterior Cortical Atrophy

114

FIGURE 6.15 Subtypes of dementia. Sources: Anusorn/Adobe Stock, Science Photo Library/Alamy Stock Photo.

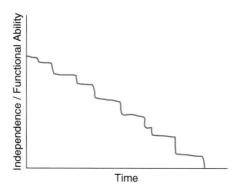

FIGURE 6.16 Stepwise decline seen in multi-infarct dementia.

Vascular Dementia

Vascular dementia occurs due to compromised blood flow to the brain, often involving small vessel atherosclerotic disease (Bir et al. 2021). This damage causes problems with memory, cognition, gait and worsening of symptoms later in the day (often called *sundowning*). When viewed retrospectively, the disease can be seen to produce a stepwise functional decline due to multiple small infarcts within the brain parenchyma (Figure 6.16). Vascular dementia shares many of its risk factors with stroke and TIA. Such patients are at high risk during any low cardiac output state or episodes of hypoxaemia.

Alzheimer's Disease

Alzheimer's disease is one of the most common types of dementia. Incidence of Alzheimer's disease increases with advancing age and is uncommon under the age of 65 years. Initial diagnosis is challenging and may be delayed. As the disease progresses, forgetfulness and memory loss, disorientation and confusion occur. Personality and mood changes may also be evident as the disease progresses and, on occasion, these may be the first symptoms to present to health professionals. The causes of Alzheimer's disease remain unclear, despite continuing investigation into disease triggers (Breijyeh and Karaman 2020). Abnormal protein plaques and neurofibrillary tangles are found in the affected brain tissue, and there is also usually widespread atrophy of the cerebral cortex. These changes are associated with a shortage of acetylcholine, loss of neuronal mass and structural changes in various areas of the brain.

Pharmacological Management

A small number of drugs may slow the rate of decline:

- Donepezil, rivastigmine and galantamine are cholinesterase inhibitors, which facilitate an increase in levels of acetylcholine.
- Memantine functions in a chemically similar way to ketamine, acting at the N-methyl-D-aspartate (NMDA) receptors. It modulates neurotransmitter activity and prevents excess entry of calcium ions into neurons.

Parkinson's Disease

Parkinson's disease mainly occurs over the age of 50 years, with an increasing prevalence over the age of 80 years. It is a progressive degenerative disease resulting from the continual loss of neurons. It primarily affects the substantia nigra within the basal ganglia. While Parkinson's disease begins as a movement disorder, it will progress to a syndrome of cognitive decline and functional loss (Figure 6.17).

In Parkinson's disease, dopaminergic neurons are damaged and die. This occurs because of a number of interplaying factors: abnormal protein formation into Lewy bodies, disruption of the blood–brain barrier, disruption to normal autophagy and alterations to cell metabolism. The symptoms of Parkinson's disease are directly attributable to the loss of these neurons, with symptoms progressing as more cells die.

Other signs and symptoms of Parkinson's disease may include:

- Confusion
- Depression
- Discoordination
- Facial masking
- Stooped posture
- Micrographia
- Muscle fatigue.

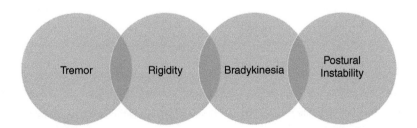

FIGURE 6.17 Cardinal signs of Parkinson's disease.

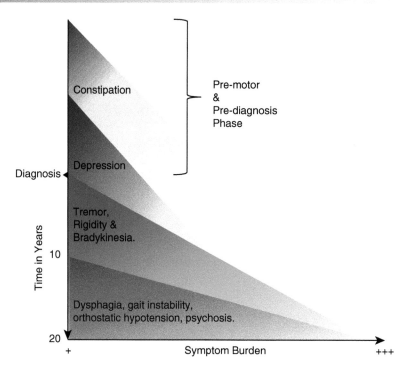

FIGURE 6.18   Development of signs and symptoms in Parkinson's disease.

While some signs and symptoms may be present for many years before diagnosis, a diagnosis is not likely to be made until the motor symptoms (Figures 6.17 and 6.18) develop. From the point of diagnosis, symptoms progress over the following 10–20 years (Figure 6.18).

Pharmacological Management

Pharmacological treatments can be grouped into a number of categories, which work by increasing the amount of circulating dopamine in the CNS:

- Levodopa (or L-dopa) is a precursor to dopamine.
- Dopamine agonists (pramipexole, rotigotine, etc.) stimulate dopamine receptors in a similar way to dopamine.
- Monoamine oxidase type B (MAO-B) inhibitors prevent the action of MAO-B, which breaks down dopamine.
- COMTs or catechol-O-methyltransferase inhibitors work by increasing the bioavailability of levodopa.
- Amantadine is a nicotinic and NMDA antagonist and dopamine agonist.

Medications Management

It is important that medication for neurological conditions such as epilepsy and Parkinson's disease are taken at the correct time each day. If timings are incorrect or a delay occurs, the serum concentration may fall below therapeutic levels and unwanted signs or symptoms will emerge.

Clinical Investigations: Magnetic Resonance Imaging

An MRI scan can provide high-quality visualisation of any soft-tissue structures within the body. It does not use ionising radiation, making it a safer option than radiographs or CT.

Seizures and Epilepsy

A seizure is clinically discernible event resulting from the uncoordinated excessive and controlled discharge of a group of neurones within the brain (Milligan 2021). Epilepsy is a common neurological condition, with an incidence of around 50 per 100 000 population and a prevalence of around 5–10 per thousand (Epilepsy Research Institute UK 2020). There is a bimodal distribution of the incidence of epilepsy, the first peak being between birth and around 20 years of age, when congenital epilepsies reveal themselves, and then a later peak where epilepsy disorders may be caused by other pathologies such as stroke (Figure 6.19).

Pathophysiology

Seizures result from an abnormal electrical discharge of neurons within the brain affecting any of the sensory, motor or autonomic neuronal functions. This abnormal discharge initially takes the form of heterogeneity of firing, followed by a hypersynchrony of these electrical discharges as a later feature linked to seizure termination (Thomas 2015). Seizure activity can result from multiple triggers. These triggers could be physiological, such as sleep deprivation, pyrexia or hypoglycaemia, or physical stimulation such as loud noises or flashing lights (Okudan and Özkara 2018). When such abnormal neuronal seizure activity occurs, it can produce a wide range of clinical signs and symptoms (NICE 2022). Seizure syndromes are diverse in their presentation and classification (Figure 6.20). While epilepsy is one cause, the aetiology of seizures is broad, encompassing environmental (e.g. heat stroke), congenital (e.g. Dravet syndrome), chemical (e.g. hypoglycaemia) and neoplastic causes among others (NICE 2022).

117

Orange Flag: Psychosocial Impact of Epilepsy

Many patients with established epilepsy will have an ambulance called for them by bystanders. While some patients with epilepsy will need to be transferred to hospital, many can be safely discharged on scene. It is helpful to remember that many patients with epilepsy are experts in their condition and will recognise whether a seizure has been normal or abnormal for them. As clinicians, we can often help them in this decision making by providing an assessment of their vital signs (for indications of a new physiological cause) and through history taking to elicit any social or environmental factors (missed medications or stressful events).

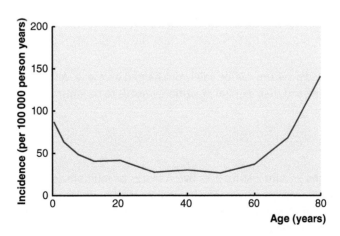

FIGURE 6.19 Incidence of epilepsy.

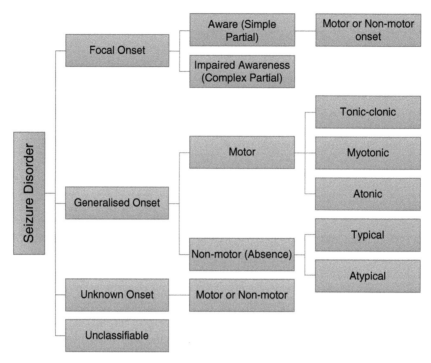

FIGURE 6.20   Seizure classification. Source: Adapted from: Fisher et al. (2017).

TABLE 6.11   The author's approach to safety netting.

Area	Advice content
General	General worsening advice
Logistical	How to access further help
Red flag	Specific signs and symptoms of worsening head injury pathology
Risk	What is the potential risk involved for the patient?

Non-conveyance

Some patients who have suffered a seizure can be safely discharged on scene. All patients discharged on scene should receive appropriate safety netting and their general practitioner needs to be informed (Table 6.11).

Status Epilepticus

Status epilepticus is a prolonged seizure lasting over five minutes or multiple seizures with incomplete resolution in between (NICE 2022). It a medical emergency requiring immediate treatment. Management in the prehospital setting follows the primary survey model of airway, breathing and circulation. The mainstay of the prehospital management of ongoing seizures is benzodiazepine therapy to terminate the seizure. If benzodiazepine is unsuccessful, enhanced care teams can provide additional pharmacological therapies (Figure 6.21).

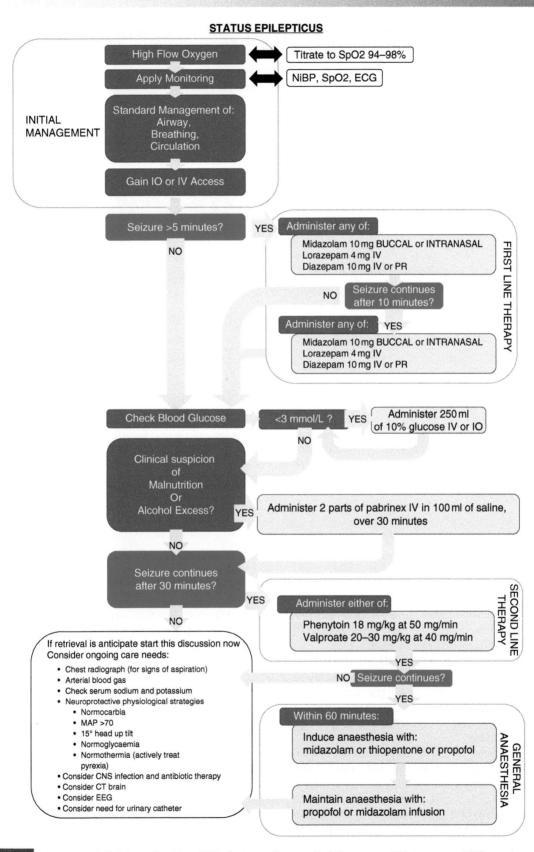

FIGURE 6.21 Management of status epilepticus. ECG, electrocardiogram; IO, intraosseous; IV, intravenous; NiBP, non-invasive blood pressure; PR, per rectum; SpO₂, oxygen saturation.

Take Home Points

- Neurological disorders are serious and can rapidly become life threatening.
- Appropriate examination will identify many serious pathologies but many patients will still require specialist imaging to reach a diagnosis.
- Conditions such as status epilepticus or significant head injury are challenging to manage in the prehospital setting, and assistance from colleagues should be sought early.

Reflective Learning Activity

The table lists some common conditions associated with the nervous system. Write some notes about each condition:

- Stroke
- Dementia
- Head injury
- Epilepsy

You could take information from this textbook or from your wider reading.

Summary

An understanding of the anatomy, physiology and pathophysiology behind various disorders informs your assessment, diagnosis and management of patients. The neurological system is one of the most complex body systems, and disorders of the brain and nerves can produce significant morbidity and mortality. Paramedics see a huge spectrum of neurological disorders, from the hyperacute to the chronic and degenerative and have a duty to provide the best care for every patient they encounter.

References

Association of Anaesthetists (2006). *Recommendations for the Safe Transfer of Patients with Brain Injury*. London: AAGBI.

Ataullah, A.H.M. and Naqvi, I.A. (2023). *Cerebellar Dysfunction*. Treasure Island, FL: StatPearls Publishing https://www.ncbi.nlm.nih.gov/books/NBK562317 (accessed 2 October 2023).

ter Avest, E., Taylor, S., Wilson, M., and Lyon, R.L. (2021). Prehospital clinical signs are a poor predictor of raised intracranial pressure following traumatic brain injury. *Emergency Medicine Journal* 38: 21–26.

Bergmans, S.F., Schober, P., Schwarte, L.A. et al. (2020). Prehospital fluid administration in patients with severe traumatic brain injury: a systematic review and meta-analysis. *Injury* 51 (11): 2356–2367.

Bir, S.C., Khan, M.W., Javalkar, V. et al. (2021). Emerging concepts in vascular dementia: a review. *Journal of Stroke and Cerebrovascular Diseases* 30 (8): 105864.

Breijyeh, Z. and Karaman, R. (2020). Comprehensive review on Alzheimer's disease: causes and treatment. *Molecules* 25 (24): 5789.

Claassen, J.A., Thijssen, D.H., Panerai, R.B., and Faraci, F.M. (2021). Regulation of cerebral blood flow in humans: physiology and clinical implications of autoregulation. *Physiological Reviews* 101 (4): 1487–1559.

Clissold, B., Phan, T.G., Ly, J. et al. (2020). Current aspects of TIA management. *Journal of Clinical Neuroscience* 72: 20–25.

Devlin, S. (2022). Not so FAST: pre-hospital posterior circulation stroke. *British Paramedic Journal* 7 (1): 24–28.

Epilepsy Research Institute UK. (2020). *Epilepsy statistics*. https://epilepsy-institute.org.uk/eri/about-epilepsy/epilepsy-statistics (accessed 2 October 2023).

Fame, R.M. and Lehtinen, M.K. (2020). Emergence and developmental roles of the cerebrospinal fluid system. *Developmental Cell* 52 (3): 261–275.

Fisher, R.S., Cross, J.H., French, J.A. et al. (2017). Operational classification of seizure types by the international league against epilepsy. *Epilepsia* 58 (4): 522–530.

Liu, S., Levine, S.R., and Winn, H.R. (2010). Targeting ischemic penumbra: part I - from pathophysiology to therapeutic strategy. *Journal of Experimental Stroke and Translational Medicine* 3 (1): 47.

Maissan, I.M., Verbaan, L.A., van den Berg, M. et al. (2018). Helicopter transportation increases intracranial pressure: a proof-of-principle study. *Air Medical Journal* 37: 249–252.

Mangold, S.A. and Das, J.M. (2023). *Neuroanatomy, Reticular Formation.* Treasure Island, FL: StatePearls Publishing https://www.ncbi.nlm.nih.gov/books/NBK556102/ (accessed 2 October 2023).

McClelland, G., Rodgers, H., Flynn, D., and Price, C.I. (2019). The frequency, characteristics and aetiology of stroke mimic presentations: a narrative review. *European Journal of Emergency Medicine* 26 (1): 2–8.

Milligan, T.A. (2021). Epilepsy: a clinical overview. *American Journal of Medicine* 134 (7): 840–847.

Nathanson, M.H., Andrzejowski, J., Dinsmore, J. et al. (2020). Guidelines for safe transfer of the brain-injured patient: trauma and stroke, 2019: guidelines from the Association of Anaesthetists and the neuro Anaesthesia and critical care society. *Anaesthesia* 75 (2): 234–246.

National Institute for Health and Care Excellence (2022). *Stroke and Transient Ischaemic Attack in over 16s: Diagnosis and initial management.* London: National Institute for Health and Care Excellence.

Okudan, Z.V. and Özkara, Ç. (2018). Reflex epilepsy: triggers and management strategies. *Neuropsychiatric Disease and Treatment* 14: 327.

Olson, D.M., Stutzman, S., Saju, C. et al. (2016). Interrater reliability of pupillary assessments. *Neurocritical Care* 24 (2): 251–257.

Sibson, L. (2017). Stroke assessment and management in pre-hospital settings. *Journal of Paramedic Practice* 9 (8): 354–361.

Stroke Association (2018). Stroke statistics. https://www.stroke.org.uk/what-is-stroke/stroke-statistics#UK%20summary (accessed 2 October 2023).

Teasdale, G., Maas, A., Lecky, F. et al. (2014). The Glasgow coma scale at 40 years: standing the test of time. *Lancet Neurology* 13 (8): 844–854.

Thomas, M. (2015). *Development of two in vitro methodologies for the study of brain network dynamics and an application to the study of seizure-evoked adenosine release.* Doctoral thesis. University of Warwick. http://webcat.warwick.ac.uk/record=b2861544~S1 (accessed 2 October 2023).

Williams, G.V. (2021). Prehospital osmotherapy in isolated traumatic brain injury: a systematic review. *Journal of Paramedic Practice* 13 (3): 114–124.

Wilson, M.H., Wise, D., Davies, G., and Lockey, D. (2012). Emergency burr holes: "how to do it". *Scandinavian Journal of Trauma, Resuscitation and Emergency Medicine* 20 (1): 1–5.

Wilson, M.H., Hinds, J., Grier, G. et al. (2016). Impact brain apnoea – a forgotten cause of cardiovascular collapse in trauma. *Resuscitation* 105: 52–58.

Zhang, S., Wang, A., Zhu, W. et al. (2022). Meta-analysis of risk factors associated with suicidal ideation after stroke. *Annals of General Psychiatry* 21 (1): 1–11.

121

Further Reading

Book, D. (2019). Disorders of brain function. In: *Essentials of Pathophysiology*, 5e, Chapter 16 (ed. C.M. Porth). Philadelphia, PA: Wolters Kluwer.

National Institute for Health and Care Excellence (2018). *Dementia: Assessment, Management and Support for People Living with Dementia and their Carers.* NICE Guideline NG97. London: National Institute for Health and Care Excellence.

National Institute for Health and Care Excellence (2023). *Head Injury: Assessment and early management. NICE Guideline NG232.* London: National Institute for Health and Care Excellence.

National Institute for Health and Care Excellence (2022). *Epilepsies in Children, Young People and Adults.* NICE Guideline NG217. London: National Institute for Health and Care Excellence.

Online Resources

Neurosymptoms.org: https://www.neurosymptoms.org/en_GB
- This is an excellent resource from Professor Jon Stone discussing functional neurological disorders.

National Institute for Health and Care Excellence: www.nice.org.uk
- Guidance on many clinical conditions.

Royal College of Emergency Medicine: www.rcemlearning.co.uk/references/neurology
- A wide range of learning resources.

Pre-Hospital Stroke Treatment Organisation: www.prestomsu.org
- Pioneering research in the area of mobile stroke units. X (Twitter): @PRESTO_MSU

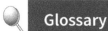

Glossary

Acetylcholine	A neurotransmitter found widely in the central and peripheral nervous systems.
Blood–brain barrier	An impermeable network of brain capillaries which acts as a filter between the brain tissue and bloodborne substances. It provides the brain with some protection from harmful toxins and metabolites.
Cerebrospinal fluid (CSF)	A clear or straw-coloured liquid which surrounds and bathes the brain.
Cerebrovascular accident	*See* stroke.
Choroid plexus	The tissue in the ventricles of the brain which produces cerebrospinal fluid.
Chronotropic	Physiological changes or medicines which change the heart rate.
Cushing's triad	A triad of irregular ventilation, bradycardia and a widening pulse pressure, which indicates a rise in intracerebral pressure.
Dementia	The loss of mental ability.
Dopamine	A neurotransmitter found in the central nervous system.
Dravet syndrome	A rare and severe form of epilepsy, associated with developmental delay.
FAST test	The 'face, arm, speech, time' test for assessing potential strokes.
Foramen magnum	A large hole in the occipital bone through which the vertebral column and spinal cord pass.
Glasgow Coma Scale (GCS)	An assessment tool designed for detecting and monitoring changes in a patient's neurological status.
Inotropic	Physiological changes or medicines which change the force of the heart's contractions.
Intracranial pressure	The recordable pressure within the skull.
Noradrenaline/norepinepherine	A neurotransmitter in the central and peripheral nervous systems.
Parenchyma	The functional tissue of an organ.
Parasympathetic nervous system (PNS)	Part of the nervous system which uses acetylcholine to moderate internal responses. Associated with a state of relaxation.
Peripheral nervous system	Cranial and spinal nerves which connect the brain and spinal cord to other parts of the body.

Reticular activating system (RAS)	Part of the brain stem.
ROSIER scale	A scoring system for identifying stroke.
Shaken baby syndrome	A complex collection of injuries seen in child abuse cases, traditionally considered as a triad of subdural haemorrhage, retinal haemorrhage and encephalopathy/cerebral oedema.
Stroke	(Also called a cerebral vascular accident.) A disease affecting the blood vessels supplying the brain. A stroke can be due to vessel occlusion or vessel disruption.
Substantia nigra	The part of the midbrain concerned with coordinating movement.
Sympathetic nervous system	Part of the nervous system which initiates response to stress through the release of norepinephrine. This assists in the 'fight or flight' response.
Ventricle	A cavity within the brain that is filled with cerebrospinal fluid.

Multiple Choice Questions

1. The GCS score is made up of the 'E, V and M' sections. What is the maximum score you can gain in each area?
   a. E6 V5 M5
   b. M5 E4 V6
   c. E4 V5 M6
   d. V5 E5 M5

2. A pathologically raised volume of cerebrospinal fluid is known as what?
   a. Herniation
   b. Elephantitis
   c. Papilloedema
   d. Hydrocephalus

3. The substantia nigra is part of what?
   a. Spinal cord
   b. Brainstem
   c. Cerebellum
   d. Basal nuclei

4. Abnormal neuronal discharge with later hypersynchrony describes which disease process?
   a. Addiction
   b. Epilepsy
   c. Parkinson's disease
   d. Migraine

5. The incidence of epilepsy has what sort of age distribution?
   a. Standard
   b. Trimodal
   c. Bimodal
   d. Uniform

6. What is cranial nerve III?
   a. Olfactory
   b. Facial
   c. Oculomotor
   d. Trigeminal

7. Which of these is NOT a cause of raised intracranial pressure.
   a. Tightly applied cervical collars
   b. Trendelenburg position
   c. Gastrointestinal infection
   d. Meningitis

8. What are the two divisions of the nervous system?
   a. Central and peripheral
   b. Automatical and sensory
   c. Central and functional
   d. Sympathetic and parabolic

9. What is the function of the trigeminal nerve?
   a. Sensory
   b. Special sensory
   c. Motor
   d. Motor and sensory

10. Memantine is structurally similar to which drug?
    a. Adrenaline
    b. Atropine
    c. Atorvastatin
    d. Ketamine

CHAPTER 7

The Cardiovascular System and Its Associated Disorders

Tom E. Mallinson

AIM

This chapter aims to provide an introduction to conditions that affect the human cardiovascular system, including their assessment and management in the prehospital setting.

LEARNING OUTCOMES

On completion of this chapter, you will be able to:

- Describe the structure and function of the components of the cardiovascular system.
- Understand conditions of the heart in terms of pump, coronary blood supply and electrical system.
- Understand pathologies affecting the vascular system.
- Understand the uses of ultrasonography in cardiac disorders.
- Understand the importance of the electrocardiogram in cardiac disorders.

Test Your Prior Knowledge
1. List the components of the cardiovascular system.
2. Describe the path blood takes through the cardiovascular system.
3. What ECG changes might you see in an occlusive myocardial infarction?
4. What disease processes affect the ability of the heart to pump blood?

Introduction

The cardiovascular system is responsible for pumping blood throughout the body, delivering oxygen and nutrients to tissues and organs while removing waste products. It consists of the heart, blood vessels and blood. An in-depth understanding of the cardiovascular system will enable you to assess and manage patients with various cardiovascular

Fundamentals of Applied Pathophysiology for Paramedics, First Edition. Edited by Ian Peate and Simon Sawyer.
© 2024 John Wiley & Sons Ltd. Published 2024 by John Wiley & Sons Ltd.

conditions effectively. This chapter explores the anatomy and function of the heart, including its chambers, valves and conduction system. The circulation of blood through the systemic and pulmonary circulatory systems are also addressed. As a paramedic, understanding the cardiovascular system is essential, as many of the patients you encounter will have cardiovascular conditions or emergencies. This chapter will provide you with a comprehensive overview of the cardiovascular system, its anatomy, physiology and common disorders that you are likely to encounter in your practice.

Gross Anatomy

The Heart

The heart is located in the mediastinum, behind the sternum and to the left side, with the lower tip sitting around 9 cm lateral between the third and sixth intercostal spaces (Figure 7.1). The average weight of the heart varies significantly, but an average male heart weighs 380 g, with an average female heart being 300 g (Westaby et al. 2023). A healthy heart measures around 12–14 cm in length and 9–11 cm in diameter.

The heart is contained within a double walled fibrous sac, which isolates the heart from surrounding structures as well as providing a degree of protection and lubrication for the heart's movement. The pericardial sac is similar to the pleural membranes (discussed in Chapter 10).

The heart comprises four distinct chambers (Figure 7.2). These chambers are divided functionally and structurally into the right and left side of the heart (Figure 7.3). The right side of the heart receives deoxygenated blood from the body (systemic circulation) via the vena cava into the right atrium. Blood progresses into the right ventricle, moving through the tricuspid valve.

On ventricular systole (contraction), deoxygenated blood is ejected from the heart through the pulmonary valve into the pulmonary artery and on to the lungs. The pulmonary artery is unusual as an artery carrying deoxygenated blood. The pulmonary artery exits the heart at the pulmonary trunk, a short stubby artery (5 cm long and 3 cm wide) before branching into the right and left pulmonary arteries. These arteries progressively divide and narrow into the pulmonary arterioles and capillary bed of the lungs. At these capillaries, gas exchange occurs and oxygenated blood begins its return journey to the left side of the heart.

Oxygenated blood returns to the heart through the left and right pulmonary veins, which bring blood from the lungs to the left atrium. Blood moves from the left atrium to the left ventricle through the bicuspid valve. This is also called the

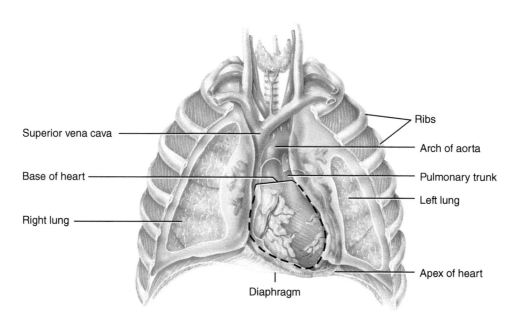

Superior vena cava

Base of heart

Right lung

Ribs

Arch of aorta

Pulmonary trunk

Left lung

Apex of heart

Diaphragm

FIGURE 7.1   Heart location.

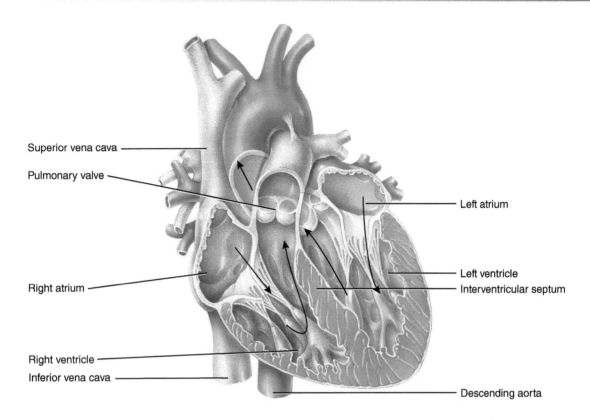

Superior vena cava

Pulmonary valve

Left atrium

Right atrium

Left ventricle

Interventricular septum

Right ventricle

Inferior vena cava

Descending aorta

FIGURE 7.2 Blood flow through the heart.

mitral valve (named because its appearance, viewed upside down, resembles the mitre, the traditional hat of Christian bishops). Blood exits the left ventricle through the aortic valve into the aorta.

At the root of the aorta are the origins of the two main coronary arteries (left and right), named from the Latin *corona*, meaning crown, seen as encircling and crowning the heart (Figure 7.4). The coronary arteries supply blood to the heart muscle (Ramanathan and Skinner 2005). The origins of these vessels lie behind the leaflets of the aortic valve. These leaflets partially cover the entrances to the coronary arteries during systole, meaning that coronary artery blood flow occurs during diastole. This is clinically important when considering tachycardias, where the diastolic time is reduced.

The left main coronary artery divides into the left anterior descending artery, which supplies the left ventricle and anterior wall of the heart, and the left circumflex artery, which supplies the lateral and posterior walls of the left ventricle (and sometimes part of the right ventricle). The right coronary artery supplies the right ventricle, part of the posterior wall of the left ventricle, part of the septum and, in 60% of people, the sinoatrial node (Figure 7.4). Deoxygenated blood from the coronary circulation drains into the coronary sinus, which in turn drains into the right atrium (Figure 7.4). A small amount is drained by the anterior cardiac vein and Thesbian veins, the former opening into the right atrium and the latter draining directly into the cardiac chambers.

The Great Vessels

The aorta, pulmonary trunk, pulmonary veins and the vena cava are often referred to as the great vessels. The aorta is the largest artery in the body. It begins at the top of the left ventricle and ascends in a cephalad direction before turning back on itself, forming the aortic arch and descending towards the abdomen. The aorta lies deep in the abdomen as a retroperitoneal structure and bifurcates around the level of the fourth lumbar vertebra into the iliac arteries. The abdominal aorta also gives rise to other large vessels including the coeliac trunk, mesenteric arteries and the paired renal arteries. These large arteries decrease in size to arterioles, then capillaries, before deoxygenated blood is returned through venules and veins to the vena cava.

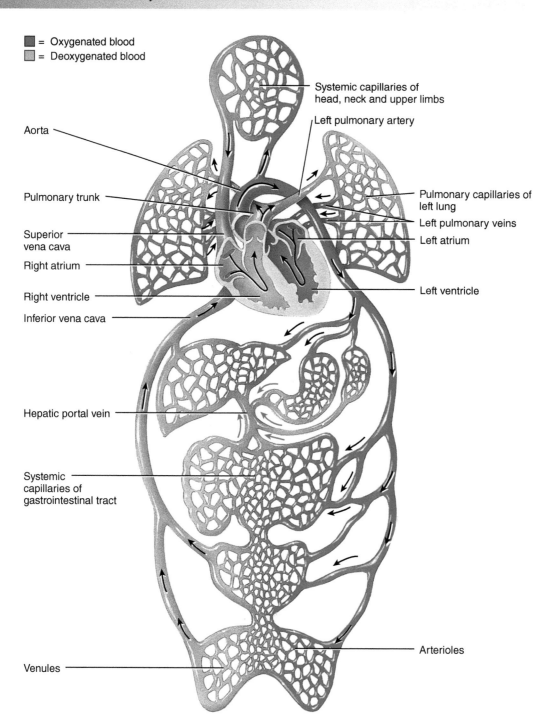

■ = Oxygenated blood
□ = Deoxygenated blood

Systemic capillaries of
head, neck and upper limbs

Aorta

Left pulmonary artery

Pulmonary trunk

Pulmonary capillaries of
left lung

Superior
vena cava

Left pulmonary veins

Right atrium

Left atrium

Right ventricle

Left ventricle

Inferior vena cava

Hepatic portal vein

Systemic
capillaries of
gastrointestinal tract

Arterioles

Venules

FIGURE 7.3   Flow of oxygenated and deoxygenated blood through the cardiovascular system.

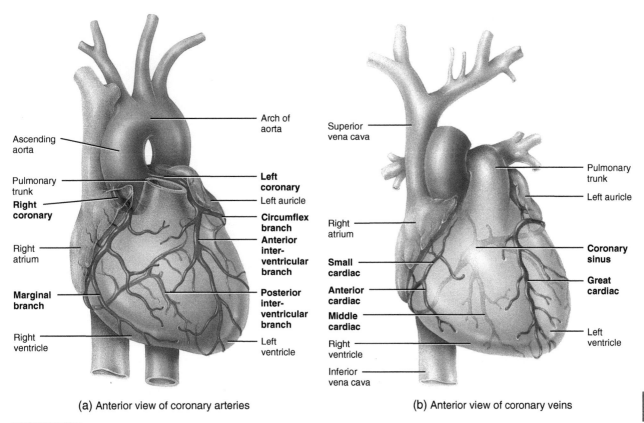

(a) Anterior view of coronary arteries

(b) Anterior view of coronary veins

FIGURE 7.4 Coronary circulation.

The vena cava is part of a relatively low-pressure system which lacks the pulsatile pressure waves of the arterial system. Normal pressure in the vena cava, referred to as central venous pressure (CVP), is around 8–12 mmHg. As a low-pressure vessel, the vena cava can be easily obstructed, for example, by the weight of a gravid uterus. Ultrasound of the vena cava is a useful method of identifying volume deficit by assessing the degree to which the vessel collapses during inspiration.

The pulmonary artery, also called the pulmonary trunk, carries deoxygenated blood from the right ventricle to the lungs. It leaves the heart as a single large vessel but splits into the right and left pulmonary arteries at the level of the carina. These arteries divide into lobar branches and then into segmental and subsegmental branches. They eventually give rise to the huge capillary beds of the alveoli, where gas transfer occurs. Oxygenated blood returns through venules and veins. The four large pulmonary veins carry oxygenated blood back from the lungs to the left atrium. From here, the oxygenated blood moves into the left ventricle and is expelled into the systemic circulation.

Reflective Learning Activity

In maternal cardiac arrest, what is the optimal method of displacing the gravid uterus to avoid vena caval compression?

Cardiac Cycle

The cardiac cycle (Figure 7.5) is a good way to understand what is happening within the heart, and to draw together the concepts of pressure changes, valve functions, blood flow and electrical activity (Table 7.1).

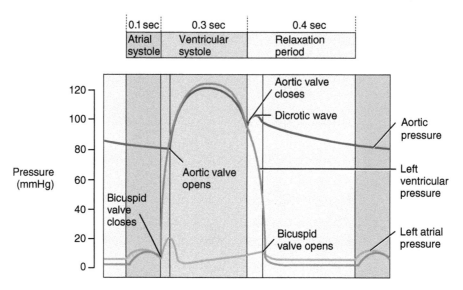

FIGURE 7.5   Cardiac cycle.

TABLE 7.1   Cardiac dynamics during the cardiac cycle.

Stage	Action	AV valves	Pulmonary and aortic valves	Blood flow	ECG finding
Ventricular diastole					
1	Isovolumic relaxation	Closed	Closed	Pulmonary and aortic valves are closed; there is no blood flow	T wave finishes
2a	Inflow: (passive ventricular filling)	Open	Closed	Blood flows into the heart filling the atria and ventricles; ventricles passively fill to 70–80% capacity	Isoelectric line between T wave and P wave
2b	Inflow: (active ventricular filling due to atrial contraction)	Open	Closed	Atrial contraction forces the remaining 20–30% of blood into the ventricles under pressure	P wave
Ventricular systole					
3	Isovolumic contraction	Closed	Closed	The ventricles are full; blood flow stops; AV valves are closed; ventricles start to contract	QRS complex; start of the T wave
4	Ejection: ventricular ejection	Closed	Open	Ventricles contract, ejecting blood into the aorta and pulmonary artery	

We start the cardiac cycle in ventricular diastole. During this phase, the heart is at rest. No areas of the heart are contracting. The ventricles passively fill with blood (flowing in from the vena cava and pulmonary veins). Ventricular volume therefore increases but pressure in the ventricles does not because they relax to accommodate the additional blood. Near the end of ventricular diastole, the atria contract (atrial systole). While they are not as muscular as the ventricles, this contraction helps push the last 20–30% of blood into the ventricles.

We now enter ventricular systole (contraction). During this stage, the ventricles rapidly contract, squeezing blood out of them into the aorta (left ventricle) and pulmonary artery (right ventricle). This causes a rapid decrease in ventricular volume, as blood is leaving, and a rise in ventricular pressure due to the ventricle squeezing the blood within it.

The volume of blood pushed out of the left ventricle is often referred to as the stroke volume (SV) and in an adult is around 95 ml (±15 ml). This ejection of blood produces a pressure wave within the systemic arterial system which produces the palpable pulses. This pressure produced by ventricular systole is measured and referred to as the *systolic blood pressure* (SVP); the residual pressure in the arteries is the *diastolic blood pressure* (DBP).

The mean (average) of these two is referred to as the mean arterial pressure (MAP) and is useful clinically, especially when providing critical care interventions:

$$MAP = \frac{(2 \times DBP) + SBP}{\beta} \tag{7.1}$$

MAP is also related to cardiac output (CO):

$$MAP = CO \times SVR \tag{7.2}$$

and systemic vascular resistance (SVR):

$$SVR = \frac{MAP - CVP}{CO} \times 80 \tag{7.3}$$

An understanding of these equations can help you understand how different disorders present clinically.

This flow of blood from the large veins through the heart and subsequently to the aorta or pulmonary artery is made possible through a number of valves in the system (Figure 7.4). Without these valves, the contraction of the ventricles (the pump) would simply push blood out in both directions. If a valve fails, significant morbidity and mortality are caused.

131

Electrical Control of the Heart

The cardiac cycle is controlled through the electrical system of the heart, the cardiac conduction system (Figure 7.6). This system coordinates contraction of the heart muscle. Fundamentally, whenever there is an electrical impulse, it stimulates muscle contraction. In relation to the heart, this simple model is complicated by two natural pacemakers and a highly insulated barrier between the atria and ventricles, pierced only by the bundle of His, a conductive passageway. In health, conduction of electricity through the heart follows a set route (Table 7.2).

While the heart has intrinsic pacemaker activity at the sinoatrial (SA) node (60–100 bpm) and the atrioventricular (AV) node (40–60 bpm), the rate and force of contraction can also be influenced by endogenous or exogenous stimuli. Sympathetic stimulation of the heart by the sympathetic nervous system (adrenergic system) increases cardiac output through an increase in both heart rate (HR) and stroke volume (SV). Cardiac output is measured in litres per minute and is calculated using the equation:

$$CO = SV \times HR \tag{7.4}$$

Parasympathetic stimulation of the heart, either by cholinergic agonists (e.g. pilocarpine), anticholinesterases (e.g. organophosphates, nerve agents) or intrinsically via the vagus nerve, results in a reduction in cardiac output. Medications that are anticholinergic in nature, such as atropine, therefore have the ability to eliminate the 'slow down' instruction from the vagus nerve and cause the heart rate to increase.

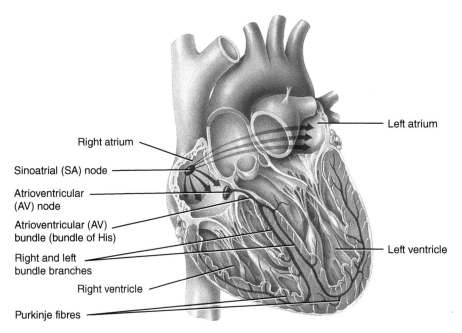

Right atrium

Sinoatrial (SA) node

Atrioventricular
(AV) node

Atrioventricular (AV)
bundle (bundle of His)

Right and left
bundle branches

Right ventricle

Purkinje fibres

Left atrium

Left ventricle

FIGURE 7.6   Conducting system of the heart.

TABLE 7.2   **Conduction of electricity through the heart.**

Node	Location	Activity
Sinoatrial	The sinus venarum of the right atrium	Generated impulse spreads through the right and left atria
Atrioventricular (AV)	Bottom and rear of the septum separating the two atria	Receives the electrical impulse which has propagated through the atria, adds a delay, and then transmits this impulse down through the bundle of His
Bundle of His	Interventricular septum	Receives the impulse from the AV node, and transmits it down to the bundle branches
Right and left bundle branches	The interventricular septum, with fascicles wrapping around the left ventricle	Facilitate onward transmission to the Purkinje fibres of the right and left ventricles. The left bundle branch further divides into the left anterior fascicle and left posterior fascicle
Purkinje fibres	The subendocardium of the right and left ventricles	Conduct electrical impulses quickly and efficiently to facilitate coordinated ventricular contraction

Minor Vessels

The minor blood vessels are all the remaining vasculature of the body. Their purpose is to deliver blood to and from all organ systems and constituent tissues (Chapter 8). The blood vessels of the human body can be considered as a vascular hourglass, with the largest diameter vessels at the top and bottom of the hourglass (Figure 7.7). Arteries and arterioles are thick walled, muscular vessels that lack valves. Pressure in the arteries fluctuates between systolic and diastolic blood pressure (Figure 7.8).

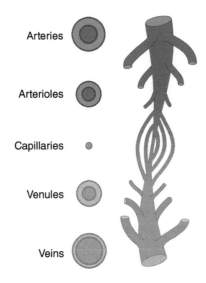

FIGURE 7.7 The vascular hourglass.

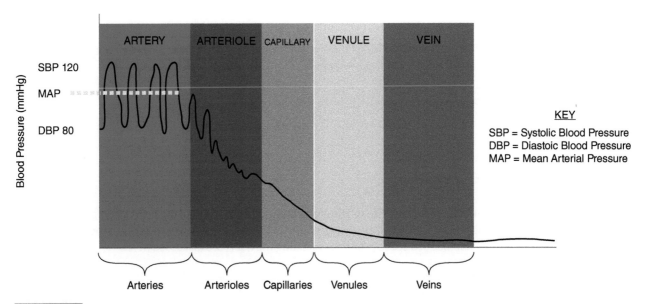

FIGURE 7.8 Pressure differential between arterial and venous systems.

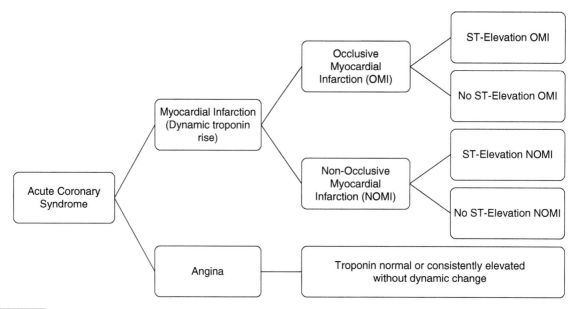

FIGURE 7.9   Classification system for acute coronary syndromes. Source: Adapted from Meyers et al. (2021).

The capillaries are the final reduction of vessel diameter, providing a network of tiny blood vessels. Capillary networks facilitate gas exchange in the lungs (Chapter 10), filtration of blood in the glomeruli (Chapter 9) and absorption of nutrients in the microvilli of the intestines (Chapter 11). They facilitate gas exchange in all metabolic tissues, delivery of nutrients and removal of waste products.

After the capillaries, blood vessel diameter increases again, initially to the venules, then the veins and eventually back to the largest veins, the vena cava and the pulmonary vein. Veins are thin walled and valved tubes full of blood at relatively low pressures (Figure 7.9). An important concept to understand the function of the systemic blood vessels is SVR, which is a measure of how much resistance these vessels are offering to the flow of blood (Eq. 7.3).

Red Flag: Systemic Vascular Resistance

Changes to SVR are significant in many disorders, for example in anaphylaxis widespread vasodilation (relaxation) significantly reduces SVR, which leads to a drop in blood pressure (MAP) and a raised heart rate to compensate.

Diseases of the Heart

It can be helpful to divide disorders of the heart into those affecting or originating within the heart's pumping mechanism, the coronary arteries or the electrical system of the heart. There are many ways in which each aspect of heart function can malfunction, and only a small number of disease processes affecting the heart are discussed here.

Snapshot 7.1   Nocturnal Breathlessness

Pre-arrival Information

A 70 year old woman has phoned 999 for acute breathlessness at 2 a.m.

On Arrival with the Patient

You are met by Mr Jayasooriya, an elderly man, who directs you upstairs to the bedroom. The window is wide open despite the chill in the air, and his wife Dr Jayasooriya is sitting upright on the edge of the bed. She is struggling to breath and occasionally coughing clear phlegm into a monogrammed handkerchief.

Physical Examination

On examination, Dr Jayasooriya's airway is patent. Auscultation of the chest reveals wet crackles in all lung zones; her heart sounds are abnormal, but you think there might be an extra sound present. You notice that Dr Jayasooriya has pitting oedema at the base of her back and up to the top of her thighs from her feet. Her abdomen is difficult to examine as she is sitting up. On asking her to lie flat, you receive a withering look as she tells you that she feels like she will die if she lies down again.

Vital Signs

Vital sign	On scene	Normal values
Temperature (°C)	36.3	36.0–37.5
Pulse (beats/min)	92	60–100
Respiration (breaths/min)	30	12–20
Blood pressure (mmHg)	163/88	100–139
O2 saturation (%)	93	95–98

Between coughing episodes, Dr Jayasooriya tells you that she is a retired anthropology professor. She has been a bit tired recently and has noticed that her ankles are swollen, but she has been trying to write a textbook and has been sitting for long periods each day and thought this was the cause.

Reflective Learning Activity

Take some time to reflect on Snapshot 7.1 and then consider the following:

1. What are your differential diagnoses here?
2. What are some specific questions you could ask which may support (or refute) your preferred differential?
3. What do you think the abnormal heart sound could be in this case?
4. Which non-parenteral medication will be of the most benefit to Dr Jayasooriya?
5. What pathophysiology links the peripheral oedema, the dyspnoea and the cardiovascular system?

Pump

Many disease processes will eventually affect the pumping action of the heart; for example, distributive shock hampers pump filling (Chapter 5), dysrhythmias affect pump function (discussed later) and various drugs will be negatively inotropic or chronotropic (Clegg and Russell 2022). Some diseases, however, are primarily related to the heart muscle structure and function in relation to pumping blood.

Red Flag: Penetrating Trauma

Any penetrating chest trauma is cardiac trauma until proven otherwise. Injuries within a central zone are especially high risk.

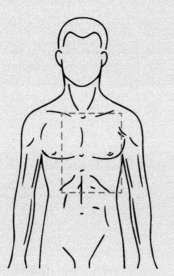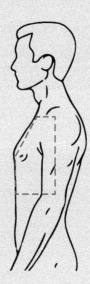

Source: Pulido et. al., (2022) / with permission of John Wiley & Sons.

Cardiac Tamponade

Cardiac tamponade occurs when there is a build-up of fluid within the fibrous pericardial sac. If this build-up occurs slowly, the sac has a small degree of stretch and may accommodate a larger amount of fluid before the ventricles become compressed and the heart pump fails. In cases of penetrating trauma, where blood accumulates rapidly between the pericardial layers, this compression of the ventricles occurs rapidly. The compression can cause a low flow state, followed by cardiac arrest, often with pulseless electrical activity as the initial arrest rhythm.

The traditional clinical signs found in cases of cardiac tamponade is Beck's triad: muffled heart sounds, low blood pressure and jugular venous distention. These may be accompanied by a sinus tachycardia and electrical alternans on ECG. Point of care ultrasound or thoracotomy will confirm a cardiac tamponade. When the tamponade is caused by blood (haemopericardium), evacuation of the clot and repair of damage to the heart will probably be required. If the accumulation is serous (i.e. from a pericarditis), needle aspiration of the fluid may be possible.

Heart Failure

Heart failure is a broad term encompassing a wide range of pathologies where the heart muscle is pumping inefficiently. This inefficiency is often due to hypertrophy – enlargement of the heart muscle due to a disease process. The ECG may provide indications that hypertrophy may be present, in the form of high amplitude QRS complexes, often referred to as voltage criteria for hypertrophy. Hypertrophy will prompt further investigation with formal echocardiography by a cardiac physiologist.

In the long term, heart failure is managed medically with an array of medications (Clegg and Russell 2022) and, in some cases, surgical correction of valvular pathology is required. Echocardiography is the key investigation for identifying and quantifying heart failure.

In the acute setting, where heart failure results in increased back pressures of blood in the pulmonary system, this rise in hydrostatic pressure may push fluid from the blood into the lung tissue and the alveoli themselves (see Chapter 10). This results in acute cardiogenic pulmonary oedema, which often presents as dyspnoea and the production of bloodstained frothy sputum. This condition is managed by the administration of glyceryl trinitrate (GTN) and providing continuous positive airway pressure (abbreviated as CPAP), a form of non-invasive ventilatory support (Mullen 2013), and sometimes administering the loop diuretic furosemide (Mursell 2009).

Medications Management: Glyceryl trinitrate

GTN is a potent vasodilator and will drop the patient's blood pressure.

Coronary Artery Disease

Disruption of blood flow through the coronary arteries can rapidly cause ischaemia and infarction to the heart muscle. The most common cause of poor coronary blood flow is the build-up of atherosclerotic plaques which narrow the lumen of the coronary arteries. This narrowing can limit blood flow, which can lead to ischaemic heart disease, where the heart muscle does not receive enough oxygenated blood. When these atherosclerotic plaques rupture, the exposed lipid deposits and released cytokines stimulate clot formation and the subsequent intraluminal thrombosis blocks blood flow (partially or completely), leading to a myocardial infarction.

Chronic Ischaemic Heart Disease

Chronic ischaemic heart disease (IHD) often presents as myocardial ischaemia, which is reliably and repeatable provoked. Provoking factors may be psychological stress or, more classically, physical exertion. The pain from this ischaemia is referred to as angina pectoris (from the Latin for choking of the chest). This reproducibility of pain with full resolution with GTN or rest allows us to define the disease as stable angina (or exertional angina). Cardiac syndrome X or microvascular angina is another form of IHD, which is less well understood. Unstable angina is a form of acute IHD or acute coronary syndrome and is far more serious.

Acute Ischaemic Heart Disease

Clinically, we divide acute coronary artery disease (acute coronary syndromes) into unstable angina and myocardial infarctions, which may be occlusive or non-occlusive (Meyers et al. 2021). Acute angina represents an insufficient supply of oxygenated blood to the myocardium, but without infarction and necrosis of heart muscle.

The term myocardial infarction represents blockage of a coronary artery and subsequent ischaemia and death to the myocardial tissue (heart muscle) distal to the blockage. Myocardial infarction is classically defined as the presence of three things:

1. Ischaemic-type chest pain lasting over 20 minutes
2. Changes on ECG
3. A dynamic rise and fall of cardiac biomarkers.

This definition has evolved in recent years to include the concepts of occlusive or non-occlusive myocardial infarction (Figure 7.9) and this is an area of continuing research. Another classification system for myocardial infarctions relates to their cause or presentation (Table 7.3; Thygesen 2018).

Myocardial infarctions can be localised in terms of territory affected and probable coronary artery involvement by assessing which leads of the ECG demonstrate the classic finding of ST segment elevation (Table 7.4). However, ST elevation is only one of many changes seen in coronary artery occlusion (Table 7.5; Mallinson 2023).

TABLE 7.3   Types of myocardial infarction.

Type	Description
1	Caused by atherothrombotic event caused by coronary artery plague rupture or erosion
2	Oxygen supply and demand mismatch without atherosclerotic plaque rupture or erosion (e.g. tachydysrhythmia, profound anaemia)
3	Sudden death of likely ischaemic cardiac origin
4	Angioplasty or angiogram related or coronary stent related
5	Cardiac surgery related: during coronary artery bypass grafting

Source: Adapted from Thygesen (2018).

TABLE 7.4   Locational of myocardial infarction.

ST segment elevation	Descriptive term	Coronary artery
I, aVL, V5, V6	Lateral	Left circumflex
II, III, aVF	Inferior	Right coronary
V1–V2	Septal	Septal left anterior descending
V1–V4	Anteroseptal	Left anterior descending
V2–V5	Anterior	Left anterior descending
V3–V6, I, aVL	Anteroseptal	Left anterior descending
V7, V8, V9	Posterior	Right coronary
V1, V4R	Right ventricle	Right coronary

TABLE 7.5 Key occlusive myocardial infarctions (OMI) presentations on ECG.

STEMI: new and persistent ST segment elevation in ≥ 2 neighbouring leads. This should be ≥ 1 mm in any lead apart from V2–V3, where the following cut-offs apply: • ≥2.5 mm in men <40 years old • ≥2 mm in men >40 years old • ≥1.5 mm in women regardless of age. New LBBB is often considered a STEMI equivalent	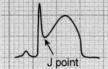	**Posterior MI**: subtle ST segment elevation in posterior leads (>0.5 mm), ST depression in anterior leads with positive R waves in V2–V3, abnormal R wave progression across the chest leads, large positive T waves in anterior leads, ischaemic changes in lateral or inferior leads. Posterior views (V7, V8, V9) are useful in identification (Figure 7.14)	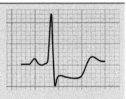
Wellens A: deeply inverted T waves inV2–V3. T waves are biphasic, with an initial positive deflection. Appropriate R wave progression and no pathological Q waves across the chest leads	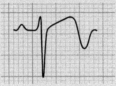	**De Winter**: tall prominent and symmetrical T waves in chest leads. No ST elevation in anterior leads with ST elevation in aVR (0.5–1 mm). May evolve into or from a classic STEMI morphology	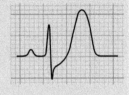
Wellens B: deeply inverted T waves in V2–V3. These are deep and symmetrical. The changes in both Wellens A and B can develop over days or weeks, even when the patient is pain free	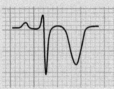	**Sgarbossa**: for patients with LBBB or paced rhythms, the modified Sgarbossa criteria are used (3 criteria); **criterion 1** – concordant ST elevation of ≥1 mm in ≥1 lead (5 points)	Any lead 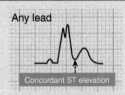 Concordant ST elevation
Shark fin: massive ST elevation in leads V1–V6, I and aVL. Early development of Q waves in aVL with ST depression in II, III and aVF. Historically referred to as 'tombstoning' as the morphology represents a proximal LAD occlusion with a strong association with ventricular fibrillation and death	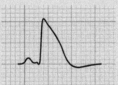	**Sgarbossa**: **criterion 2** – concordant ST depression of ≥1 mm in ≥1 lead of V1–V3 (3 points)	V1-3 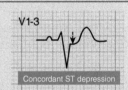 Concordant ST depression
South African flag: represents a high lateral STEMI. ST elevation localised to leads I and aVL and possibly V2, with ST depression in lead III	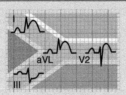	**Sgarbossa**: **criterion 3** – excessive discordant ST elevation in ≥1 lead with ≥1 mm of elevation, being >25% of the depth of the preceding S wave (2 points) *A total Sgarbossa score of ≥3 has a high specificity for myocardial infarction but a low sensitivity*	Any lead 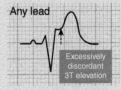 Excessively discordant 3T elevation

LAD, left anterior descending; LBBB, left bundle branch block; MI, myocardial infarction; STEMI, ST-elevation myocardial infarction.

Key Investigations: Electrocardiogram

An electrocardiogram provides a visual representation of the electrical activity within the heart, which provides information about different anatomical regions (Yue and Chan 2022). Application of 12 thoracic electrodes, in addition to the four limb electrodes (Figure 7.10), will produce an 18-lead diagnostic ECG and paramedics should be confident in placing these electrodes and interpreting the subsequent ECG waveforms (American Academy of Orthopaedic Surgeons 2023; Sanders 2012).

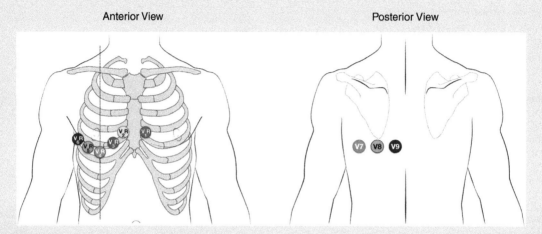

Anterior View   **Posterior View**

FIGURE 7.10   Electrode positions for 12- to 15-lead and 18-lead ECGs (not shown are the limb leads). Source: Chiu-Sun Yue 2000/ with permission of Elsevier.

Key Investigation: Cardiac Markers

A blood test to measure cardiac markers is a key investigation in the differential diagnosis of acute coronary syndromes (Williams 2022). These are proteins that play key roles in muscle contraction and are released in muscle cell death. The most commonly used cardiac marker is troponin. Currently, cardiac marker testing is predominantly done in hospital; however, it is also being trialled in the prehospital environment (Williams 2022).

Red Flag Alert: Chest Pain

Chest pain with a normal ECG can still be a significant cardiac event. Without normal troponin levels, you cannot rule out a myocardial infarction.

Treatment

The treatment of IHD is considered in terms of primary prevention, secondary prevention and acute treatment. Primary prevention is concerned with reducing someone's risk of experiencing angina or a myocardial infarction. Medications such as statins, blood pressure medications and dietary changes are used. Secondary prevention is to reduce the risk for people who have already experienced angina or a myocardial infarction. Management then includes all the primary prevention strategies, with additional medications to inhibit platelet aggregation, such as aspirin and clopidogrel (Clegg and Russell 2022).

Orange Flag Alert: Depression

Depression is common in patients with acute coronary syndrome and correlates with worse outcomes.

Acute treatment of a myocardial infarction centres on reperfusion therapy, either through pharmacological or physical means. Pharmacological treatment takes the form of thrombolysis, the administration of drugs to break down clots (Clegg and Russell 2022). These treatments break down blood clots occluding coronary blood flow. Thrombolysis is also indicated in the treatment of large pulmonary emboli or those causing cardiac arrest (Deakin 2021). In the prehospital setting, administering thrombolytics intra-arrest for a pulmonary embolism or myocardial infarction may be life saving, but seeking senior medical advice can be beneficial (Hitt and Pateman 2015). Unfortunately, these drugs are non-selective so can break down blood clots elsewhere in the body, causing unwanted bleeding.

Medications Management: Aspirin

Aspirin administered for acute coronary syndrome should be chewed not swallowed. This is to avoid first-pass metabolism and ensure rapid onset of action.

The physical treatment option is angioplasty. This involves cannulating a distal artery, often the right-side radial artery. Once a patent cannula is placed, a long angioplasty catheter is threaded into a coronary artery under x-ray guidance. A balloon is then inflated to compress the atherosclerotic plaque and restore blood flow through the coronary artery, a stent can be left in place to keep the artery open.

Reflective Learning Activity

If you were en route to a cardiac catheterisation laboratory with a patient experiencing a heart attack and they went into cardiac arrest, would your local cath lab still accept them?

Prior to accessing reperfusion therapy, either thrombolysis or angioplasty, a number of other steps can be taken to improve outcomes from myocardial infarction (Clegg and Russell 2022; Peate et al. 2022). Aspirin is a cyclooxygenase (or COX) inhibitor, which blocks the formation of thromboxane-A2 in platelets, reducing their ability to form blood clots (see Chapter 8). Other, similar antiplatelet drugs may also be given, such as clopidogrel or prasugrel (Hollier et al. 2021). In addition to these drugs, GTN is administered in an attempt to dilate the coronary arteries and increase blood flow to the myocardium. Analgesia is also provided, often in the form of opiates, either morphine, diamorphine or fentanyl.

Medications Management: Oxygen

In acute coronary syndrome, oxygen is only administered where the patient is hypoxaemic, as oxygen is a potent vasoconstrictor and hyperoxaemia exacerbates myocardial ischaemia.

Snapshot 7.2   Palpitations

Pre-arrival Information

A 33-year-old woman is experiencing palpitations and feels too unwell to stand up. She is at her home in a residential street.

Primary Survey

Danger: the scene is safe.
Response: the patient is normally responsive.
Catastrophic haemorrhage: there is no catastrophic bleeding.
Airway: patent.
Breathing: respiratory rate is increased at 22 breaths/minute.
Circulation: palpable radial pulses are rapid and weak.
Disability: alert and orientated to person, place and time.
Exposure: the patient is in a warm home.

Scenario

Sethina is 33 years of age and was feeling fine today until she sat down at her desk to do some writing and felt her heart beating fast. She felt like she was going to pass out, and lay on the floor before this could happen; she then phoned 999. She feels faint, short of breath and describes her chest feeling really uncomfortable.

Examination

On general examination, Sethina is a slim woman with mild nail clubbing. She has equal bilateral air entry on auscultation of her lungs, with a soft and non-tender abdomen.

Vital Signs

Vital sign	On scene	Normal values
Temperature (°C)	36.8	36.0–37.5
Pulse (beats/min)	174	60–100
Respiration (breaths/min)	22	12–20
Blood pressure (mmHg)	78/44	100–139 (systolic)
O$_2$ saturation (%)	95	95–98

Electrocardiogram

Tachycardia at a rate of 174 beats/minute. The QRS complexes are narrow (< 120 ms). The rhythm is regular and you think there is a P wave before every QRS but it is hard to tell at this rate.

Reflective Learning Activity

Reflect on Snapshot 7.2 and consider the following:

1. What cardiac dysrhythmia is presented in this case?
2. Can you name five systemic causes of this presentation?
3. How could you treat this without medication?
4. As a paramedic, what interventions would you likely be offering to this patient, and which medications might you use?
5. Do any enhanced care teams or clinicians in your locale offer additional interventions which would benefit this patient?

Electrical

A number of disruptions to the normal electrical rhythm can affect patients. Many of these events will disrupt the functional abilities of the heart as a pump and lead to cardiogenic shock. The heart rhythm can be too fast (tachydysrhythmia), too slow (bradydysrhythmia) or disordered in another way (dysrhythmia or sometimes *arrythmia*).

Tachydysrhythmias may present with palpitations, dizziness, shortness of breath or collapse. They create two problems to normal heart function. First, there is inadequate time for the ventricles to fill before the heart contracts. This results in less blood being pumped out of the heart with each heartbeat. Second, due to the rapid heart rate, there is reduce relaxation time between beats. The relaxation time (diastole) is when the coronary arteries receive their blood supply. As a result, tachydysrhythmias result in direct myocardial ischaemia, in addition to the heart muscle already having an increased oxygen demand as it is working harder to pump too quickly.

Management of inappropriate tachycardias is usually through addressing the underlying cause (e.g. fluid depletion, pyrexia). In some cases, however, cardioversion is required. Cardioversion is the medical term for restoring the heart to its normal rhythm. This can be achieved with vagal manoeuvres or medications, often with adenosine as a first-line option for narrow complex tachycardias, such as supraventricular tachycardiac (Clegg and Russell 2022; Sharp 2015), amiodarone for broad complex tachycardias or using electricity in the form of direct current cardioversion.

Orange Flag Alert: Hyperventilation Syndrome

Hyperventilation syndrome (or panic attacks) can mimic or cause narrow complex tachycardia. Equally, experiencing a tachydysrhythmia can cause panic and anxiety. Be on guard for both diagnoses.

Slow heart rates may be a natural physiological bradycardia when seen in fit and healthy individuals. However, there is a huge array of other causes for pathological bradydysrhythmias (Sidhu and Marine 2020). Common causes encountered in prehospital care include cardiac ischaemia, hypothermia, carotid sinus hypersensitivity or as an adverse effect of drug therapy (Clegg and Russell 2022). A complete heart block will also result in the ventricular rate (pulse rate) dropping to the natural rate of the pacemaker at the AV node (40–60 beats/min). Absolute bradycardia is the term used for a heart rate below 40 beats/minute, and will nearly always require treatment. Prehospital management of bradycardias causing impaired cerebral perfusion include atropine or external cardiac pacing (Association of Ambulance Chief Executives and Joint Royal Colleges Ambulance Liaison Committee, 2022).

Medications Management: Atropine

Atropine given at doses below 500 μg in adults can cause unwanted bradycardia.

There are many other types of cardiac dysrhythmia (Till 2021) and it is beyond the scope of this chapter to cover them all. A collection of cardiac dysrhythmias which occur due to conduction problems at the AV node are collectively known as the AV blocks. These are important to recognise and to understand which are more dangerous for your patient (Table 7.6).

The last two rhythms of vital importance in prehospital care are ventricular fibrillation (VF) and ventricular tachycardia (VT), as VF always requires immediate defibrillation, as does VT when there is no pulse, to revert the heart to a rhythm compatible with life (Figures 7.11 and 7.12).

TABLE 7.6   Heart blocks.

AV block		Description	Diagram
First degree	First-degree heart block	Consistently prolonged PR interval > 200 ms	
Second degree	Mobitz type 1 (wenckebach)	Intermittent conduction failure at the AV node. The PR interval is prolonged with each beat, until a QRS complex is missed	
Second degree	Mobitz type 2[a]	Intermittent conduction failure at AV node. PR interval remains consistent but occasionally a QRS complex is missing	
Third degree	Complete heart block[a]	Complete electrical dissociation between atria and ventricles. P waves are regular and QRS complexes are regular, but they are independent from one another	

[a] High risk of asystole.

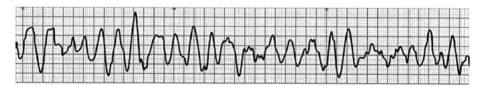

FIGURE 7.11   Ventricular fibrillation.

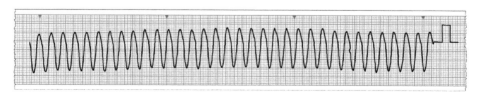

FIGURE 7.12   Ventricular tachycardia (may be pulsed or pulseless).

Diseases of the Vasculature

Aortic Dissection

In some patients, the wall of the aorta can weaken and split or bulge to form an aneurysm. In these cases, the aorta can completely rupture, resulting in an extremely poor prognosis. A rupture of the abdominal aorta, for example, has a mortality of around 80–90%. A high index of suspicion and rapid transportation to a suitable receiving hospital is key to reducing this (Smith 2011).

Red Flag: Blood Pressure

A systolic blood pressure difference greater than 20 mmHg between the arms in a patient with chest pain may indicate a thoracic aortic aneurysm. This is a surgical emergency.

Aortic Compression

In cases of significant trauma, there may be benefit in compressing the aorta. This has two main benefits: it isolates the proximal portion of the body, essentially reducing the amount of tissue and organs requiring perfusion and also provides a means to stop exsanguination from significant bleeding in the lower limbs or pelvis. Prehospital occlusion of the descending aorta can be undertaken through retrograde endovascular aortic occlusion (known as REBOA) and external or internal abdominal aortic compression.

Peripheral Vascular Disease

145

Peripheral vascular disease is a medical condition characterised by the narrowing or occlusion of the blood vessels outside the heart, brain and great vessels. This narrowing or blockage causes reduced blood flow and subsequent ischaemia. The most common cause is atherosclerosis. Symptoms vary and may include leg pain, numbness, paraesthesia, temperature changes or the development of leg ulcers. Peripheral vascular disease is predominantly managed through medical means. This takes the form of optimising risk factors, such as reducing high blood pressure and hypercholesterolaemia. Narrowed or occluded vessels can also be surgically bypassed or opened using angioplasty.

Clinical Investigations: Angiogram

A core test is acquiring an angiogram. This is where contrast is injected into blood vessels and then radiographic images (plain radiograph or CT) are acquired. This demonstrates narrowing of blood vessels or 'filling defects' (Figure 7.13).

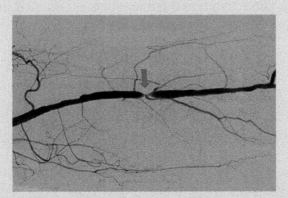

FIGURE 7.13 Angiography demonstrating a significant filling defect indicated by the arrow. Source: Natalie et.al. (2018)/John Wiley & Sons, Inc.

Venous Thrombosis

A deep vein thrombosis (DVT) most commonly occur the in the veins of the leg, but can also develop in the arms. In some cases, a venous thrombosis in the calf may propagate and spread proximally, resulting in thrombosed femoral or iliac veins and in some cases even involving the vena cava. These thrombi limit the drainage of blood from a limb, leading to collateral veins becoming dilated and varicosed as they provide venous drainage from the limb. Portions of the thrombus may also break free and travel to the heart. There, these portions will travel through the right side of the heart and into the lungs, where they form a pulmonary embolus. In cases where there is a hole between the right and left sides of the heart (e.g. patent foramen ovale), such a travelling blood clot can move into the systemic circulation and then cerebral circulation causing a stroke. The presence of a DVT can be rapidly identified by ultrasound and is part of point of care ultrasound training.

Reflective Learning Activity

The following table lists some common conditions associated with the cardiovascular system. Write some notes about each condition:

- Myocardial infarction
- Tachydysrhythmia
- Cardiac tamponade
- Aortic aneurysm

You could use information from this textbook and from wider reading of journal articles and clinical practice guidelines.

Take Home Points

- The heart can experience problems with its pump or its electrical control.
- Rapid prehospital administration of antiplatelets saves lives in acute coronary syndromes.
- Cardiac problems can deteriorate into cardiac arrest. Prepare for this eventuality and you will not be taken by surprise.

Summary

This chapter has provided an introduction to the anatomy and physiology of the cardiovascular system and disease processes which affect this organ system. To diagnose and manage these conditions effectively, clinicians need to have a good understanding of the underpinning anatomy and physiology.

References

American Academy of Orthopaedic Surgeons (2023). *Nancy Caroline's Emergency Care in the Streets*, 9e. Burlington, MA: Jones & Bartlett Learning.

Association of Ambulance Chief Executives; Joint Royal Colleges Ambulance Liaison Committee (2022). *JRCALC Clinical Guidelines*. Bridgwater: Class Professional Publishing.

Clegg, L. and Russell, F. (2022). Medications used in the cardiovascular system. In: *Fundamentals of Pharmacology for Paramedics*, 167–181. Chichester: Wiley.

Deakin, E.A. (2021). *Special Circumstances Guidelines*. London: Resuscitation Council UK.

Hitt, A. and Pateman, J. (2015). Intra-cardiac arrest thrombolysis in the pre-hospital setting: four cases worth considering. *Journal of Paramedic Practice* 7 (1): 26–30.

Hollier, R., Sealy, M., Ross, N., and Ebbs, P. (2021). Prehospital clopidogrel use and STEMI management: a review. *Journal of Paramedic Practice* 13 (6): 1–10.

Mallinson, T. (2023). Additional rules for reading an electrocardiogram. *Journal of Paramedic Practice* 15 (3): 95–97.

Meyers, H., Bracey, A., Lee, D. et al. (2021). Comparison of the ST-elevation myocardial infarction (STEMI) vs. NSTEMI and occlusion MI (OMI) vs. NOMI paradigms of acute MI. *Journal of Emergency Medicine* 60 (3): 273–284.

Mullen, R. (2013). Ambulance CPAP saves lives: why don't we use it? *Journal of Paramedic Practice* 5 (12): 672–677.

Mursell, I. (2009). Drug regimes for acute cardiogenic pulmonary oedema. *Journal of Paramedic Practice* 1 (4): 140–144.

Peate, I., Evans, S., and Clegg, L. (2022). *Fundamentals of Pharmacology for Paramedics*. Chichester: Wiley.

Pulido, J.A., Mariana, R., Jessica, E. et al. (2022). "Predicting mortality in penetrating cardiac trauma in developing countries through a new classification: Validation of the Bogotá classification." *Health Science Reports* 5 (6): e915.

Ramanathan, T. and Skinner, H. (2005). Coronary blood flow. *Continuing Education in Anaesthesia, Critical Care and Pain* 5 (2): 61–64.

Sanders, M. (2012). *Mosby's Paramedic Textbook*. Burlington, MA: Elsevier/Mosby.

Sharp, A. (2015). Pre-hospital treatment of supraventricular tachycardia: a literature review. *Journal of Paramedic Practice* 7 (12): 618–628.

Sidhu, S. and Marine, J. (2020). Evaluating and managing bradycardia. *Trends in Cardiovascular Medicine* 30 (5): 265–272.

Smith, N. (2011). Management of the ruptured abdominal aortic aneurysm: challenges facing paramedics. *Journal of Paramedic Practice* 3 (7): 360–365.

Thygesen, K. (2018). "Ten commandments" for the fourth universal definition of myocardial infarction 2018. *Circulation* 40 (3): 226–226.

Till, C.L. (2021). *Clinical ECGs in Paramedic Practice*. Bridgwater: Class Professional Publishing.

Westaby, J., Zullo, E., Bicalho, L. et al. (2023). Effect of sex, age and body measurements on heart weight, atrial, ventricular, valvular and sub-epicardial fat measurements of the normal heart. *Cardiovascular Pathology* 63: 107508.

Williams, G. (2022). Prehospital point-of-care biomarkers: missing link in acute myocardial infarction? *Journal of Paramedic Practice* 14 (3): 119–125.

Yue, C. and Chan, W. (2022). Use of 18-lead electrocardiogram in diagnosing right ventricular and Posterior Wall involvement in patients with acute inferior myocardial infarction. *Journal of the Hong Kong College of Cardiology* 8 (2): 43–48.

Further Reading

Gander, B. (2020). Prehospital amputation: a scoping review. *Journal of Paramedic Practice* 12 (1): 6–13.

Nutbeam, T. and Boylan, M. (2013). *ABC of Prehospital Emergency Medicine*. Chichester: Wiley.

Peate, I., Evans, S., and Clegg, L. (2022). *Fundamentals of Pharmacology for Paramedics*. Chichester: Wiley.

Porter, K. (2010). Prehospital amputation. *Emergency Medicine Journal* 27 (12): 940–942.

Proctor, A., Eaton, G., and Francis, J. (2023). *Primary Care for Paramedics*. Bridgwater: Class Professional Publishing.

Till, C. (2021). *Clinical ECGs in Paramedic Practice*. Bridgwater: Class Professional Publishing.

Willis, S., Hill, R., and Peate, I. (2021). *Clinical Cases in Paramedicine*. Chichester: Wiley.

Online Resources

Life in the Fast Lane: *ECG Library*. https://litfl.com/ecg-library (accessed 3 October 2023).

Resuscitation Council UK: www.resus.org.uk (accessed 3 October 2023).

Glossary

Angiography	Obtaining radiographic (x-ray) views of vessels by injecting contrast into them.
Angina pectoris	Condition producing pain in the chest (and possibly neck, shoulders).
Asystole	An ECG trace lacking electrical cardiac activity.
Atrioventricular (AV) node	Part of the cardiac electrical conduction system.
Bicuspid valve	*See* Mitral valve
Bradycardia	A slow heart rate, usually ; less than 60 beats/minute.
Bradydysrhythmia	Inappropriately slow heart rate.
Bundle of His	Part of the cardiac electrical conduction system which links the atria to the ventricles.
Cardiac tamponade	Compression of the heart by large amounts of fluid within the pericardial sac.
Clopidogrel	Antiplatelet drug.
Coronary	Relating to the vessels surrounding the heart and supplying the myocardium.
Diastole	Period of time when the heart muscle is relaxing (opposite of systole).
Dysrhythmia	Disordered heart rhythm.
Echocardiogram	Use of ultrasound to image the heart.
Electrocardiogram	Recording of the electrical impulses of the heart.
Heart attack	*See* Myocardial infarction.
Ischaemia	Restriction in blood flow to tissue or organs.
Infarction	Injury or death of tissue resulting from lack of blood supply.
Mitral	Relating to the mitral valve or resembling a mitre (hat).
Mitral valve	One way valve dividing the left atrium and left ventricle, also known as the bicuspid valve.
Myocardial infarction	Damage sustained to the myocardium due to inadequate oxygen supply.
Myocardium	Heart muscle.
Occlusive myocardial infarction	Heart attack due to a blocked coronary artery.
Purkinje fibres	Distal component of the cardiac electrical conduction system; specialised myocardial fibres which rapidly conduct electrical impulses.
Q wave	The first negative deflection of the QRS complex on an ECG.
R wave	The first positive deflection of the QRS complex on an ECG.
S wave	A negative wave occurring after a positive wave; represents final depolarisation of the ventricles.
Systole	Contraction of heart muscle.
T wave	Positive deflection on the ECG after the QRS complex representing ventricular repolarisation.
Tachycardia	A fast heart rate, usually considered to be over 100 beats/minute.
Tachydysrhythmia	An inappropriately fast heart rate.
Troponin	Marker of cardiac injury found in the blood.
Varicosity	Dilated and tortuous vessels.
Ventricular fibrillation	Disorganised depolarisation of the ventricles.
Ventricular tachycardia	Organised rapid depolarisation of the ventricles, which may or may not produce a pulse.

Multiple Choice Questions

1. How many heart valves are there?
   a. 2
   b. 3
   c. 6
   d. 4

2. Which heart block is also known as Wenckebach?
   a. 1st-degree AV block
   b. 2nd-degree type 1
   c. Complete heart block
   d. 2nd-degree type 2

3. Which cardiac valve is also known as the mitral valve?
   a. Tricuspid
   b. Bicuspid
   c. Aortic
   d. Pulmonary

4. The Sgarbossa criteria are used to detect myocardial infarctions in patients with what pre-existing condition?
   a. Electrical alternans
   b. Hypothermia
   c. Angina
   d. Left bundle branch block

5. In the cardiac cycle, the beginning of ventricular systole coincides with which of the following?
   a. T wave
   b. P wave
   c. QRS complex
   d. U wave

6. Haemorrhage from prehospital amputation can be controlled with tourniquet application and what else?
   a. Alginate dressings
   b. Perivascular adrenaline injection
   c. Arterial clamping
   d. Venous embolisation

7. At what stage of the cardiac cycle does ventricular pressure exceed aortic pressure?
   a. Late diastole
   b. Early diastole
   c. Coinciding with the P wave
   d. Systole

8. Which of the following describes a type 2 myocardial infarction?
   a. Sudden cardiac death of a presumed cardiogenic aetiology
   b. Infarction secondary to cardiac surgery, percutaneous angiography or stent insertion
   c. Oxygen supply and demand mismatch without atherosclerotic plaque rupture or erosion
   d. Isovolumetric myocardial ischaemia secondary to a systemic autoimmune or inflammatory disease

9. Elevated troponin in a patient's blood indicates what?
    a. Angina
    b. Aortic dissection
    c. Atrial stretch
    d. Damaged myocardium

10. Coronary arteries supply blood to what?
    a. Carotid sinus
    b. Myocardium
    c. Internal mammary artery
    d. Aorta

CHAPTER 8

The Blood and Associated Disorders

David Yore

AIM

The aim of this chapter is to understand the importance of blood in the human body.

LEARNING OUTCOMES

On completion of this section you will be able to:

*   Describe the normal composition of blood.
*   List the functions of red blood cells, white blood cells and platelets.
*   Discuss common blood conditions and diseases and identify risk factors associated with the diseases.
*   Describe care management for patients in haematological emergencies.

Test Your Prior Knowledge
1.   What is the percentage breakdown of blood between plasma, red blood cells and white blood cells?
2.   List the functions of red blood cells, white blood cells and platelets.
3.   Name at least four factors effecting coagulation and what we can do prehospitally to counter them.

Introduction

As a paramedic, you will often respond to haematological emergencies. They can be difficult to assess and challenging to treat in the prehospital setting; however, interventions made can be lifesaving (Caroline 2014). A well-grounded understanding of disorders of the blood and the haematopoietic tissues is essential for any prehospital practitioner to treat these patients effectively. Blood is a connective tissue that contains cells and cell fragments. It is not physically connected to nor gives mechanical support to any structures of the body but is rather called a connective tissue, as it consists of blood cells surrounded by a non-living fluid matrix called blood plasma. It has the same origin as that of any other

Fundamentals of Applied Pathophysiology for Paramedics, First Edition. Edited by Ian Peate and Simon Sawyer.
© 2024 John Wiley & Sons Ltd. Published 2024 by John Wiley & Sons Ltd.

connective tissue types and is essentially the fluid of life – without it, we would not be able to live. Blood regulates the pH of our body, restricts fluid loss during injury, provides defence against pathogens and toxins and regulates body temperature.

Functions of Blood

Blood has several functions within the human body, all of which play very important roles:

- *Respiration*: blood transports the oxygen from the lungs to the tissues throughout the body and returns carbon dioxide from the tissues to the lungs.
- *Defence*: blood carries cells and antibodies which protect the body from any foreign infection or organisms.
- *Excretion*: blood transports the waste products of cell metabolism to the excretory organs.
- *Nutrition*: blood carries nutrients from the digestive tract to cells throughout the body.
- *Regulation*: blood transports hormones to the necessary organs and sends excess heat which is built up to the surface of the body to be released.

Each of these functions is essential to life and, once we understand this, we can then understand how blood disorders and injuries can be so detrimental to our patients.

Composition of Blood

Blood can be split up into different sections, which can be seen during centrifugation (Figure 8.1). Blood is composed of erythrocytes (red blood cells), thrombocytes (platelets), leucocytes (white blood cells) and plasma, a yellow-coloured fluid due to the different particles that are dissolved in it (Figure 8.2).

Plasma

Most of the plasma found in the blood is composed of water (91%). It also contains waste products, hormones, gases, nutrients and dissolved blood proteins, all of which have their own purposes. There are three principal types of plasma proteins, and together they make up approximately 7% of the plasma. These proteins stay in the blood vessels, as they are too large to diffuse through the capillaries (Waugh and Grant 2018).

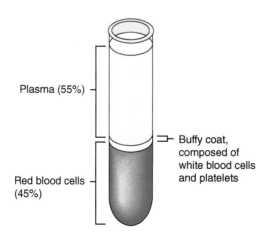

Plasma (55%)

Buffy coat, composed of white blood cells and platelets

Red blood cells (45%)

FIGURE 8.1   Components of blood separated by centrifugation. Source: Peate (2019)/John Wiley & Sons.

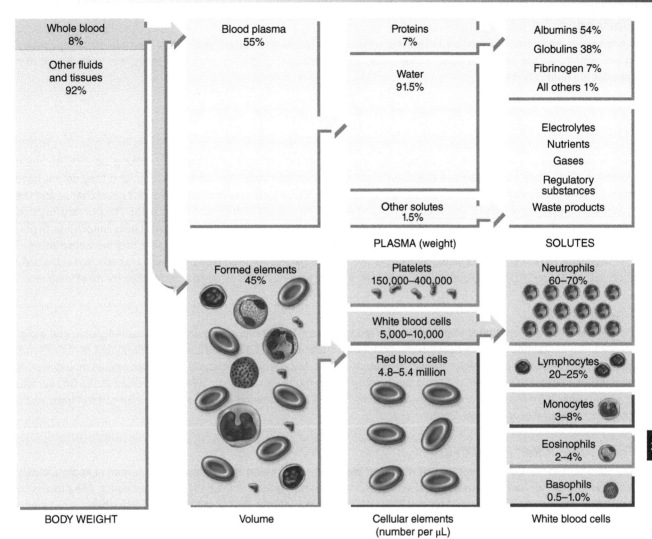

FIGURE 8.2 The composition of blood cells Source: Elling and Elling (2015)/Jones & Bartlett Learning.

Albumins

Approximately 60% of proteins are albumins, which are used to maintain osmotic pressure and also act as carrier molecules for other substances such as hormones and lipids (Waugh and Grant 2018).

Globulins

Globulins are the next most common plasma protein found in the plasma. They are divided into three groups, depending on their function:

1. Alpha globulin
2. Beta globulin
3. Gamma globulin.

The alpha and beta globulins are formed in the liver and their role is to transport lipids and fat-soluble vitamins. Gamma globulins are also known as immunoglobulins, which are complex structures that play a vital role in immunity. They prevent diseases such as measles and tetanus (Waugh and Grant 2018).

Fibrinogen

Fibrinogen is the last main component of plasma which can be found in the blood. Without this component being present in our system, we are unable to make a blood clot. When fibrinogen and other plasma proteins are removed, all that remains is a fluid called serum.

Red Blood Cells

Also known as erythrocytes, red blood cells are the most dominant type of blood cell, making up 99% of blood (Caroline 2014). They are shaped like biconcave discs and are unique cells that are enucleated, and they do not have mitochondria or ribosomes present (Figure 8.3). The biconcave shape increases the surface area for gas exchange and the thinness of the centre of the cell allows easy entry and entry for the gases (Waugh and Grant 2018). The primary function of red blood cells is to transport oxygen and carbon dioxide (approximately 20%). As they do not have mitochondria present to produce energy, they use anaerobic respiration and this does not use up any oxygen that they are transporting.

In general, red blood cells last up to four months, and approximately two million red blood cells are destroyed in the body every second (Mader 2011). Red blood cell counts are taken to diagnose many diseases and evaluate their course of treatment.

Haemoglobin

Haemoglobin is a protein that is found within the red blood cell. It contains a globular protein called globin and a pigmented iron-containing complex called haem (Waugh and Grant 2018). Each molecule of haemoglobin contains fours globin chains and four haem units, each with one atom of iron. As each atom can combine with an oxygen molecule, this means that a single haemoglobin molecule can carry up to four molecules of oxygen (Waugh and Grant 2018). On average, approximately 280 million haemoglobin molecules are carried in a red blood cell, so one red blood cell will transport a billion molecules of oxygen (Peate 2019).

Formation of Red Blood Cells

The stem cells in the red bone marrow are where red blood cells are formed from. They have a lifespan of approximately 120 days (due to not having a nucleus) and account for approximately 25% of the body's total cell count. The process by which they are formed is called *erythropoiesis*. Both folic acid and vitamin B_{12} are required for the synthesis of red blood cells (Waugh and Grant 2018).

154

8 µm

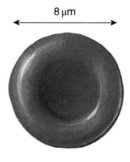

Surface view

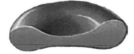

Sectioned view

FIGURE 8.3   A red blood cell.

Transportation of Gases

The primary function of red blood cells is to transport oxygen from the lungs to the tissues and organs around the body. In the alveoli of the lungs, oxygen combines with each of the four oxygen-binding sites of the haemoglobin molecule to form oxyhaemoglobin, and the molecule becomes saturated. This is then transported by the blood to the tissues where it is needed. When the oxygen content of the blood changes, so does its colour. Oxygen-rich blood is bright red due to the high levels of oxyhaemoglobin in it compared with blood with poorer oxygen levels, which is dark blue in colour as the molecule is not fully saturated. The oxyhaemoglobin molecule releases its oxygen under certain conditions (Waugh and Grant 2018):

- *Low pH*: tissues which are metabolically active (e.g. muscles during exercise) release acid waste products and so the local pH is reduced.
- *Hypoxia*: where oxygen levels are low, oxyhaemoglobin breaks down and releases oxygen to the tissues. As tissue oxygen demand rises, so the supply rises to match it. Where oxygen levels are high in contrast, such as in the lungs, the formation of oxyhaemoglobin is favoured.
- *Temperature*: as tissues metabolise, their temperature rises. They have higher than normal oxygen needs, resulting in a higher oxygen supply to the active tissue.

As well as transporting oxygen from the lungs to the tissues of the body, red blood cells also transport carbon dioxide from the tissues to the lungs in three ways:

1. 10% is dissolved in plasma.
2. 20% combines with the haemoglobin of the red blood cell to form carbaminohaemoglobin.
3. 70% combines with water to form carbonic acid, which is converted to bicarbonate and hydrogen ions.

155

Control of Erythropoiesis (Production of Red Blood Cells)

Red blood cell numbers are constant because the bone marrow produces erythrocytes at the rate at which they are destroyed (Waugh and Grant 2018). The primary stimulus to increase red blood cell production is hypoxia. This can result from anaemia, hypovolaemia, poor blood flow, reduced oxygen concentration of inspired air or lung diseases. If any of these conditions are present, erythropoietin production occurs.

Blood Groups

The surface of red blood cells carries a range of different proteins called antigens, which are recognised by the immune system of the body (Elling and Elling 2015). Antibodies are present in the plasma of the blood. They react with the antigens of the red blood cell. Antibodies are specific to certain antigens and, when they combine, they form a link to connect red blood cells to each other – agglutination of the red blood cells occurs (Peate 2019). In the ABO system, the presence of A or B antigen gives type A or type B blood; the presence of both A and B gives type AB blood while their absence gives type O blood (Table 8.1; Figure 8.4). For blood transfusions, blood types must be matched between a donor and a recipient for a safe transfusion. As blood group AB make neither anti-A nor anti-B antibodies, they are sometimes referred to as the universal recipients.

Another important system to note is the Rh (rhesus) system. Like the antigens, patients who are Rh negative cannot receive blood from an Rh positive donor, although the opposite is fine. Approximately 85% of people have the rhesus factor. Each of the four types of blood can be Rh positive or negative, giving a total of eight possible combinations, which are the eight know common blood types.

TABLE 8.1   Blood groups.

Blood group	Gives to these groups	Receives from these groups
O−	All	O− only
O+	AB+, A+, B+, O+	O−, O+
A−	AB−, AB+, A+, A−	O− and A−
A+	AB+ and A+	O−, O+, A−, A+
B−	B−, B+, AB−, AB+	O− and B−
B+	B+, AB+	O−, O+, B−, B+
AB−	AB−, AB+	O−, A−, B−, AB−
AB+	AB+ only	All

Source: Irish Blood Transfusion Service n.d.

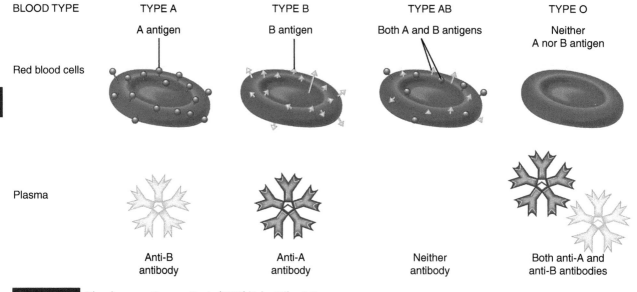

FIGURE 8.4   Blood groups. Source: Peate (2019)/John Wiley & Sons.

White Blood Cells

White blood cells, or leucocytes, have an important function in defence and immunity in the body. There are approximately 5000–10 000 white blood cells in every cubic millimetre of blood (Peate 2019). There are different types of white blood cells, and each has a different function. The primary function of all white blood cells is to fight infection. The number of white blood cells can increase in infections to approximately 25 000 per cubic millimetre of blood. An increase in white blood cells is known as *leucocytosis* and an abnormally low level of white blood cells is called *leukopenia* (Peate 2019). In contrast to red blood cells, leucocytes do have nuclei and are able to move across blood vessel walls into the tissues. The two main types of leucocytes are named according to their appearance; Granulocytes have large cytoplasmic granules that are easily seen with a light microscope, whereas agranulocytes are leucocytes that lack those granules. Granulocytes are again split down into three types – neutrophils, eosinophils and basophils. Agranulocytes are divided into monocytes and lymphocytes.

Neutrophils

Neutrophils are the most common type of white blood cell found in the blood, accounting for approximately 60–65% of granulocytes. They destroy bacteria, antigen–antibody complexes and foreign matter (Elling and Elling 2015). The number of neutrophils in the blood increases in:

- Pregnancy
- Leukaemia
- Infection
- Metabolic disorder (e.g. acute gout)
- Inflammation
- Myocardial infarction.

Eosinophils

Like neutrophils, eosinophils also migrate from blood vessels. They function in the body's allergic response and are increased in people with allergies. Certain parasitic infections also result in an increase in the number of eosinophils present in the blood. Eosinophils contain lysosomal enzymes and peroxidase, which are toxic to parasites and result in the destruction of the organisms (Peate 2019).

Basophils

Basophils are the least common of all the granulocytes. They contain elongated lobed nuclei. In inflamed tissues, they become mast cells and secrete granules containing heparin, which inhibits blood clotting, and histamine, which increases tissue inflammation. They play an important role in providing immunity against parasites (Peate 2019).

157

Lymphocytes

Lymphocytes are the smallest of the agranulocytes. They originate in the bone marrow but migrate through the blood to the lymphatic tissues. Lymphocytes account for 25% of leucocytes and are mostly found in the lymphatic tissue, such as the lymph nodes, spleen, tonsils and thymus. Two types of lymphocytes can be found in the body – T cells and B cells. These cells are named in connection with where they originate in the body. T lymphocytes originate from the thymus gland, whereas B lymphocytes originate in the bone marrow. B cells produce and secrete antibodies that bind and destroy foreign antigens whereas T cells interact directly with antigens, producing the cellular immune response (Elling and Elling 2015).

Monocytes

Monocytes account for 5% of the agranulocytes in the blood. They develop in the bone marrow and are among the first line of defence in the inflammatory process. Monocytes migrate out of the blood into the tissues in response to an infection. Through a process called phagocytosis, they surround microbes and digest them. They are vital in immunity and inflammation by destroying specific antigens (Peate 2019).

Platelets and Blood Clotting

Platelets are also known as thrombocytes. They are small cells consisting of cytoplasm surrounded by a plasma membrane that are essential for clot formation. They are produced in the red bone marrow and their lifespan is approximately five to nine days (Standfield 2011). Despite having no nucleus, their cytoplasm is packed with granules containing a variety of substances that promote blood clothing, which causes haemostasis (cessation of bleeding). Approximately one-third of platelets are stored within the spleen, as opposed to the circulatory system, which acts as an emergency store that can be released as required to control excessive bleeding.

Haemostasis

Haemostasis is the body's internal blood clotting mechanism. When there is damage to a blood vessel, there are a series of processes that occur to stop the loss of blood and start the healing process. The worse a vessel wall is damaged, the faster coagulation begins. There are three primary components in this process: platelet aggregation, vasoconstriction and coagulation (Waugh and Grant 2018).

Platelet Aggregation

Platelets are highly specialised to recognise injury to a blood vessel. The adherent platelets stick to each other and release chemicals such as adenosine diphosphate (ADP), which attracts more platelets to the site of injury. The additional platelets then stick to the ones that are already there, and they too release chemicals. This results in a large volume of platelets arriving at the site of damage, which quickly form thrombi. These thrombi subsequently undergo contraction and consolidation to prevent blood loss and promote wound healing (Berndt et al. 2014). This formation is usually complete within six minutes of injury.

Vasoconstriction

When platelets locate a damaged blood vessel, their surface becomes sticky and they adhere to the damaged wall. They then release serotonin, which causes constriction of the blood vessels, resulting in a reduction or complete cessation of blood flow through the vessel. The vessel itself also releases other chemicals such as thromboxane, which also causes vasoconstriction (Waugh and Grant 2018).

Coagulation

If a vessel is damaged to such a degree that the above mechanisms cannot control the bleeding, them the complex process of coagulation begins. The clotting phase involves numerous clotting factors (Table 8.2), most being synthesised in the liver.

Two pathways have been identified that trigger a blood clot – the intrinsic pathway and the extrinsic pathway. The extrinsic pathway occurs when blood vessels are ruptured and tissue damage takes place. It is a rapid clotting system. The intrinsic pathway is slower and is activated when the inner walls of the blood vessels are damaged.

Environmental factors that can treated in the prehospital field can influence coagulation. The 'lethal triad' of hypothermia, acidosis and coagulopathy is a well-known concept in patients with trauma. Anaesthesia, (Forrest et al. 2014) explains that 'the major issue is coagulopathy, and the other factors contribute to its severity'. They discuss the importance of maintaining as close to normal physiology as possible and state, 'we should go to considerable lengths to keep the casualty as warm as possible'. Hypothermia, volume loss, acidosis and delayed scene time are all factors that can have significant impacts on coagulation and ultimately patient outcomes.

TABLE 8.2 Blood clotting factors.

Number	Factor
I	Fibrinogen
II	Prothrombin
III	Thromboplastin
IV	Calcium
V	Proaccelerin, labile factor
VII	Serum prothrombin conversion accelerator
VIII	Antihemophilic factor
IX	Christmas factor, thromboplastin component
X	Stuart power factor
XI	Plasma thromboplastin antecedent
XII	Hagerman factor
XIII	Fibrin-stabilising factor

Hypothermia

By removing the patient quickly from a cold or exposed environment and by using simple treatments such as blankets, warm intravenous fluids, heat packs, foil blankets and heaters, we can help to reduce hypothermia in patients, thus reducing its effects on coagulation.

Volume Loss

Practitioners should cease the bleed at source, if possible, limit crystalloid resuscitation, adopt permissive hypotension and activate the major haemorrhage policy (Forrest et al. 2014). Conditions such as disseminated intravascular coagulopathy may result in trauma: uncontrolled haemorrhage occurs as a result of the severe reduction of clotting factors due to the blood loss (Caroline 2014).

Acidosis

As with hypothermia, treatments such as oxygen therapy can help to reduce respiratory acidosis. Early blood sampling is needed to determine the severity of acidosis, which needs to be treated as early as possible. The effects of acidosis on coagulation are greater than hypothermia. Both conditions further increase the severity of trauma-induced coagulopathy (Forrest et al. 2014).

Delayed Scene Time

Worldwide standards agree that delayed arrival on scene is one of the major factors in patient mortality, with standards recommending that time to trauma scene be less than 10 minutes (Ashburn et al. 2020). Sampalis et al. (1993) found that hospital time in excess of 60 minutes was associated with a threefold increase in mortality. As practitioners, we must reduce on-scene arrival times as much as possible and transport patients to the most appropriate facility at the earliest opportunity, while continuing to treat and monitor them throughout.

Snapshot 8.1   Dangerous Areas of Bleeding

Pre-arrival Information

You receive a call to a 32-year-old man who has been involved in a road traffic collision. Patrick was pulling out of a junction onto a major road when he was hit side on by a pickup truck travelling at 75 mph.

On Arrival with the Patient

On your arrival, you are met by a police officer, who seems panicked and tells you that your patient is very poorly. Your scene survey shows a significant mechanism of injury, with the centre point of impact being the driver side door. The only information you are told is that he was initially talking and complaining of pain in his stomach but has since become unresponsive.

Primary Survey

Airway: snoring sounds – treated with trauma-jaw thrust and oropharyngeal airway to good effect.
C-spine: active spinal motion restriction in place via fire department personnel.
Breathing: equal rise and fall of the chest, air entry upon all fields on auscultation. Elevated respiration rate.
Circulation: delayed capillary refill. Weak radial pulse – fast and regular. Skin pale and clammy. No significant external haemorrhage.
Disability: unresponsive on the AVPU scale.

Vital Signs

Vital sign	Observation	Normal range
Pulse (beats/min)	130 regular	80–100 regular
Respiration rate (breaths/min)	24	12–20
SpO$_2$ (%)	94	94–98
Capillary refill (s)	>2	<2
Blood pressure (mmHg)	86/40	120/80
Eyes	1 – no response	4 – spontaneously
Verbal	2 – incomprehensible sounds	5 – orientated
Motor	5 – localises to pain	6 – obeys commands
Total GCS score	8	15
Temperature (°C)	35.4	37
Pupils	Equal, round, sluggish reaction	Equal, round, reactive

Secondary Survey

Head: small abrasions to face. Pupils equal and sluggish to react. Facial bones intact.
Neck: contusions on right hand side. No subcutaneous emphysema. Trachea in normal anatomical position.
Chest: no paradoxical movement, bruising to left hand side of ribcage. Normal breath sounds on auscultation.
Abdomen: transverse contusion noted. Rigidity present in all regions.
Pelvis: unstable.
Extremities: left mid-shaft femur fracture. Delayed capillary refill in all four limbs. Absent pulse on left foot.

Now reflect on the information in Snapshot 8.1 and consider the following:

1. What injuries could the patient suffering from?
2. What interventions can paramedics make to reduce further deterioration of the patient?
3. Would you take the patient to the nearest emergency department or to a major trauma centre?

Areas of Internal Bleeding of Concern

The circulatory system is a closed looped system through which the blood is circulated by the heart through blood vessels to supply the body's organs with oxygen and nutrients. As paramedics, we often see both internal and external bleeding. It is important that we are aware of the dangerous areas of internal bleeding in the body and how we can treat them in the prehospital setting.

Almost any organ or blood vessel can be damaged by trauma, causing internal bleeding. As discussed above, the body has its own compensatory mechanisms to combat any loss in volume or damage to the blood vessel but, in prehospital care, it is often the case that the body cannot compensate for the severity of the injury that has occurred.

The most important first step is to *recognise* that the patient is haemorrhaging, either internally or externally. It is by prompt recognition that prehospital interventions will make the most positive outcome to the patient. This is done through a thorough primary assessment, detailed physical examination and taking an in-depth history of the events that have occurred and the mechanism of injury that has resulted in the injuries found. It is through our understanding of anatomy and pathophysiology that we build a collective diagnosis of what we think might be occurring in the patient.

In relation to external haemorrhage, it is important to identify what type of bleeding is occurring: capillary, veinous or arterial (Figure 8.5). Capillary bleeding is slow with an even flow. Venous bleeding is steady and dark red in colour (due to the lack of oxygen in the blood) and arterial bleeding is spurting, has a pulsating flow and is bright red in colour, as it is oxygen rich (Figure 8.2; Caroline 2014). Capillary bleeding is caused by abrasions to the skin and usually will have slowed or even stopped before the arrival of prehospital care. Venous bleeding is from deeper areas within the bodies tissues and is usually not life threatening unless the injury is severe or blood loss is not controlled. Arterial bleeding is caused by an injury that has damaged an artery. This is the most difficult blood type to control.

161

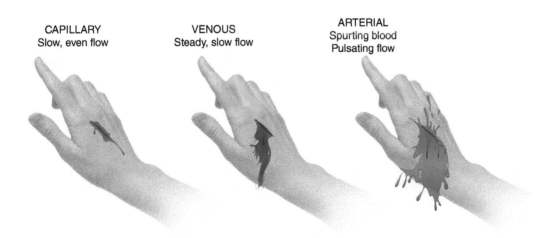

CAPILLARY
Slow, even flow

VENOUS
Steady, slow flow

ARTERIAL
Spurting blood
Pulsating flow

FIGURE 8.5 Types of bleeding.

The vital signs that we can see during the condition of shock, such as low blood pressure, rapid pulse rates and cool clammy skin, are not definitions of shock; they are merely systemic manifestations of the entire pathological process. The acute loss of blood volume from haemorrhage causes an imbalance in the relationship of the volume of fluid in the body, compared with the size of the vessels through which the fluid travels. The average 70-kg human has approximately five litres of circulating blood volume. The chest, abdomen, retroperitoneal space and long bones are all areas in which large volumes of blood can accumulate that need to be addressed at the earliest opportunity. Shock is covered more in depth in Chapter 5.

Chest Injury: Haemothorax

The primary physiological function of the thorax is to maintain oxygenation and ventilation via the lungs and circulation via the heart and blood vessels (Caroline 2014). A significant increase can be seen in mortality and morbidity in patients in whom there was a failure to recognise the potential for thoracic injury or whose treatment was delayed or inappropriate. Each pleural space can accommodate approximately 3000 ml of fluid.

Clinical Presentation
- Ventilatory insufficiency – hypoxia, agitation, anxiety, tachypnoea, dyspnoea.
- Hypovolemic shock – tachycardia, hypotension, pale/clammy skin.

Abdominal Trauma

Unrecognised abdominal injury is one of the major causes of preventable death in trauma. Owing to the limitations of prehospital assessment, any patient we come across with suspected abdominal injuries is best managed by prompt transport to an appropriate facility. If blood is lost in the abdominal cavity, regardless of its source, it can contribute to or be the primary cause of haemorrhagic shock.

Injuries to the abdomen can be caused by blunt or penetrating trauma. Penetrating traumas such as stab wounds or gunshots are more easily identifiable than blunt trauma. It is good practise visualising the path of potential trajectory of the penetrating object, as this can help to identify possible injured internal organs.

Blunt trauma injuries can be more challenging to recognise as they can often be internal. The spleen and liver can bleed easily if damaged and blood loss from these organs can occur at a rapid rate. An increase in the intra-abdominal pressure produced by compression can also rupture the diaphragm, causing the abdominal organs to move upwards into the pleural space. This can then compromise the expansion of the lungs and, in turn, can affect both respiratory and cardiac function.

Red Flag Alert: Intra-abdominal Bleeding

The most reliable indication of intra-abdominal bleeding is the presence of hypovolemic shock from an unexplained source.

Clinical Presentation
Most severe abdominal injuries will present as abnormalities that are identified in the primary survey of the patient, primarily when looking at breathing and circulation. The classification of shock generally corresponds to the findings of the breathing, circulation and disability findings:

- Severe pain
- Rigid abdomen
- Hypotension

- Tachycardia
- Significant mechanism of injury.

Pelvic Fractures

Haemorrhage from injuries such as pelvic fractures can accumulate up to five litres of fluid into the retroperitoneal space. Haemodynamically unstable open pelvic fractures have mortality rates as high as 70%. This is discussed in more depth in Chapter 15.

Clinical Presentation
- Pelvic pain
- Profound hypovolemia
- Pelvic instability
- Contusions and lacerations
- Haematuria.

Long Bones

Long-bone (femur) fractures are discussed in more depth in Chapter 15. It is important to be aware that the thighs of the human body can hold large volumes of blood in patients who are bleeding internally. The bleeding needs to be treated at the earliest opportunity.

Clinical Presentation
- Extreme pain
- Shortening of the injured limb
- Bulging around the site of injury
- Delayed or absent pedal pulses.

Care and Management of Internal Bleeding

Significant internal bleeding can often be difficult to control. Unlike external haemorrhage, internal haemorrhaging can be more difficult to stop and, in most cases, requires surgical intervention. Despite being difficult to manage, we can still provide meaningful interventions in the prehospital field, which have been proven to improve patient outcomes and reduce fatalities in patients who are in haematological emergencies.

Splinting

Internal haemorrhage is primarily controlled by immobilisation, which also has the added benefit of providing pain relief. The intention of splinting is to provide support and prevent any movement of the broken bone ends. As well as providing good pain relief, splinting also reduces the risk of further damage and controls bleeding by aiding clots to form where blood vessels have been damaged (Caroline 2014). Any injured area should be moved as little as possible during the application of a splint. There are several types of splints available for different areas of the body, but all serve the same purpose: to immobilise the limb, to prevent further injury and to aid the body's natural clotting system to stop the bleeding. In the prehospital setting, it is common to use pelvic binders (Figure 8.6), traction splints for mid-shaft femur fractures, rigid splints for the limbs and a vacuum mattress for full body immobilisation.

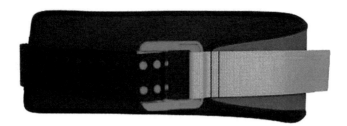

FIGURE 8.6   Pelvic binder. Source: SAM MEDICAL / https://www.sammedical.com/products/pelvic-binder?variant=17074974916697 / last accessed under March 19, 2022.

Intravenous Access

Obtaining intravenous access enables the prehospital provider to administer both pain-relieving medication and medications that aid in the body's natural clotting system. It also allows the prehospital provider to have immediate access should the patient's condition deteriorate into cardiac arrest (Caroline 2014). A patient in a haematological emergency needs prehospital blood transfusions or alternative medication, such as tranexamic acid (TXA), to be administered to them in the prehospital field. This drug aids in the body's natural clotting mechanisms and/or replaces the blood that has been lost due to the injury or illness from which the patient is suffering.

There are obvious complications with prehospital blood transfusion, so it is essential that the right blood group is administered to patients.

Medications Management: Tranexamic Acid

TXA is a medicine which helps to control bleeding. It is classed as an anti-haemorrhagic and an anti-fibrinolytic. It is often used in the prehospital setting for the treatment of suspected significant internal or external haemorrhage associated with trauma or postpartum haemorrhage (PHECC 2021). Studies have shown that TXA is safe to use in the prehospital setting post-injury and administration of prehospital TXA within one hour from injury to patients at risk of haemorrhage is associated with 30-day survival benefit, lower incidence of multiple organ failure and lower transfusion requirements (Li et al. 2021).

Rapid Transportation

Any patient who is in a haematological emergency from infection or trauma needs rapid transportation to the appropriate medical facility. Patients who have bleeding in dangerous areas of the body are at high risk of mortality if they do not receive the appropriate treatment in an appropriate time frame (Caroline 2014). As prehospital providers, it is our responsibility to ensure that these patients receive the most appropriate treatment and are transferred to the most appropriate facility where possible. However, at times, a patient may have to go to their closest emergency department to be stabilised before they can be transported to a major trauma centre.

Other Treatments

Sometimes patients who are bleeding in these dangerous body areas also require other interventions or treatments in the prehospital field. Needle thoracocentesis in the case of tension pneumothorax is has been proven to be lifesaving. Supplemental oxygen administration has also been proven to improve outcomes in patients who are bleeding in dangerous body areas.

Pain relief and fluid therapy are two important treatments; however, it is imperative that the prehospital provider does not increase on scene time for these treatments. Ideally, patients with significant haemorrhage need blood transfusions in the prehospital setting, but if this is not available, fluid therapy such as sodium chloride or Hartmann's solution can be given to ensure that the patient has a palpable radial pulse.

Snapshot 8.2   Sickle Cell Anaemia

Pre-arrival Information

You are called to a 36-year-old woman who is complaining of shortness of breath and moderate abdominal pain.

On Arrival with the Patient

On your arrival, you meet a slim black woman sitting on the couch holding her stomach. She states that she has a history of sickle cell anaemia but has not had an episode like this for a prolonged time. She is extremely anxious and tells you that she is finding it difficult to catch her breath.

Primary Survey

Airway: patent
Breathing: equal rise and fall of the chest, shallow depth and laboured.
Circulation: weak and fast radial pulse. Skin pale and sweating profusely.
Disability: alert on the AVPU scale.

Vital Signs

Vital sign	Observation	Normal range
Pulse (beats/min)	112 regular	80–100 regular
Respiration rate (breaths/min)	28	12–20
SpO$_2$ (%)	90	94–98
Capillary refill (s)	>2	<2
Blood pressure (mmHg)	106/42	120/80
Eyes	4 – spontaneously	4 – spontaneously
Verbal	5 – orientated	5 – orientated
Motor	6 – obeys commands	6 – obeys commands
Total GCS score	15	15
Temperature (°C)	38.7	37
Blood glucose (mmol/l)	4.5	4–7
Pupils	Equal, round, reactive	Equal, round, reactive

Secondary Survey

During your secondary survey, the patient points at her left upper quadrant when you ask where her pain is, and states that she has vomited twice since calling the ambulance. She also states that she cannot warm up and is having difficulty breathing.

Anaemia

Anaemia is a reduction in red blood cells and/or haemoglobin in the body. It is usually associated with some sort of underlying disease but can also be caused from acute or chronic blood loss. Anaemia results in a reduction of the body's ability to transport oxygen to the tissues, causing hypoxia (Peate 2019). The most common causes of anaemia are excessive loss of blood through haemorrhage, destruction of red blood cells, deficient red blood cell production due to red bone marrow failure, lack of intake of iron, folic acid or vitamin B_{12}, infections such as malaria, and pregnancy (Peate 2019). There are three common types of anaemia: microcytic (small red blood cells), macrocytic (large red blood cells) and normocytic (normal-sized red blood cells).

Iron Deficiency Anaemia

Iron deficiency anaemia is the most common type of anaemia. It affects 2–5% of adult men and post-menopausal women (Caroline 2014). Iron is essential for production of young red blood cells in the body. As iron is a component of haem, as discussed above, a deficiency of iron leads to decreased haemoglobin synthesis, which results in the reduction of oxygen transport. Common causes include gastrointestinal blood loss, menstrual bleeding, and blood loss due to frequent donations of blood or diagnostic tests for patients who are hospitalised for long periods of time.

Sickle Cell Anaemia

Sickle cell is where the red blood cell takes the shape of a sickle, resulting in them becoming easier to be destroyed, causing anaemia (Figure 8.7). It is caused by defective haemoglobin cells. In sickle cell anaemia, when the red blood cells are initially developing their membranes, they become deformed and rigid. This causes the cells to become lodged in small blood vessels, leading to formation of a thrombus. This reduction in blood flow or complete blockage results in a lack of oxygen to parts of the body (Waugh and Grant 2018). There is no cure for most people with sickle cell anaemia, although treatments can relieve pain and help to prevent further problems associated with the condition. Longer-term problems can also arise due to poor perfusion, such as cardiac disease, kidney failure, retinopathy, poor tissue healing and slow growth in children (Waugh and Grant 2018). Patients who are pregnant, have an infection or are dehydrated are often predisposed to a sickle cell crisis because of intravascular clotting and ischaemia.

Orange Flag Alert: Sickle Cell

Patients with sickle cell can often feel stigmatised for their condition. It is important to treat them with dignity and respect, as we do with all patients.

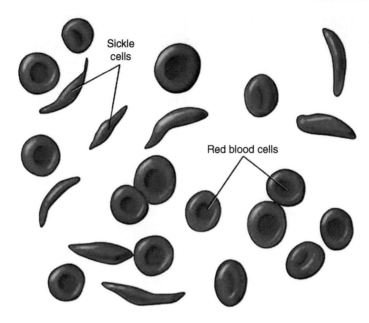

FIGURE 8.7 Sickle cell anaemia blood cells.

Assessment of Patients with Anaemia

The primary and secondary assessments should be the same for all patients we encounter, but we may want to ask more specific questions if we suspect anaemia in the patient. Most commonly, patients with anaemia tend to complain of feeling lethargic, having no energy, or feeling as if they have overexerted themselves (Caroline 2014). They can also develop an angina-type chest pain, which happens because of a reduction in oxygen availability to the myocardium itself.

Care and Management of Patients with Anaemia

As anaemia is a condition in which there is a reduction in haemoglobin levels in the body, it is important that we monitor the airway and breathing of our patients closely and administer high-flow oxygen where necessary. In cases where patients are complaining of chest pain, it is important that we do not simply diagnose the pain as a symptom of their anaemia. We must obtain a complete 12-lead ECG to rule out any myocardial infarction or other cardiovascular complication that could be causing this pain. If there is a reduction in blood pressure, intravenous fluid therapy could be warranted (Caroline 2014).

In patients who present with an epistaxis and a history of anaemia, it is often the case that the haemorrhage will not stop with the use of direct pressure alone, and administration of a nasal pack may be necessary. Patients with sickle cell anaemia can often be in severe pain due to the reduction of blood flow or complete cessation of oxygen going to the area of the body that the sickle cells have blocked. In these cases, it is appropriate to treat with relevant pain management as per local guidelines if it is not contraindicated (Caroline 2014). In a sickle cell crisis, oxygen administration can help with pain in patients who are having an acute episode.

It is important that patients whom we are suspect or know are suffering from anaemia of any kind go to the relevant care facility for further investigations and treatments to be carried out. A full blood count is required, as well as tests for the levels of different vitamins and minerals present in the body. Often, a full physical examination is required by a medical doctor and, where necessary, an examination of the patient's bone marrow can take place.

Snapshot 8.3   Sepsis

Pre-arrival Information

You are called to an 81-year-old man who was unable to be roused by his carer this morning. He was last seen yesterday morning after recently getting his urinary catheter changed and was complaining of feeling hot and tired.

On Arrival with the Patient

On your arrival, you are brought into a bedroom where you find a slim man who appears unresponsive. The carer states that she cannot wake him and that, despite a significant medical history, he is normally quite independent. She is quite upset as the he does not have any family.

Primary Survey

Airway: patent
Breathing: equal rise and fall of the chest, shallow depth and fast.
Circulation: weak and fast radial pulse. Skin pale and sweating profusely.
Disability: pain responsive on the AVPU scale.

Vital Signs

Vital sign	Observation	Normal range
Pulse (beats/min)	120 regular	80–100 regular
Respiration rate (breaths/min)	24	12–20
SpO$_2$ (%)	93%	94–98
Capillary refill (s)	>2	<2
Blood pressure (mmHg)	84/42	120/80
Eyes	2 – to pain	4 – spontaneously
Verbal	2 – groaning	5 – orientated
Motor	4 – normal flexion	6 – obeys commands
Total GCS score	8	15
Temperature (°C)	39.1	37
Blood glucose (mmol/l)	8.2	4–7
Pupils	Equal, round, reactive	Equal, round, reactive

Secondary Survey

During your secondary survey, you notice that the patient's catheter bag is not filling and there is a pus-like substance at the insertion site. You are handed his regular medication and a home care plan which shows a significant medical history of kidney problems, previous bowel cancer, hypertension, chronic obstructive pulmonary disease, hyperlipidaemia, coronary stents and a myocardial infarction.

Reflective Learning Activity

Reflect on the information In Snapshot 8.3 and consider the following:

1. What condition is the patient suffering from?
2. What interventions can paramedics make to help improve the patients condition?
3. Are there prehospital medications available that may be of benefit here?

Sepsis

Sepsis is a life-threatening reaction to an infection. It happens when your immune system overreacts to an infection and starts to damage your body's own tissues and organs. The basis of septic shock and systemic inflammatory response syndrome (SIRS) is a complex process of inflammatory response and multisystem organ failure. Relative hypovolaemia develops in sepsis because the vasculature in the body dilates. As practitioners we must be very mindful of sepsis, especially in patients with inadequate immune responses such as patients with diabetes, liver disease or HIV/AIDS, neonates, older adults, pregnant women and people with alcohol dependency. If not recognised early, this can have devastating consequences to the patient and result in organ failure and ultimately death. In sepsis, complex interactions occur between the pathogen and the body's defence system. The initial response results in leaking capillaries, vasodilation, fluid shifts and microthrombi formation (Caroline 2014, p. 922). In some patients this then progresses to an uncontrolled and unregulated inflammatory-immune response, resulting in hypoperfusion to the cells due to the opening of arteriovenous shunts, tissue destruction and organ death. This results then in multiple organ disfunction syndrome and often death.

Once the inflammatory response is initiated in the body, a complex cascade of events, both local and systemic occur (Caroline 2014, p. 730). White blood cells, platelets, mast cells and plasma cells all participate in tissue inflammatory reactions. Mast cells release a variety of substances during inflammation, such as histamine and serotonin which both increase vascular permeability and cause vasodilation. It is from our understanding of such reactions that we know that during infection, neutrophils scour the body to destroy infectious pathogens, but during sepsis these begin to attack the body's own tissues and organs. It can cause abnormal blood clotting that results in small clots or burst blood vessels that damage or destroy tissues.

Assessment of Patients with Markers of Systemic Inflammatory Response Syndrome

As with all patients we encounter, patients who we suspect are presenting with sepsis should be firstly examined using the primary and secondary assessments. We should suspect SIRS in any patient who is generally unwell with a suspected infection and a temperature lower than 36°C or above 38°C (AMLS 2017) as well has at least one other criteria including pulse rate > 90 beats/minute, respiration rate more than 20 breaths/minute, acute confusion or increased blood glucose level (> 7.7 mmol) in a person without diabetes (PHECC 2021).

It is by a thorough history taking and obtaining a complete set of vital signs that we confidently screen for sepsis in our patients. The Robson Prehospital Severe Sepsis screening tool has a 75% success rate in identifying sepsis (AMLS 2017, p. 159).

Other tools which can be used to identify sepsis but are not always widely available in the prehospital setting include capnography, serum glucose levels, serum lactate levels, ultrasonography and central venous pressures.

Treatment of Sepsis

Sepsis is a life-threatening condition and as such, prehospital treatment of septic shock must be aggressive. Practitioners should ensure adequate oxygenation and rapid fluid infusion. The goal of fluid resuscitation in septic patients is to restore perfusion to the tissues and organs of the body. If a patient's status deteriorates, we must reassess the primary survey and ensure that no further airway management interventions are required. Other treatments include:

- Paracetamol administration if clinically indicated in pyrexia patients.
- Broad spectrum antibiotics (until a more targeted antibiotic can be used when the results of blood cultures are available).
- Oxygen therapy to maintain saturations as per local guidelines.
- Vasopressor or inotrope infusion titrated to effect where available where regular fluid resuscitation is ineffective.

We should also ensure that we have pre-alerted the receiving facility for an incoming patient with suspected septic shock, so they can prepare as required and ensure optimal patient treatment. Patients in severe sepsis are acutely unwell, so we should always be mindful of the possibility of the need for cardiopulmonary resuscitation.

External Considerations

We must be mindful of external considerations when we are discussing the blood and its associated disorders. Many patients we encounter in the prehospital field are on numerous medications, many of which can influence how the blood works and its clotting factors. Atrial fibrillation is an extremely common cardiac rhythm. Many of the elderly patients we encounter have a history of this condition, which comes with associated risks of clots. Clots put these patients at higher risks of stroke, so many such patients are treated with warfarin or novel oral anticoagulants, both being blood-thinning medications.

When we are dealing with patients who are bleeding either internally or externally and we are aware that these patients take these medications daily, it is important that we understand the complexities involved in treating them. Patients who are on these medications have increased bleeding time and are at far higher risks of, for example, intracranial haemorrhage in the case of a simple fall. They should be treated with the utmost care and brought to the appropriate facility in a timely manner. In the prehospital field, we do not have the ability to rule intracranial haemorrhage in or out and it is important that these patients are not left at home.

Intracranial Bleeding

We should suspect internal bleeding in the brain in any patient who has had trauma to the head and/or is showing any signs of acute neurological impairment. Clinical presentations range from nausea and vomiting, confusion, seizures, dizziness, headaches, abnormal speech to complete loss of consciousness and ultimately death (Caroline 2014). Obviously, it is not only patients who have had trauma who can present with intracranial bleeding, but also those who are on non-vitamin K oral anticoagulants or warfarin. From a prehospital perspective, assessments such as blood pressure and a pupil assessment can be good indicators of intracranial bleeding when coupled with the clinical presentation present and the history of the event preceding the injury. As practitioners, we must be vigilant of any increase in intracranial pressure, which is the pressure within the cranial vault (Caroline 2014). Early signs of an increase in this pressure can be vomiting and headaches, and in later stages, can be Cushing's triad of hypertension (with a widening pulse pressure), bradycardia and irregular respirations (Caroline 2014).

Clots are far more common in cerebral vascular accidents than in haemorrhages. It is important that we find out quickly whether patients are on any blood thinners, as this can alter their treatment pathways.

Treatment of Intracranial Haemorrhage

From a prehospital perspective, there is little we can do for a patient who is having an acute intracranial haemorrhage. In hospital, this can often be reversed by treatments such as craniotomies or medications. Stroke patients who are taking these blood thinning medications can often have poor outcomes due to the complications of trying to reverse the adverse effects off their prescribed medications. Patients who are on the newer novel oral anticoagulants, such as apixaban, can have difficulty in having their medications reversed. Patients who are on warfarin, however, can be treated in hospital with vitamin K (Hanley 2004), which has been proven to have good outcomes in patients with haemorrhagic stroke. Our role as prehospital practitioners is to identify the clinical presentation that points towards an intracranial haemorrhage, manage the condition as best we can and promptly transport the patient to the relevant primary care facility, ideally one which has a neurological centre. We can manage clinical presentations of these patients such as a headache, nausea/vomiting and seizures with intravenous paracetamol, antiemetics and anticonvulsants in the prehospital field, but we cannot treat intracranial haemorrhage outside of the hospital. As for external bleeding, these conditions are far more difficult to manage to stop the haemorrhage.

Finally, as prehospital practitioners, we must also be aware of other blood disorders that we can often come across in our prehospital care. It is important that we understand these conditions and are aware of the complications which can arise from them. Common disorders and diseases apart from those mentioned above include leukaemia, vitamin K deficiency and haemophilia.

Red Flag Alert: Intracranial Haemorrhage

The only way in which we can determine the severity of intracranial haemorrhage is by radiological assessments. This is time critical, and the patient needs to have a CT (computed tomography) scan at the earliest opportunity to improve their outcome.

Leukaemia

Leukaemia is cancer of the body's blood-forming tissues, including the bone marrow and the lymphatic system. It results in the uncontrolled increase in the production of leucocytes. Unlike other cancers, leukaemia does not form into a mass that can be seen in radiological imaging such as x-ray. In the UK, leukaemia is the 12th most common cancer in adults, with two principal types being found: acute and chronic leukaemia. Each of these is further subdivided:

- Acute myeloid leukaemia (AML)
- Acute lymphoblastic leukaemia (ALL)
- Chronic myeloid leukaemia (CML)
- Chronic lymphoblastic leukaemia (CLL).

Risk factors for these leukaemias include exposure to radiation, smoking, age, previous cancer treatments and diseases that affect the immune system (Peate 2019).

Pathophysiology of Leukaemia

The production of white blood cells occurs in the bone marrow. From here, the cells pass from the bone marrow, into the bloodstream and then the lymphatic system (Peate 2019). White blood cells are involved in various functions of the body's immune system, as outlined above, which protects the body against infections. Acute leukaemia is more aggressive and develops rapidly. It is more often found in the younger age group. Leukaemic cells are immature and poorly differentiated; they proliferate rapidly, have a long lifespan and do not function normally (Peate 2019). Leukaemia itself can cause anaemia, thrombocytopenia (reduction of platelets in the blood) and leukopenia (a decrease in the white blood cells) while also been known to produce an extremely high white blood cell count.

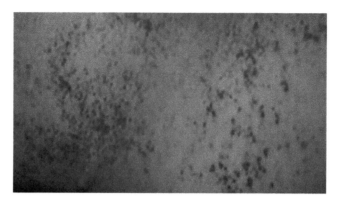

FIGURE 8.8   Petechiae. Source: Watson (2023)/Healthline Media LLC.

Clinical Presentation

Leukaemia presents itself differently in patients, depending on the stage of the leukaemia and the patient's current treatment. Typically, patients with leukaemia complain of fatigue, headaches, dyspnoea and or can have signs of neurological defects (Caroline 2014). If the patients are undergoing current chemotherapy or radiotherapy for their condition, they are also at higher risk of infection, so a thorough assessment of all history and vital signs is required. At times, these patients may be reluctant to call an ambulance as they do not like going into hospitals any more than is necessary, so they can often present with significant signs of septic shock and need to be treated immediately. Signs of bleeding in patients with cancer which can often be overlooked are petechia (Figure 8.8), ecchymosis and bruising (Belfance and Limmer 2014).

Treatment

As with all patients, airway support and oxygen therapy should be commenced as appropriate. There may also be a need for fluid therapy and analgesia, depending on the patient's presentation (Caroline 2014).

If the patient is presenting with signs of septic shock, they should be administered intravenous antibiotics as per local guidelines as early as possible. If they are to be transported to hospital, especially if they are unwell, it is important to find out the patient's and family's wishes about what to do should the patient go into cardiac arrest. If they do not wish to be transported to hospital, you should liaise with the ambulance control centre for on-call advice, palliative care teams, the patient's general practitioner and other health care professionals, as required.

Orange Flag Alert: Mental Health Support

Patients with leukaemia typically require continual positive support as they often have a negative outlook towards their medical condition. Their support network may also require reassure and guidance, as they may be unsure about the condition and why their loved-one might be deteriorating.

Haemophilia

Haemophilia is a haematological disorder in which clotting does not occur or is insufficient (Caroline 2014). It is primarily classified into two types.

1. Type A is due to low levels of factor VII (antihemophilic globulin and antihemophilic factor).
2. Type B is associated with a deficiency of factor IX (plasma thromboplastin component).

Caroline (2014) discusses how the levels of factors VIII and IX determine the severity of the disease. Spontaneous intracranial haemorrhage is common in haemophilia and is a major cause of death in these patients.

Clinical Presentation

Haemophiliacs can suffer from acute and chronic bleeding, which can occur at any time. This bleeding can at times be life threatening and at other times of no acute concern to the paramedic.

With patients suffering from haemophilia, it is important we are on the lookout for signs of acute blood loss. Signs such as pale skin, weak pulses and hypotension are of great concern to the practitioner looking after these patients. One should also take note of any haemorrhage of unknown origin, such as epistaxis, haemostasias, haematuria or melaena (Caroline 2014). In these patients, any blood loss can result in a reduced blood oxygen level (SpO$_2$) reading as there is a decrease in the oxygen carrying capacity of the blood.

Red Flag Alert: Bleeding in Haemophilia

Any injury or illness which can cause bleeding must not be dismissed in any patient with haemophilia. This could be fatal to a haemophilia patient.

Treatment

As with all patients in a haematological emergency, treat findings as appropriate. Often, people who have certain diseases are more informed about the condition than we are, so it is important that we ask them any necessary questions. In an acute episode of bleeding, the patient requires the replacement of the missing clotting factor through intravenous administration. We should treat bleeding in these patients in the same way that we do with any other external bleeding, with direct pressure and pad/bandages. However, with patients with haemophilia, one should have a much higher concern regarding internal bleeding. For example, in many patients, some swelling following a fall is not a major cause for alarm; however, in a patient with haemophilia, the concern is that the swelling is not caused by oedema but from a broken blood vessel which is now bleeding into the joint or tissue (Greenhaus 2020).

The most important treatment we can give as prehospital providers is to ensure timely transport to an appropriate facility. Prehospital interventions such as the administration of TXA can be used to treat haemophilia. TXA binds to a protein called plasminogen in the blood. Plasminogen is normally converted to an enzyme called plasmin, which degrades clots and digests or degrades clotting factors. By binding to plasminogen and preventing its conversion to plasmin, TXA increases the amount of clotting factor in the blood and encourages clot formation, as newly forming clots are not being digested as quickly by plasmin. TXA can be used alone in treating mild or moderate haemophilia or in combination with clotting factors in severe haemophilia.

173

Summary

This chapter has discussed some of the most dangerous areas of the body in which bleeding can occur that we may encounter in the prehospital field. As prehospital providers, we need to have a good underpinning knowledge of these areas, how they are best treated and what pertinent interventions we can make to help provide positive outcomes to our patients. We also discussed different blood disorders and the pathophysiology behind these conditions. It is by our knowledge that we can identify these conditions and make the correct decisions in relation to our patient's care. It is our duty to ensure that each of our patients receives the most accurate information possible in relation to their disease or condition and that we provide the necessary care.

References

Ashburn, N.P., Hendley, N.W., Angi, R.M. et al. (2020). Prehospital trauma scene and transport times for pediatric and adult patients. *Western Journal of Emergency Medicine* 21 (2): 455–462.

Belfance, B. and Limmer, D. (2014). EMS response to the cancer patient. *EMS World* (October). https://www.hmpgloballearningnetwork.com/site/emsworld/article/11653565/ems-response-cancer-patient (accessed 4 October 2023).

Berndt, M., Metharom, P., and Andrews, R. (2014). Primary haemostasis: newer insights. *Haemophilia* 20 (Suppl 4): 15–22.

Caroline, N. (2014). *Emergency Care in the Streets*, 7e. Burlington, MA: Jones & Bartlett Learning.

Elling, B. and Elling, K. (2015). *Anatomy & Physiology for the Prehospital Provider*, 2e. Burlington: Jones & Bartlett Learning.

Forrest, M., Lax, P., and van der Velde, J. (ed.) (2014). *Anaesthesia, Trauma and Critical Care Course Manual 2014*, 8e. Warrington: ATACC Group.

Greenhaus, D. (2020). Hemophilia: when the bleeding won't stop. *EMS World* (June). http://hmpgloballearningnetwork.com/site/emsworld/article/1224422/hemophilia-when-the-bleeding-wont-stop (accessed 4 October 2023).

Hanley, J.P. (2004). Warfarin reversal. *Journal of Clinical Pathology* 57 (11): 1132–1139.

Irish Blood Ttansfusion Service. (n.d.) Blood group basics. https://www.giveblood.ie/learn-about-blood/blood_group_basics (accessed 4 October 2023).

Li, S.R.M. et al. (2021). Early prehospital tranexamic acid following injury is associated with a 30-day survival benefit. *Annals of Surgery* 3 (274): 419–426.

Mader, S. (2011). *Understanding Human Anatomy and Physiology*, 5e. Boston, MA: McGraw Hill.

Peate, I. (2019). *Fundamentals of Applied Pathophysiology: An Essential Guide for Nursing and Healthcare Students*, 3e. Chichester: Wiley.

PHECC (2021). *Clincial Practice Guidelines: Advanced Paramedic*, 7e (updated 2023). Naas, Ireland: Pre-Hospital Emergency Care Council.

Sampalis, J.S., Lavoie, A., Williams, J.I. et al. (1993). Impact of on-site care, prehospital time, and level of in-hospital care on survival in severely injured patients. *Journal of Trauma* 34 (2): 252–261.

Standfield, C. (2011). *Principles of Human Physiology*, 4e. Boston, MA: Benjamin Cummings.

Watson, S. (2023). What causes petechiae? *Healthline* (25 August). https://www.healthline.com/health/petechiae (accessed 4 October 2023).

Waugh, A. and Grant, A. (2018). *Ross and Wilson Anatomy and Physiology in Health and Illness*, 13e. Edinburgh: Elsevier.

Further Reading

National Association of Emergency Medical Technicians (2014). *Prehospital Trauma Life Support*, 8e. Burlington, MA: Jones & Bartlett.

National Association of Emergency Medical Technicians (2017). *AMLS Advanced Medical Life Support: An assessment-based approach*, 2e. Burlingtown, MA: Jones and Bartlett Learning.

Peate, I. and Evans, S. (ed.) (2021). *The Fundamentals of Anatomy and Physiology for Nursing and Healthcare Students*, 3e. Oxford: Wiley.

Waugh, A. and Grant, A. (2018). *Ross and Wilson Anatomy and Physiology in Health and Illness*, 13e. Edinburgh: Elsevier.

Online Resources

NHS England. Symptoms: sepsis. https://www.nhs.uk/conditions/sepsis (accessed 30 October 2023).

Nickson, C. (2020). Trauma! pelvic fractures II. *Life in the Fast Lane* 3 November. https://litfl.com/trauma-pelvic-fractures-ii (accessed 3 October 2023).

Glossary

Adenosine diphosphate	Molecular store of chemical energy for chemical reactions.
Agglutination	The clumping of antigenic particles.
Antibody	Defensive blood protein used by B-lymphocytes in response to the presence of an antigen.
Antigen	A substance that stimulates the body's immunological defences.
Blood groupa	Any of various classes into which human blood can be divided according to immunological compatibility, based on the presence or absence of specific antigens on red blood cells.
Bone marrow	The soft fatty vascular tissue found in the interior cavities of bones that is a major site of blood cell production.
Capillary	A tiny blood vessel between an arteriole and a venule, which has leaky walls to allow exchange of substances between the blood and the tissues.
Centrifugation	The process by which blood is separated into it separate components by rotating at high speed.
Coagulation	Blood clotting.
Contusion	A bruise.
Erythrocyte	Another name for a red blood cell.
Erythropoiesis	The production of red blood cells.
Haematological emergency	An acute life-threatening condition in haematological disease.
Haematopoietic Tissues	Bone marrow, peripheral blood and certain lymphoid tissue.
Haemoglobin	Part of an erythrocyte. It binds to oxygen giving blood its red colour.
Haemostasis	The stopping of blood flow.
Hormone	A substance produced by an endocrine glad and transported in blood to stimulate specific cells or tissue into action.
Hypotension	Abnormally low blood pressure.
Hypoxia	Inadequate levels of oxygen in the tissues.
Leucocytes	White blood cells
Leukaemia	Cancer of the bone marrow that prevents the normal manufacture of red and white blood cells and platelets, resulting in anaemia, increased susceptibility to infection and impaired blood clotting.
Molecule	A particle containing two or more atoms which are connected by chemical bonds.
Pathogens	A micro-organism capable of causing disease.
Permissive hypotension	The act of maintaining a blood pressure lower than physiological levels in a patient who has suffered from haemorrhagic blood loss. It is used to maintain adequate vasoconstriction and organ perfusion.
pH	A measure of the acidity or alkalinity of a solution.
Plasma	Clear, straw-coloured liquid portion of the blood.
Platelets	Small cell fragments found in blood involved in blood clotting.
Sepsis	The destruction of tissues by disease causing bacteria or their toxins.
Shock	A clinical syndrome resulting from inadequate tissue and organ perfusion because of decreased blood volume or circulatory stagnation.
Sickle cell disease	A hereditary blood disease that mainly affects people of African ancestry. It is characterised by the production of abnormal haemoglobin in red blood cells, distorting them into characteristic sickle shapes, which may block small blood vessels causing severe pain.
Vasoconstriction	The constriction of blood vessels, which increases blood pressure.

Multiple Choice Questions

1. Which of these is not a function of the blood?
   a. Respiration
   b. Excretion
   c. Regulation
   d. All of the above are functions

2. What is the most common blood group?
   a. A
   b. B
   c. O
   d. AB

3. In sickle cell anaemia, the red blood cell count is:
   a. Reduced
   b. Increased
   c. Normal
   d. Zero

4. How many classifications are there for haemorrhagic shock?
   a. One
   b. Two
   c. Three
   d. Four

5. Sickle cell anaemia is genetic: true or false?
   a. True
   b. False

6. An abnormally low platelet count is known as:
   a. Leukaemia
   b. Lymphoma
   c. Thrombocytopenia
   d. Anaemia

7. Which of the following is not a dangerous area of bleeding?
   a. Femur
   b. Lower limbs
   c. Head
   d. Chest

8. Which is the more common type of haemophilia?
   a. Type A
   b. Type B
   c. Both are equally common

9. If bleeding is spurting and bright red, it is:
   a. Capillary bleeding
   b. Arterial bleeding
   c. Venous bleeding
   d. All the above

10. Proteins make up what percentage of the plasma of the blood?

    a. 3%

    b. 7%

    c. 10%

    d. 14%

CHAPTER **9**

The Renal System and Associated Disorders

Liam Rooney

AIM

The aim of this chapter is to investigate and explore some common renal disorders, relate them to normal physiology and examine treatment modalities available to paramedics.

LEARNING OUTCOMES

After completing this chapter, you will be able to:

- Understand the normal anatomy and physiology of the renal system.
- Expand your knowledge of some renal disorders you may encounter as a paramedic.
- Understand and remember terminology used to describe urine output.
- Develop an understanding on the effects of medications on renal function.

Test Your Prior Knowledge

1. Name all parts of the renal system.
2. Name four common renal disorders.
3. What effect can renal impairment have on other body systems?
4. What is the difference between acute kidney injury and chronic kidney disease?
5. What type of traumatic injuries to the renal system would a paramedic expect to encounter?

Introduction

The renal system, also known as the urinary system, plays an important role in maintaining homeostasis of water and electrolyte concentrations in the body. Cells consume oxygen and nutrients during metabolic activity and produce waste products such as carbon dioxide, urea and uric acid. These waste products can be toxic if they accumulate, so must be

Fundamentals of Applied Pathophysiology for Paramedics, First Edition. Edited by Ian Peate and Simon Sawyer.
© 2024 John Wiley & Sons Ltd. Published 2024 by John Wiley & Sons Ltd.

expelled from the body. While the respiratory system expels carbon dioxide, the renal system disposes of most other waste, including the nitrogenous compounds urea and uric acid, excess ions and, sometimes, excreted drugs. It does this by removing waste products from blood and excreting them in urine by micturition. The renal system also helps to regulate blood composition, pH, volume and pressure. It also maintains blood osmolarity and produces hormones (Waugh and Grant 2018).

The renal system (Figure 9.1) consists of:

- Two kidneys, which secrete urine.
- Two ureters, which carry urine from the kidneys to the urinary bladder.
- The urinary bladder, which collects and stores urine.
- The urethra, through which urine is excreted.

Kidneys

The kidneys are bean-shaped organs, typically 11–12 cm long, 5–7 cm wide, 3 cm thick and weighing 135–150 g. They are positioned just above the waist between the peritoneum and the posterior wall of the abdomen, in the retroperitoneal space, one on each side of the vertebral column between the levels of the 12th thoracic vertebra and the 3rd lumbar vertebra, giving them some protection by the lower ribcage. The right kidney is slightly lower than the left, due to the space occupied superiorly by the liver.

External Structure

The external structure of the kidney is shown in Figure 9.2. The indentation on the concave medial border of each kidney is called the renal hilum or renal hilus. This is where the ureters, nerves, lymphatic vessels and blood vessels emerge from the kidneys. Three layers of tissue cover and surround each kidney:

- *Renal fascia* – a thin outer layer of connective tissue that anchors the kidney to the abdominal wall and surrounding structures.
- *Adipose tissue* – the middle layer of fatty tissue surrounding the renal capsule.
- *Renal capsule* – a smooth inner layer of tissue that is continuous with the outer layer of the ureter.

179

Internal Structure

The internal structure of the kidney is shown in Figure 9.2. The renal cortex is the outermost part of the kidney, a reddish-brown layer of tissue immediately below the renal capsule surrounding the renal pyramids. The medulla consists of pale, cone-shaped renal pyramids. The base of each pyramid faces the renal cortex, while the apex points towards the renal hilum and is called a renal papilla. Together, the renal cortex and renal medulla constitute the parenchyma of the kidney. Within this parenchyma, there is an abundance of blood vessels and more than one million microscopic structures called nephrons. Filtrate from the nephron passes through large papillary ducts in the renal papilla and into cuplike structures called the minor and major calyces. As no further reabsorption can take place in the calyces, the filtrate becomes urine. From here, the urine drains into a large cavity called the renal pelvis, then to the ureter and on to the bladder (Tortora and Derrickson 2017).

Nephrons

Nephrons filter blood, perform selective reabsorption and excrete unwanted waste products from the filtered blood. Although small in mass, the kidneys receive 20–25% of cardiac output via the right and left renal arteries. Renal blood flow through both kidneys equates to approximately 1200 ml/minute in adults. Each nephron is about 3 cm long and

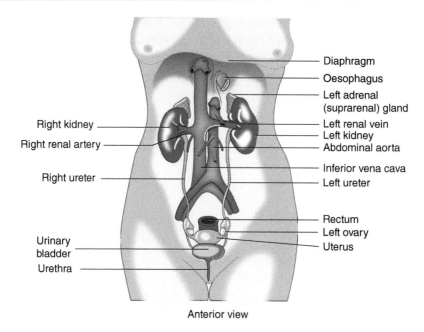

Anterior view

FIGURE 9.1   Renal system, anterior view (female). Source: Peate (2018).

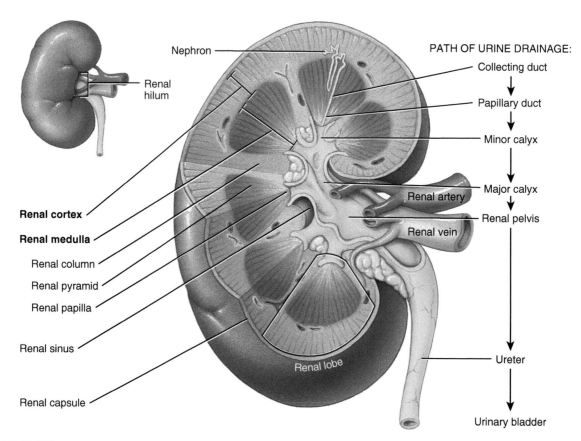

FIGURE 9.2   Anatomy of the kidney (anterior view, right kidney). Source: Tortora and Derrickson (2017).

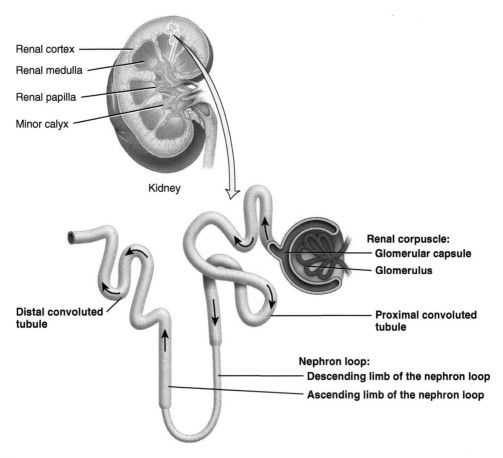

Renal cortex

Renal medulla

Renal papilla

Minor calyx

Kidney

Renal corpuscle:
Glomerular capsule
Glomerulus

Distal convoluted
tubule

Proximal convoluted
tubule

Nephron loop:
Descending limb of the nephron loop
Ascending limb of the nephron loop

FIGURE 9.3 Components of a nephron. Source: Tortora and Derrickson (2017).

181

loops through the renal medulla, giving the pyramids their distinctive striated appearance. Nephrons are divided into several sections (capsules), each of which has a different function. The renal corpuscle consists of the glomerular (Bowman's) capsule, a cup-shaped capsule that surrounds a collection of capillaries, called the glomerulus. Blood is filtered in the glomerular capsule and the filtrate is passed into the renal tubule, which consists of three sections (Figure 9.3):

- The cells lining the *proximal convoluted tubule* actively reabsorb water, nutrients and ions from the filtrate into the interstitial fluid surrounding the renal tubule.
- The *nephron loop* (*loop of Henle*), is divided into descending and ascending loops, the ascending loop being thicker than the descending, which results in less reabsorption in this part of the nephron.
- The *distal convoluted tubule* is where active secretion of ions and acids and selective reabsorption of water, sodium, and calcium ions occur (Peate 2018).

Multiple nephrons drain into collecting ducts, which unite into papillary ducts and empty into minor and major calyces through the renal pelvis and excrete via micturition. The number of nephrons is constant from birth. If nephrons become diseased or injured, new ones do not form; the remaining nephrons adapt and deal with the additional load. In fact, declining kidney function may not become apparent until function is less than 25% of normal due to this adaptability. Removal of one kidney, for example, stimulates hypertrophy of the remaining kidney; nephrons become larger and are eventually able to filter blood at 80% of the rate of two kidneys (Tortora and Derrickson 2017).

Renal Physiology

Metabolised cellular waste, control of water and electrolyte levels and the excretion of hydrogen ions to maintain pH balance makes up the composition of urine. To form urine, there is an exchange of substances between the nephron and the blood in the renal capillaries. The following three processes are performed:

1. *Filtration* is the first step of urine production. Water and other solutes move across the semipermeable wall of the glomerulus, where they are filtered into the glomerular capsule and then into the renal tubule. The composition of this filtrate will be adjusted as it moves through the other sections of the renal tubule. Molecules too large to filter here, such as blood cells, platelets, plasma proteins and some drugs, remain in the capillaries.

2. *Selective reabsorption* – most reabsorption of the filtrate back into the blood takes place in the proximal convoluted tubule. Substances such as sodium, calcium, potassium and chloride are reabsorbed to maintain fluid and electrolyte balance and the blood pH. However, if these substances are excess to the body's requirements, they are excreted in the urine. Some 60–70% of the filtrate reaches the nephron loop. By the time that it reaches the distal convoluted tubule, only 15–20% of the original filtrate remains. The composition of this filtrate is now very different. More electrolytes are reabsorbed here, especially sodium, so the fluid entering the collecting ducts is now quite dilute. The main function of the collecting ducts is to reabsorb as much water as the body requires.

3. *Secretion* – any substance not removed by filtration, either because of the short time they remain in the glomerulus or because the molecules are too large to pass through the semipermeable wall, are secreted into the renal tubule by the peritubular capillaries which surround the convoluted tubules length. These substances include hydrogen ions, ammonium ions, potassium ions, creatinine and certain drugs, such as penicillin and aspirin (Waugh and Grant 2018; Lazenby 2011).

Composition of Urine

Adults normally pass approximately 1–1.5 l of urine each day. Fluid intake, blood pressure, diet, body temperature, mental state and overall general health all influence urine volume. Urine is approximately 95% water and 5% solutes and electrolytes. Typical solutes present in urine include urea (from the breakdown of protein), creatinine (from the breakdown of creatine in muscle fibres), uric acid (from the breakdown of nucleic acids), urobilinogen (from the breakdown of haemoglobin) and small quantities of other substances such as fatty acids, pigments, enzymes and hormones. The amber colour of urine is due to the pigmented substance urobilin, which is generated from haemolysis when some urobilinogen is converted to urobilin.

When disease alters kidney function or body metabolism, substances not normally present may appear in urine, or normal solutes may appear in abnormal quantities. Examples would be glucosuria (excessive glucose), which may indicate diabetes mellitus, or haematuria (red blood cells), which may indicate a pathological condition, such as kidney stones.

Regulating Blood Pressure: the Renin–Angiotensin–Aldosterone System

The renin–angiotensin–aldosterone system is a series of reactions occurring in the kidney to aid in the regulation of blood pressure. Figure 9.4 outlines the process.

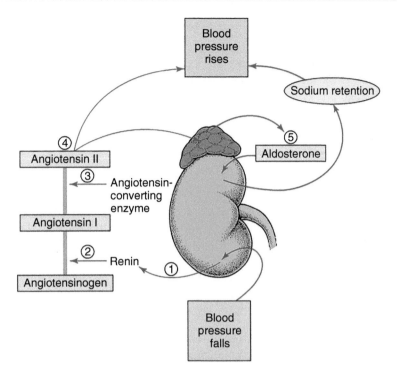

FIGURE 9.4 Steps involved in the regulation of blood pressure through the renin–angiotensin–aldosterone system. (1) When systolic blood pressure falls to 100 mmHg or lower, the kidneys release the enzyme renin into the circulatory system. (2) Renin splits angiotensin, a large protein which circulates in the bloodstream, into pieces. One of these pieces in angiotensin I. (3) This is split by angiotensin-converting enzyme. One of these pieces, angiotensin II is a very potent and active hormone. (4) Angiotensin II causes vasoconstriction, increasing blood pressure. (5) It also initiates the release of the hormone, aldosterone from the adrenal glands and the antidiuretic hormone (vasopressin) from the pituitary gland. Both hormones cause the kidneys to retain sodium. This increased sodium causes water to be retained, therefore, increasing blood volume and blood pressure. Source:MerckManual.https://www.merckmanuals.com/home/multimedia/figure/regulating-blood-pressure-the-renin-angiotensin-aldosterone-system.

Ureters

Ureters carry urine from the kidneys to the urinary bladder. They are hollow muscular tubes about 25–30 cm in length and vary in diameter between 1 and 10 mm along their course from the renal pelvis to the urinary bladder. The ureters enter the urinary bladder obliquely through the posterior muscle wall of the bladder. This physiological arrangement means as urine accumulates in the bladder and pressure increases, the ureter openings are compressed preventing backflow of urine back towards the kidneys. When this physiological valve is not working properly, microbes from urine may travel back up the ureters, causing infection in one or both kidneys.

The ureters have three layers:

- Inner layer of transitional epithelium
- Middle layer of smooth muscle
- Outer layer of fibrous connective tissue.

This smooth muscle propels urine along the ureters by peristalsis, several times a minute, emptying small amounts of urine into the urinary bladder each time (Tortora and Derrickson 2017).

Urinary Bladder

The urinary bladder is a hollow, distensible muscular organ located in the pelvic cavity posterior to the symphysis pubis. In males, it is directly anterior to the rectum, and in females it lies anterior to the vagina and inferior to the uterus. The bladder is roughly pear shaped but as it becomes distended with urine it becomes more spherical. Capacity varies between 350 and 600 ml.

The urinary bladder has three layers (Figure 9.5):

- Inner layer of transitional epithelial mucosa
- Middle layer of smooth muscle and elastic tissue call the detrusor muscle
- Outer layer of loose connective tissue, covered by the peritoneum.

Discharge of urine (micturition) occurs through a combination of voluntary and involuntary muscular contractions. When the volume of urine in the bladder exceeds 200–400 ml, stretch receptors in the bladder wall transmit nerve impulses to the spinal cord and trigger a spinal reflex known as the micturition reflex. This reflex causes contraction of the detrusor muscle and relaxation of the internal urethral sphincter muscle. Filling of the urinary bladder instigates a desire to urinate before the micturition reflex occurs. Although voiding of the bladder is a reflex, as children, we learn to initiate and stop it voluntarily. Through this learned control of the external urethral sphincter muscle and some pelvic floor muscles, we can initiate urination or delay it for a limited period (Tortora and Derrickson 2017).

Urinary Incontinence

There are several types of urinary incontinence, and all have slightly different pathophysiological causes (NHS England 2023):

- *Stress incontinence* is usually the result of the weakening of or damage to the muscles used to prevent urination – the pelvic floor muscles and the urethral sphincters. Incontinence occurs when physical pressure is placed on the bladder (e.g. coughing or laughing).

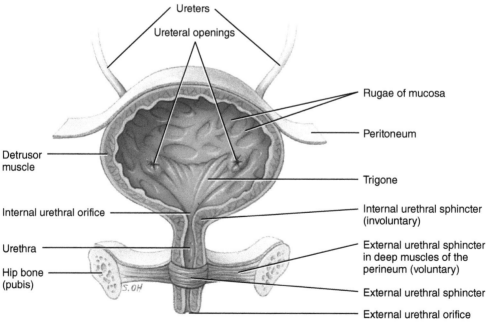

Anterior view of frontal section

FIGURE 9.5   Layers of the urinary bladder. Source: Peate (2018).

- *Urge incontinence* is usually caused by overactivity of the detrusor muscles. These muscles normally control the storage and discharge of urine from the bladder. When this occurs, one may feel an intense pressure or urge to urinate.
- *Overflow incontinence* is often caused by an obstruction or blockage in the bladder. The blockage prevents the bladder from emptying fully, causing urine to leak.
- *Continuous incontinence* happens when the bladder is not be able to store urine at all, causing continuous leakage. This may be caused by a birth defect, a spinal injury or a bladder fistula.

There are some conditions which may increase the chance of urinary incontinence developing, such as:

- Pregnancy and vaginal birth
- Obesity
- Familial history
- Age
- Brain and spinal cord disease.

Urethra

The urethra is a small tube leading from the internal urethral orifice and drains urine from the body. In males, the urethra is approximately 20 cm in length and passes through three distinct regions: first through the prostate, then through the peritoneum and the pelvic diaphragm, and finally through the through the penis (Figure 9.6). The female urethra is shorter at approximately 4 cm long and is bound to the anterior vaginal wall. The external urethral orifice is located between the

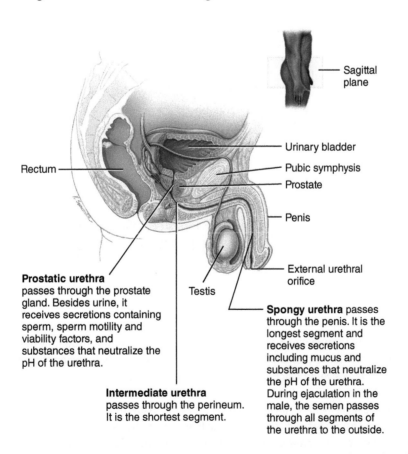

FIGURE 9.6 Sagittal section through the pelvis showing the male urethra. Source: Tortora and Derrickson (2017).

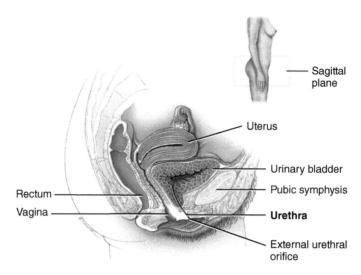

FIGURE 9.7   Sagittal section through the pelvis showing the female urethra. Source: Tortora and Derrickson (2017).

clitoris and the vaginal opening (Figure 9.7). While it is a common duct for both urinary and reproductive systems in males, the urethra is entirely separate from the female reproductive system.

Disorders of the Renal System

As discussed earlier, the renal system plays an important role in maintaining homeostasis of numerous other body systems, so it follows that a range of systemic diseases and diseases of other organ systems may manifest in the kidneys. For example, chronic kidney disease (CKD) is a common presentation in patients with long-standing diabetes, hypertension and some autoimmune disorders. Patients may be completely asymptomatic until quite advanced kidney failure is present. As the internal structures of the kidneys have no pain receptors, pain will only be present in those disorders that involve the renal capsule, ureter, urinary bladder and urethras. Early-stage kidney disease may present with urine abnormalities, and as disease progresses, systemic symptoms and signs of lost renal function may be diagnosed, such as oedema, fluid overload, anaemia or electrolyte imbalance. A wide range of chronic complications due to the nature of the presenting renal disease may be seen in patients, and it is important for the paramedic to recognise these complications to understand the pathophysiological basis behind the many different presentations of kidney disease (McPhee and Hammer 2019). Table 9.1 lists common signs and symptoms of renal disorders.

Renal Calculi

Renal calculi or kidney stones are formed when crystals of salts, normally in solution, solidify in any part of the urinary tract. They are quite common with more than 1 in 10 people affected and usually between the ages of 30 and 60 years. While both men and women may develop calculi, they are more prevalent in men. While small calculi may be easily passed through urination, larger stones may become lodged in the urinary tract and may need to be broken up or surgically removed. Causes of renal calculi includes low water intake leading to low urine output, a high-protein, low-fibre diet, recurring urinary/kidney infections, metabolic conditions, such as gout or hyperparathyroidism and raised pH of urine. Some medications are also known to increase the risk of developing renal calculi. These include, aspirin, antacids, diuretics, some antibiotics, some antiviral medications and certain antiseizure medications (NHS England 2022).

TABLE 9.1   Common signs and symptoms of disorders of the urinary system.

Sign/symptom	Definition and description
Oliguria	Urine output of less than 400 ml/d
Anuria	Absence of urine
Dysuria	Pain on passing urine, often described as a burning sensation
Polyuria	Passing unusually large amounts of urine
Nocturia	Passing urine at night while sleeping
Incontinence	Involuntary loss of urine
Frequency	The need to pass urine frequently, usually in small amounts
Urgency	Sudden compelling need to urinate
Haematuria	Presence of blood in the urine
Proteinuria	Presence of protein in the urine
Glycosuria	Presence of glucose in the urine
Ketonuria	Presence of ketones in the urine

Source: Waugh and Grant (2018).

Patients with renal calculi will commonly present with haematuria and acute, severe flank pain that will often radiate to the abdomen and groin. It is sometimes described as being colicky pain, referring to the spasm-like pain caused by muscle contractions around a partial or complete blockage of the urinary tract. Nausea and vomiting are often reported. If there is an infection present, patients may present with fever, chills or other systemic signs of infection. Prehospital management should include intravenous hydration, if required, analgesia and antiemetic medications (Leslie et al. 2022).

Snapshot 9.1

Pre-arrival Information

A 48-year-old man in a city centre hotel is complaining of constant right-sided flank pain.

Control and Dispatch Information

Time of call: 3.30 a.m.
Information received: 48 year-old man, vomiting and abdominal/back pain
Resources tasked: ambulance (2 × paramedics)
On scene: 3.45 a.m.
Depart scene: 4:30 a.m.
At hospital: 4:38 a.m.

On Arrival with the Patient

On arrival, you are taken to a hotel room by the manager, where you find the patient in considerable distress sitting on the side of the bed, currently vomiting into a small bin. Appropriate personal protection equipment for dealing with this patient would include gloves, mask and eye protection for maximum infection control.

Background Information

The patient is visiting the city for a stag weekend. He has been drinking alcohol heavily for the previous two days. Pain started 12+ hours ago and has progressively worsened. He began vomiting one hour previously. He hasn't eaten since 6 p.m. His last alcohol intake was at 11 p.m.

Patient Assessment

Primary survey reveals an alert patient with a patent airway, respiratory rate 20+, pulse tachycardic, strong radial pulse.

Vital Signs

Initial vital signs measured at 3:50 a.m.

Vital sign	Observation	Normal range
Pulse (beats/min)	110 tachycardic	80–100 regular
Respiration rate (breaths/min)	23	12–20
SpO$_2$ (%)	98 (room air)	94–98
Capillary refill (s)	<2	<2
Blood pressure (mmHg)	160/80	120/80
Eyes	4	4 – spontaneously
Verbal	5	5 – orientated
Motor	6	6 – obeys commands
Total GCS score	15	15
Temperature (°C)	36.8	37
Pupils	4+/4+	Equal, round, reactive
Blood glucose (mmol/l)	6.4	
Pain score	10/10	

Allergies: no known allergies.
Medications: allopurinol, atorvastatin, OTC antacids.
Past medical history: gout, hypercholesterolaemia.
Last intake: water at 3 a.m.

On Examination

Respiratory: Increased work of breathing, normal bilateral breath sounds, respiration rate 23 breaths/minute, symmetrical chest movement.
Cardiovascular: No cyanosis, pale, diaphoretic, normal heart sounds. 12-lead ECG reveals sinus tachycardia.
Abdominal: reports unrelenting right-sided flank pain, coming in waves. Denies dysuria, reports haematuria. Significant nausea with two episodes of vomiting. No abdominal distension, examination unremarkable, right flank tenderness. Unable to find a comfortable position.

Repeat observations:

Vital sign	4.05 a.m.	4:20 a.m.
Pulse (beats/min)	Pulse 115 regular	105 regular
Respiration rate (breaths/min)	22	22
SpO_2 (%)	98%	98
Blood pressure (mmHg)	162/84	155/78

Reflective Learning Activity

Reflect on the information in Snapshot 9.1 and consider the following:

1. What is your working diagnosis for this patient?
2. Outline your treatment plan for this patient that will manage his pain, his nausea and vomiting, and his comfort levels.
3. What would be an appropriate analgesic in this instance?
4. What is the most likely cause of his renal calculus?
5. Why is this disorder so painful?

Medications Management: Ibuprofen

Paramedics have a wide choice of analgesic medications in their armamentarium. The choice they make must be an educated one, especially in those patients with renal impairment. Non-steroidal anti-inflammatory drugs such as ibuprofen, a medication widely used by paramedics, should be avoided in patients with impaired renal function. Ibuprofen may cause the retention of sodium, potassium and fluid in patients who have not previously suffered from renal impairment, because of its effect on renal perfusion. This may lead to oedema, hypertension or cardiac insufficiency in susceptible patients. Patients already prescribed diuretics, ACE (angiotensin-converting-enzyme) inhibitors or beta blockers, and the elderly have an increased risk of developing renal toxicity with ibuprofen use. In those patients who may be dehydrated or elderly patients with impaired kidney function, ibuprofen use can exacerbate this impairment, possibly leading to acute renal failure, although it is usually reversible.

189

Medication Management: Antiemetics

Antiemetic medication is used to manage, prevent and treat nausea and vomiting. Paramedics may have use of one or more antiemetics, depending on their jurisdiction. Cyclizine and ondansetron are two common antiemetic drugs. They are both administered parenterally, either, intramuscularly, intravenously or subcutaneously.

Cyclizine is an H_1 histamine receptor antagonist; it is non-drowsy and has an antiemetic effect within two hours of administration. While cyclizine is not known to have a detrimental effect on renal impairment, it should be used with caution in patients with severe heart failure or acute myocardial infarction, as it may result in a reduction of cardiac output due to increases in heart rates.

Ondansetron is a potent serotonin (5HT3) receptor antagonist. It has no significant impact on renal function; however, it is of interest to note that in patients with moderate to severe CKD, elimination half-life of the drug is increased, but is clinically insignificant. It should, however, be used with caution in patients with a history of cardiac conduction problems, such as, long QT syndrome.

Urinary Tract Infections

Urinary tract infections (UTIs) can occur anywhere in the genitourinary tract. They may lead to inflammation of the kidneys (pyelonephritis), the urinary bladder (cystitis) or the urethra (urethritis). UTIs are more common in females due to their shorter urethras, except in the very young and the elderly, where both sexes are equally susceptible. Most infections will enter at the urethra and spread upwards. Factors that may predispose patients to UTIs include catheterisation, any cause of obstruction (calculi, tumour, enlarged prostrate, pregnancy) or congenital abnormalities (Berkowitz 2007).

- *Cystitis* symptoms can include dysuria, increased urinary frequency and urgency, haematuria, suprapubic discomfort and cloudy urine with an offensive smell.
- *Urethritis*, which is most often the result of sexual transmission, will have similar symptoms.
- *Pyelonephritis* is usually caused by bacteria spreading upwards from the bladder but may also be bloodborne. This bacterial infection causes small abscesses to form in the renal pelvis and calyces. This will lead to destruction of nephrons; kidney function will depend on how much healthy tissue remains when the infection subsides. Symptoms will include malaise, pyrexia, flank and/or back pain, vomiting and rigours, and patients are often systemically unwell (Wyatt et al. 2020).

Paramedics should be aware of the potential for sepsis in the management of patients presenting with a UTI, especially with acute pyelonephritis. Treatment should include oxygen, intravenous fluid therapy, parenteral antimicrobials and paracetamol for pyrexia, always remembering to follow local protocols (PHECC 2021).

Snapshot 9.2

Pre-arrival Information

An 88-year-old man has had an altered level of consciousness since morning; he is normally alert. He has had reduced urine output for two days, with possible urinary retention.

Control and Dispatch Information

Time of Call: 12:30 p.m.
Information received; 88 year-old man, altered level of consciousness
Resources tasked: ambulance (2 × paramedics)
On scene: 12:40 p.m.
Depart scene: 1:10 p.m.
At hospital: 1:22 p.m.

Background Information

The patient lives at home with his carer; he is bedridden in a downstairs room. He has a home carer call twice per day. He was recently discharged from hospital, where he was treated for a chest infection, and has completed a course of antibiotics. He is normally alert and communicative. He has had reduced urinary output for two days, no catheter in place. Onset of confusion since morning, with reduced oral intake. His home care team became concerned when they called at 11 a.m., they contacted the patient's son, who rang for ambulance when he arrived at the house. The patient has been well previously, with normal food and fluid intake up to now.

Patient Assessment

Primary survey reveals a patient who responds to verbal stimuli, with a patent airway. Initial vitals taken at 12:50 p.m.

Vital Signs

Vital sign	Observation	Normal range
Pulse (beats/min)	68 strong carotid, weak radial	80–100 regular
Respiration rate (breaths/min)	10	12–20
SpO$_2$ (%)	98 (room air)	94–98
Capillary refill (s)	<2	<2
Blood pressure (mmHg)	84/59	120/80
Eyes	3	4 – spontaneously
Verbal	1	5 – orientated
Motor	5	6 – obeys commands
Total GCS score	9	15
Temperature (°C)	35.8	37
Pupils	3+/3+	Equal, round, reactive
Blood glucose (mmol/l)	7.2	

Allergies: no known allergies.
Medications: calcium carbonate tablets, galantamine, memantine, bumetanide, bisoprolol, pantoprazole.
Past medical history: Alzheimer's disease, hypertension, heart failure.
Last intake: 30–40 ml fluid intake since morning.

On Examination

Respiratory: shallow breathing, normal breath sounds upper lobes, diminished breath sounds lower, respiration rate 10 breaths/minute, symmetrical chest movement.
Cardiovascular: no cyanosis, normal colour, no peripheral oedema, neck veins normal, normal heart sounds. 12-lead ECG reveals sinus rhythm with first-degree Atrio-Ventricular block.
Abdominal: Some lower distention, rigid in hypogastric region with grimace on palpation.

Repeat observations:

Vital sign	1 p.m.	1.15 p.m.
Pulse (beats/min)	72 regular	70 regular
Respiration rate (breaths/min)	12	15
SpO$_2$ (%)	98	98
Blood pressure (mmHg)	91/57	93/59

Reflective Learning Activity

Reflect on the information in Snapshot 9.2 and consider the following:

1. What is your working diagnosis for this patient?
2. Would any of his medication have an influence on masking symptoms?
3. Outline your treatment plan for this patient using your own protocols, to manage his symptoms.
4. With the patient's oliguria and urinary retention, what will be required in the emergency department to relieve these issues?

Medication Management: Ceftriaxone

Ceftriaxone is a third-generation broad-spectrum antibiotic, which works on a selection of both Gram-positive and Gram-negative bacterial infections. It can be administered both intramuscularly and intravenously, depending on the jurisdiction. It presents in powder form and requires reconstitution prior to administration. Antimicrobial treatment is an important part of sepsis treatment. In many countries, the 'give three, take three' concept of sepsis treatment is practised: give oxygen, give intravenous fluids, give antibiotics, take blood cultures, take blood for lactate testing, measure urine output. Prehospital practitioners can easily 'give three', as currently taking blood for either point-of-care testing or in-hospital testing is uncommon. If these six procedures are carried out within the first hour following sepsis recognition, the associated mortality rate is reported to be reduced by as much as 50% (Smyth et al. 2016).

Glomerular Disease

There are several conditions which may cause damage to the kidney glomeruli, either as a direct result of kidney disease or indirectly because of disease elsewhere in the body.

- *Glomerulonephritis* is inflammation of the kidney which involves the glomeruli. A common cause of this condition is a reaction to toxins produced by streptococcal bacteria that have recently infected another part of the body, especially the throat. This inflammation results in the glomeruli filling with blood, resulting in blood cells and plasma passing into the filtrate. As a result, the patient will symptoms including oliguria, profound haematuria and proteinuria. This can lead to permanent damage and chronic renal failure.
- *Nephrotic syndrome* is a condition indicated by proteinuria and high levels of blood cholesterol. Albumin is the main protein lost, as it is the smallest and most common. When the daily albumin loss exceeds the amount produced by the liver, there is a significant fall in the total plasma protein level. This leads to widespread oedema, especially around the eyes, ankles, feet and abdomen. Renal blood flow is reduced, which stimulates the renin–angiotensin–aldosterone system, increasing reabsorption of water and sodium, further reducing blood osmotic pressure, increasing the oedema. This cycle continues once albumin continues to be lost. Nephrotic syndrome is associated with some disorders of unknown origin and also systemic disorders, such as diabetes mellitus, lupus, some cancers and AIDS (Norman and Franks 2023).

Diabetic Nephropathy

Diabetes is one of the leading causes of kidney failure, as well as having a detrimental effect on other body systems (see Chapter 12). The disease damages large and small blood vessel throughout the body, including the kidneys. Diabetic nephropathy occurs when there is progressive damage of glomeruli and nephrotic syndrome, reduced glomerular filtration rate (GFR), arteriosclerosis of the renal arteries and arterioles, causing renal ischaemia and hypertension. The condition carries high morbidity and mortality (Varghese and Jialal 2022).

GFR is the volume of filtrate formed by both kidneys in one minute. The GFR of a healthy adult is about 125 ml/minute, which equates to around 180 l/day. Almost all the filtrate is reabsorbed within the renal tubules, with less than 1% (1–1.5 l) excreted as urine. The varying volumes and concentrations of urine are due to the selective reabsorption of some filtrate constituents and tubular secretion of others. The estimated GFR (eGFR) is used to assess how well the kidneys are functioning. Blood is tested to establish the levels of creatinine, which is normally excreted by the kidneys. Higher levels of creatinine in the blood indicate reduced kidney function. The eGFR is calculated from the age, sex and levels of creatinine. While eGFR is not measured by paramedics, it is important to understand the concept and the implications of overall eGFR on kidney health.

Acute Kidney Injury

Acute kidney injury (AKI) may occur as a complication of other conditions not necessarily associated with the kidneys. AKI is common, serious and potentially very harmful. There are up to 100 000 deaths yearly associated with AKI in the United Kingdom, with over 65% of AKI cases occurring in the community. It is therefore important for paramedics to be aware of the potential for AKI in patients presenting with any causative factors. There are many causes of AKI and most occur in patients with long-term illnesses, but AKI can affect anyone.

The possible causes of AKI include:

- Pre-renal injury: hypovolaemia (haemorrhage, burns), cardiogenic shock, sepsis, medications.
- Renal injury: damage to the kidney itself, acute nephritis, acute tubular necrosis, glomerulonephritis.
- Post-renal injury: obstruction of the renal system, renal calculi, tumour of the bladder, uterus or cervix, enlarged prostrate, fibrosis (Wyatt et al. 2020).

Some of the causes of acute tubular necrosis, which is one of the most common causes of AKI, include:

- *Ischaemia* – trauma, haemorrhage, burns, severe shock, dehydration, myocardial infarction, prolonged and complex surgery, especially in older patients.
- *Drugs* – nephrotoxic medications (e.g. non-steroidal anti-inflammatory drugs, ACE inhibitors, lithium compounds, paracetamol overdose).
- *Haemoglobinaemia* – accumulation of haemolysed red blood cells (e.g. malaria, incompatible blood transfusion).
- *Myoglobiaemia* – accumulation of myoglobin released from damaged muscle (e.g. following crush injuries).

Paramedics should consider AKI in any patient over 65 years with a history of kidney disease, those on nephrotoxic medications, any patients systemically unwell (sepsis). Assess for signs of dehydration, vomiting, diarrhoea and reduced urine output.

Chronic Kidney Disease

The onset of CKD is generally slow and asymptomatic, progressing over several years. The most common cause is diabetes mellitus, followed by hypertension, glomerulonephritis, with less common causes such as polycystic kidney disease, obstruction and infection. Patients suffering episodes of AKI have an increased risk of developing CKD and end-stage renal disease. Patients with CKD should be tested regularly for their eGFR and albumin/creatinine levels. These results will determine how damaged the kidneys are and what stage of CKD the patient is at. Table 9.2 outlines the stages of CKD in relation to their eGFR.

TABLE 9.2   Stages of chronic kidney disease (CKD) in relation to percentage of estimated glomerular filtration rate (eGFR).

CKD stage	Description of kidney function	eGFR (%)
1	Kidney function is normal, but investigations find signs of kidney disease	<90
2	Slightly reduced kidney function with investigations suggesting kidney disease	60–90
3	Moderately reduced kidney function	30–60
4	Severely reduced kidney function	15–30
5	Severe or end-stage kidney failure, kidneys have lost almost all their function	<15

When eGFR falls to below 20% of normal, reabsorption of water is greatly reduced. This results in the production of up to 10 l of urine per day and polyuria. Reduced eGFR leads to accumulation of waste products in the blood, particularly urea and creatinine, which results in a condition known as uraemia. Signs and symptoms that may be present include nausea, vomiting, gastrointestinal bleeding, pruritus, anaemia and hypertension. Patients in stage five of CKD will die without interventions such as dialysis or transplant (Wyatt et al. 2020).

Dialysis

Patients on dialysis may be transported inter-hospital by paramedics or may present with dialysis-related complications between dialysis sessions. *Pulmonary oedema* may occur due to non-compliance with diet and fluid restriction. Prehospital treatment with diuretics will be ineffective; treatment includes oxygen and sublingual nitrates while transportation for immediate dialysis needs to be arranged. *Pre-dialysis hyperkalaemia* may present with neuromuscular symptoms (paralysis, muscle spasm, weakness) or arrhythmias including cardiac arrest.

Red Flag Alert: Vascular Access

Vascular access for dialysis is crucial, the preferred choice being an arteriovenous fistula. This is made by connecting a vein to a nearby artery, normally in the patient's arm, creating a large blood vessel with a fast blood flow. This fistula needs to be protected at all costs. They should never be occluded with blood pressure cuffs or tourniquets and should not be used for vascular access except in a life-threatening emergency. They are a common source for infection which will generally present with acute viral illness symptoms (Wyatt et al. 2020).

Tumours

Kidney tumours are usually malignant; benign tumours are uncommon. *Renal adenocarcinomas* are more common in men over 50 years. Clinical features include haematuria, back or flank pain, anaemia, weight loss and fever. *Nephroblastoma (Wilms' tumour)* is one of the most common malignant tumours in children under 10 years. Clinical presentations include haematuria, hypertension, abdominal pain and, occasionally, intestinal obstruction (Waugh and Grant 2018).

Bladder tumours may be malignant or benign. Males are more at risk than females and age profile is comparable to kidney cancers. Smokers account for almost half of all cases and people exposed to certain chemicals used in the leather, dye, rubber and aluminium industries also face an increased risk. Early identification and quick treatment results in a favourable prognosis for these patients (Tortora and Derrickson 2017).

Ageing and the Renal System

Ageing influences all body systems. In the renal system, kidneys shrink, have a decreased blood flow and filter less blood due to a reduction of and damage to glomeruli. Renal blood flow and filtration rate decline by approximately 50% between the ages of 40 and 70 years. The elderly are at risk of dehydration as thirst decreases with age, and they are more sensitive to fluid balance alterations. Kidney disorders such as acute and chronic kidney inflammation and renal calculi become more common. Elimination of drugs becomes less efficient with reducing kidney function, which could potentially lead to accumulation and toxicity. Urinary bladder changes result in a reduction in size and capacity and a weakening of the muscles. Incontinence is common: 15% women and 10% men over the age of 65 years will be affected to some extent, and these figures double by the age of 85 years (Davis et al. 2020). Prostate enlargement is common in older men and may cause urinary retention and micturition problems. UTIs are more common in the elderly, indeed, paramedics should suspect UTI in the elderly patient without obvious infection elsewhere if they present with two or more of the following symptoms: dysuria, urgency, frequency, urinary incontinence, flank or suprapubic pain, haematuria and new-onset confusion or worsening of existing confusion. Antibiotic therapy should be started for these patients because of the high risk of developing sepsis (Wyatt et al. 2020).

Trauma

Renal Trauma

Most kidney injuries are caused by direct blunt abdominal trauma, the kidney being crushed against the paravertebral muscles or between the 12th rib and the spine. Indirect trauma, such as falls from height, may tear major blood vessels or rupture the ureter at its junction with the kidney. Penetrating injuries tend to be more severe and less predictable than blunt traumas. They may produce major tissue damage to the parenchyma, blood vessels and collecting system (Singh and Sookraj 2023). Paediatric patients are particularly prone to renal trauma due to ribs being softer than adults as they have not yet completely ossified. Patients may present with flank pain/tenderness, and there may be visible bruising or abrasions. Pharmacological and non-pharmacological support is required, with prompt transport to the emergency department for imaging and prospective surgery.

Bladder/Urethral Trauma

The bladder may rupture as a direct blow to the lower abdomen. These injures often occur to patients with distended bladders. Bone fragments from a fractured pelvis may also penetrate the bladder or tear the urethra. Haematuria or the inability to pass urine, bruising and low abdominal tenderness are some common clinical features (Wyatt et al. 2020).

Summary

The renal system consists of the kidneys, ureters, bladder and urethra. There are disease processes which may affect one or multiple parts of the renal system. As a paramedic, you will unquestionably be involved in the care and management of patients with complex medical needs. Renal disorders often coexist with other comorbidities, such as cardiovascular

195

disease and diabetes. Those patients with advanced kidney disease may also experience psychological upset, as their disease is not curable and may lead to death. Being aware and supportive of both the patient and teir family will enable you to be become a balanced practitioner.

References

Berkowitz, A. (2007). *Clinical Pathophysiology Made Ridiculously Simple*, 47–71. Miami, FL: Medmaster.

Davis, N., Wyman, J., Gubitosa, S., and Pretty, L. (2020). Urinary incontinence in older adults. *AJN, American Journal of Nursing* 120 (1): 57–62.

Lazenby, R. (2011). *Handbook of Pathophysiology*, 4e, 737–791. Philadelphia, PA: Wolters Kluwer Lippincott Williams and Wilkins.

Leslie, S., Sajjad, H., and Murphy, P. (2022). *Renal Calculi*. Treasure Island, FL: StatPearl Publishing.

McPhee, S. and Hammer, G. (2019). *Pathophysiology of Disease: An Introduction to Clinical Medicine*, 8e, 1097–1158. New York, NY: McGraw-Hill.

NHS England. (2022). *Kidney stones.* https://www.nhs.uk/conditions/kidney-stones (accessed 4 October 2023).

NHS England. (2023). *Urinary incontinence.* https://www.nhs.uk/conditions/urinary-incontinence (accessed 4 October 2023).

Norman, J.C. and Franks, M. (2023). *Pathophysiology: The Renal System*. Sacramento, CA: NetCE. https://www.netce.com/coursecontent.php?courseid=2066&productid=7807&scrollTo=chap.1 (accessed 4 October 2023).

Peate, I. (2018). *Fundamentals of Applied Pathophysiology: An Essential Guide for Nursing and Healthcare Students*, 3e, 248–277. Hoboken, NJ: Wiley Blackwell.

PHECC (2021). *Clinical Practice Guidelines: Advanced Paramedic*, 7e (updated 2023). Naas, Ireland: Pre-Hospital Emergency Care Council.

Singh, S. and Sookraj, K. (2023). *Kidney Trauma*. Treasure Island, FL: StatPearls Publishing.

Smyth, M., Brace-McDonnell, S., and Perkins, G. (2016). Identification of adults with sepsis in the prehospital environment: a systematic review. *BMJ Open* 6 (8): e011218.

Tortora, G. and Derrickson, B. (2017). *Principles of Anatomy and Physiology*, 15e, 993–1035. Hoboken, NJ: Wiley.

Varghese, R. and Jialal, I. (2022). *Diabetic Nephropathy*. Treasure Island, FL: StatPearls Publishing.

Waugh, A. and Grant, A. (2018). *Ross & Wilson Anatomy and Physiology in Health and Illness*, 13e, 369–393. Philadelphia, PA: Elsevier.

Wyatt, J., Taylor, R., de Wit, K., and Hotton, E. (2020). *Oxford Handbook of Emergency Medicine*, 5e. Oxford: Oxford University Press.

Further Reading

Hammer, G.D. and McGee, S.J. (2019). *Pathophysiology of Disease: An introduction to clinical medicine*, 8e. New York, NY: McGraw-Hill Education.

Nutbeam, T. and Boylan, M. eds. *ABC of Pre-Hospital Emergency Medicine. Chichester: Wiley Blackwell.*

Rennke, H. and Denker, B. (2020). *Renal Pathophysiology: The Essentials*, 5e. Philadelphia, PA: Wolters Kluwer.

Online Resources

NHS England. Diagnosis chronic kidney disease: https://www.nhs.uk/conditions/kidney-disease/diagnosis

Think Kidneys: www.thinkkidneys.nhs.uk

NHS resource raising awareness of kidney disease for healthcare professionals.

Glossary

Albumin	Protein made by the liver; helps to maintain blood osmotic pressure, stopping fluid leaking form blood vessels to surrounding tissue.
Armamentarium	The medicines, equipment and techniques available to a medical practitioner.
Fistula	A connection between two body parts, such as artery to vein.
Genitourinary	Both urinary and genital body systems.
Haemolysis	The break down of red blood cells.
Homeostasis	A state of balance among all the body systems needed for the body to survive and function correctly.
Hypertrophy	The enlargement of an organ or tissue due to an increase in the size of the cells.
Malaise	General body weakness, feeling ill.
Micturition	Urination.
Myoglobin	Protein supplying oxygen to cells of muscles.
Parenchyma	The functional tissue of an organ as distinguished from the connective and supporting tissue.
Parenteral	Medication administered via routes other than the mouth and alimentary canal.
Peritoneum	The lining of the abdominal cavity covering the abdominal organs.
Pruritus	Severe itching of the skin.
Retroperitoneal	Situated behind the peritoneum.

Multiple Choice Questions

1. The right kidney is positioned slightly lower than the left due to which organ?
   a. The space occupied superiorly by the gallbladder
   b. The space occupied inferiorly by the colon
   c. The space occupied superiorly by the liver
   d. The space occupied inferiorly by the liver

2. The path of urine drainage from the kidneys to the urethra is:
   a. minor calyx → major calyx → collecting duct → papillary duct → renal pelvis → ureter → urinary bladder
   b. collecting duct → papillary duct → minor calyx → major calyx → renal pelvis → ureter → urinary bladder
   c. collecting duct → papillary duct → renal pelvis → minor calyx → major calyx → ureter → urinary bladder
   d. urinary bladder → ureter → renal pelvis → major calyx → minor calyx → papillary duct → collecting duct

3. What is the name given to the nephron loop within the renal tubule?
   a. The loop of Henry
   b. The loop of Bowman
   c. The loop of Filtrate
   d. The loop of Henle

4. How much urine does a healthy adult pass each day?
   a. 2–2.5 l
   b. 1–1.5 l
   c. 500–750 ml
   d. 3–4 l

5. A person passing abnormally high amounts of urine is known to have what condition?
   a. Polyuria
   b. Anuria
   c. Oliguria
   d. Dysuria

6. How are kidney stones formed?
   a. crystals of potassium, normally in solution, solidify in any part of the urinary tract
   b. Crystals of salts, normally in solution, solidify in any part of the urinary tract
   c. High levels of urea and creatinine in filtrate
   d. Taking too many antacids

7. A common cause of glomerulonephritis is a reaction to toxins produced by which bacterial infection?
   a. Staphylococcus
   b. *Clostridium difficile*
   c. *Escherichia coli*
   d. Streptococcus

8. Which of the following is an example of pre-renal injury?
   a. Sepsis
   b. Renal calculi
   c. Bladder tumour
   d. Heart failure

9. A patient with stage 2 chronic kidney disease would be expected to have an eGFR of what percentage?
   a. <90%
   b. 60–90%
   c. 30–60%
   d. 15–30%

10. Paediatric patients may be more prone to renal trauma because?
    a. They are smaller than adults
    b. They are more prone to blunt force trauma
    c. Their rib cage does not provide as much protection as it does in adults
    d. Their anatomy is different from that of adults

CHAPTER 10

The Respiratory System and Associated Disorders

Ian Macleod and Simon Sawyer

AIM

This chapter aims to reviews the anatomy and physiology of the respiratory system and to explore the pathophysiology and prehospital management of common respiratory system diseases.

LEARNING OBJECTIVES

After completing this chapter, you will be able to:

- Understand the anatomy and physiology of the respiratory system.
- Discuss the processes involved in ventilation and respiration.
- Understand the pathophysiology of common disease processes impacting the respiratory system which are encountered in the prehospital environment.
- Discuss prehospital management of asthma, chronic obstructive pulmonary disorder and upper airway obstructions.

Test Your Prior Knowledge
1. Name the major anatomical structures and their locations in the respiratory tract.
2. What is the difference between ventilation and respiration?
3. What is the difference between the effects of salbutamol and ipratropium on the airways?
4. Which of adrenaline's effects can be of use to a patient in respiratory distress?

Fundamentals of Applied Pathophysiology for Paramedics, First Edition. Edited by Ian Peate and Simon Sawyer.

Introduction

The respiratory system incorporates a group of structures that warm, humidify, filter and conduct air from the atmosphere to the alveoli, where gas exchange occurs between the lungs and the blood. Controlled by the central nervous system, the respiratory system acts both autonomically and voluntarily to facilitate a range of biological functions, such as breathing, talking, eating and even swimming.

The respiratory system works in conjunction with many other bodily systems; for example, it works with the immune systems to protect the body from inhaled pathogenic materials, with several lines of defence preventing infection through breathing. The respiratory system works in conjunction with the cardiovascular system to deliver oxygen from the environment to the cells for energy production and to remove carbon dioxide, the metabolic waste product.

There are two main anatomical divisions of the respiratory system: the *upper respiratory tract*, incorporating the nasal cavity, larynx and pharynx (those elements above the thorax) and the *lower respiratory tract*, composed of the trachea, primary bronchi, bronchioles and alveoli (the elements of the system within the thorax). The respiratory system may also be divided in terms of function: the *conducting zone*, which provides a path for air to move in, out and through the lungs, and the *respiratory zone*, where the vital function of oxygen and carbon dioxide exchange takes place (Figure 10.1).

Any disease process that impacts on the respiratory system is a significant threat to homeostasis, given our constant need to oxygenation to sustain life. The average person will take about 40 million breaths every year. If a person lives to 80 years, their respiratory system will have reliably performed over three billion breaths, never once failing (well, only failing once, at the very end). Quite a feat!

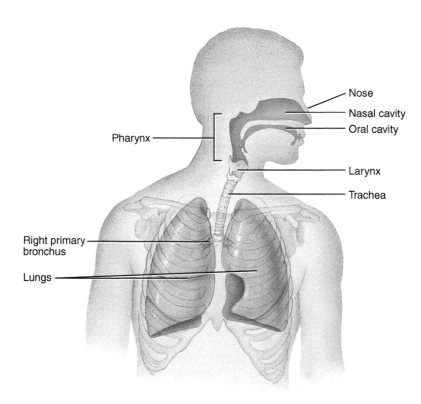

Anterior view showing organs of respiration

FIGURE 10.1   Gross anatomy of the respiratory system.

Anatomy and Physiology

The Upper Respiratory Tract

Air can enter the respiratory tract through the mouth, although it most usually enters through the nose, where it travels along two parallel nasal cavities in which small hairs attempt to collect and entrap particles from the air in aggregates of mucus (snot) for expulsion. Highly vascular folds in the mucous membranes, called turbinates, warm and humidify the air, preventing potentially dry or cold air from irritating the lower airways. Four pairs of sinuses surrounding the nose contribute to the filtration and preparation of air for inhalation; these hollow pockets also aid in speech and serve as protective mechanisms to the delicate features of the head and face.

The pharynx, generally known as the throat, conducts air from the nasal cavity and food from the mouth to the trachea and oesophagus, respectively. Eustachian tubes join the middle ear and pharynx, allowing air movement to balance pressures within the ears.

The larynx sits below the pharynx, anatomically divided at the point of the epiglottis and incorporating the vocal cords and glottis. The epiglottis is a small nape of muscle tissue which closes over the trachea during swallowing to prevent materials from entering and occluding the airways. Owing to its position and function, the potential for the epiglottis and surrounding tissues to become infected and swell may result in significant obstruction to airflow. The vocal cords serve the functions of vibrating to articulate sound, and can snap closed when encountering foreign particles, further preventing entry of foreign materials into the lungs. Composed of a cartilaginous skeleton, the larynx incorporates ligaments and muscle to facilitate its primary functions; these structures make the larynx prominent in the neck and give rise to the term *voice box*.

The Lower Respiratory Tract

From the larynx, air enters the trachea, or windpipe, an approximately 12-cm long, 2-cm diameter tube (in adults) that is reinforced by 16–20 cartilaginous rings, preventing collapse of the structure under low or relatively negative pressure. These cartilaginous rings are C-shaped and are open at the posterior, where the trachea sits against the oesophagus. These incomplete rings allow for expansion of the trachea with breathing, and of the oesophagus during swallowing. The open ends of these rings are held in place and manipulated through control of the trachealis muscles.

A bifurcation at the inferior end of the trachea splits air into the left and right primary bronchi at a point called the carina. The angles of departure from the trachea to these primary bronchi are not equal; As can be seen from Figure 10.1, the right bronchus is wider, shorter and more vertically oriented due to the additional right-sided lung lobe (three lobes on the right, with two on the left, allowing space for the heart). This is of significance in the management of foreign body obstruction; the object may be propelled into the right lung through positive pressure in some cases.

The respiratory tree divides into smaller airways many times over in the same way that branches of a tree split off many times. Large secondary and tertiary bronchi conduct air to and through the lung lobes before dividing out into bronchioles. There are about 25 generations of conducting bronchiole, each becoming progressively narrower, directing air into the terminal bronchioles and finally the respiratory bronchioles.

The bronchiole wall is composed of smooth muscle, which allows for muscular constriction, narrowing the airway, increasing resistance and reducing air movement, and for relaxation-induced dilation, increasing the flow and volume of air movement. Sympathetic and parasympathetic innervation controls this dilation and constriction though the tissue may spasm and constrict in response to a local stimulus, mediated by beta-adrenoceptors in the cells of smooth muscle.

The respiratory bronchioles are continuous with the alveoli, small air sacs constituting the terminus of the airways and the primary point of gas exchange (Figure 10.2). These bunched alveolar sacs are highly numerous (about 300 million) and are lined with a substance called surfactant, which helps break the tension between the walls of the deflated alveoli and aids diffusion of gases into the blood.

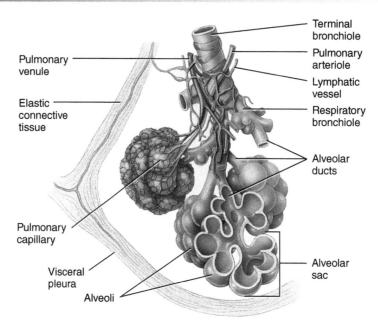

Diagram of a portion of a lobule of the lung

FIGURE 10.2   Anatomy of the alveoli.

Tightly adjacent to the alveoli are capillaries arising from the pulmonary arteries and collecting to form the pulmonary veins. These pulmonary capillaries are supplied by arteries which constrict in response to low alveolar oxygen level. This reflex helps to ensure blood is diverted to areas of the lung with higher oxygen content. This mechanism plays a critical role in influencing fetal circulation and transition to breathing. A tight junction enables movement of gases through the alveolar and capillary walls between the air and the blood, specifically the haemoglobin component of blood.

Respiratory Muscles

The diaphragm is a double dome-shaped muscle anchored to the lumbar vertebrae, sternum (at the xiphoid process) and ribcage and by a central tendon to the pericardium. This central tendon separates these two dome-shaped segments into their left and right elements. Anatomically, the diaphragm separates the thorax and abdomen, meaning that the rise and fall of the diaphragm during breathing shifts the abdominal contents upwards and downwards, which influences the mechanisms of trauma. Three hiatuses breach the diaphragm, the *aortic hiatus*, permitting passage of the aorta and thoracic duct, the *caval hiatus*, allowing the phrenic nerve and inferior vena cava to pass, and the *oesophageal hiatus*, which communicates with the oesophagus and vagus nerves. The diaphragm is innervated by the phrenic nerve, which originates at C3, 4, 5 of the vertebral column.

Accessory muscles may be engaged to aid the diaphragm when obstruction inhibits normal breathing; generally, muscle activation is a component of inspiration, but there are accessory expiratory muscles. The muscles activating the ribcage include the intercostals, the subcostals and transversus thoracis, in combination with the sternocleidomastoid and scalene. These muscle groups expand the ribcage, further reducing intrathoracic pressure. The abdominal muscles, the *rectus abdominis*, contract to increase intraabdominal pressure, which exerts an upwards force on the diaphragm, aiding the expiration of air (as do the internal intercostals), noting that this does not overcome the effects of obstructive airways pathologies. Innervation of the intercostal and abdominal muscles originates in the thoracic spine, meaning that high spinal injuries may result in loss of control of the ribcage, but retention of diaphragm control (arising in the cervical spine).

Ventilation

The mechanical act of drawing air in and out of the lungs, inhaling and exhaling respectively, is known as ventilation. A lining, the visceral pleura, adheres to the outer surface of the lung and is nestled inside a second lining, the parietal pleura, which is continuous with the inside of the thorax and top surface of the diaphragm. A small amount of fluid between these two pleurae enables the layers to slide over one another without causing damage to the changing shape and size of the tissues.

As the diaphragm flattens, it draws the parietal pleura downwards; the film of fluid between pleural layers creates a tension so that both move together. As the visceral pleura is drawn downwards (and outwards by the ribcage), the volume within the lungs increases, causing the pressure to reduce. This results in a pressure gradient, where atmospheric pressure exceeds intrathoracic pressure and air moves into the airways and throughout the lung tissue, the phase known as *inhalation*.

When the diaphragm relaxes, it returns to its resting, domed shape; the lung volume is reduced and pressure rises. This time, the pressure gradient is such that intrathoracic pressure exceeds atmospheric pressure, and air moves out of the lung tissues, through the airways and exits the body. This phase of ventilation is called *exhalation*.

The requirement for a pressure gradient to facilitate ventilation helps us to understand how high altitude, diving and chest wall injuries all can affect the ability to effectively self-ventilate.

Inhalation is an active, muscular process; the respiratory muscles and accessory muscles can work to generate a negative pressure and draw air into the lungs. Exhalation is primarily a process of relaxation and while several muscles can work to aid exhalation, they cannot generate the force required to exhale in some severe obstructive respiratory emergencies, such as asthma (discussed later). This effect results in gas trapping and breath stacking.

The ventilation ratio describes the duration of inhalation compared with exhalation and is normally 1:2 in healthy individuals (i.e. one second of inhalation to two seconds of exhalation). Several factors may cause this ratio to vary. Total lung capacity is approximately 6 l in healthy adults (Delgado and Bajaj 2022), although with each cycle of ventilation only a relatively small volume of air is moved; this is known as the tidal volume and is roughly 10 ml for every kilogramme of body weight. The average adult tidal volume is 700 ml. Inspiratory reserve volume and expiratory reserve volume define the quantities of air that could be moved through deepest inhalation or exhalation, respectively; residual volume is the remaining air which cannot be exhaled. These concepts are presented visually in Figure 10.3.

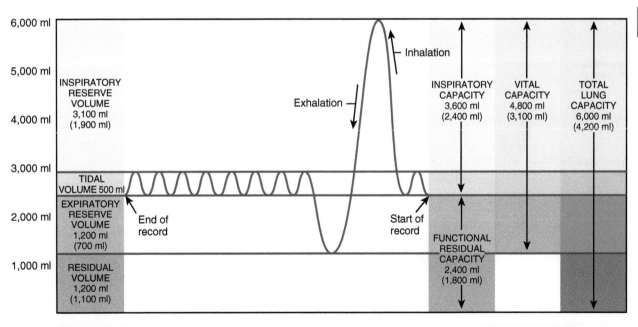

FIGURE 10.3 Total lung capacity by inspiration and expiration cycle.

Breathing is controlled through complex mechanical and neurochemical processes, stimulated primarily by carbon dioxide levels in the blood and coordinated by three regions of the brainstem. Receptors detect stretch within the airways, which determines volume, and irritation caused by pathogenic material. Chemoreceptors detect arterial oxygen levels in the peripheries and pH in the central nervous system, the latter constituting about 85% of respiratory drive (Brinkman et al. 2023). Acidity and alkalinity directly correspond to carbon dioxide levels; in response, respiratory rate and depth increase in the presence of high CO_2 and the related acidic state or decrease as CO_2 is reduced and blood turns alkaline.

Respiration

Ventilation in the process of moving air to and from the lung tissue. At the border of the alveoli and capillaries, the process of respiration, or gas exchange takes place, through the process of diffusion (Figure 10.4). At this point, the single-cell thickness alveolar and capillary walls bring air and blood within 1 µm of one another (Dezube 2023).

Diffusion occurs because of a concentration gradient. The air in our lungs, taken from the atmosphere, is approximately 21% oxygen (at sea level and assuming that the air is free from contaminants). The blood returning to the lungs from systemic circulation is relatively deoxygenated, as our body has just taken up oxygen into the tissues. Because of this relative difference, oxygen diffuses from the alveoli into the blood in the capillaries, binding to haemoglobin molecules. This oxygenated blood is then transported to the tissues by way of the blood stream, and the whole process repeats itself over and over, for your entire life.

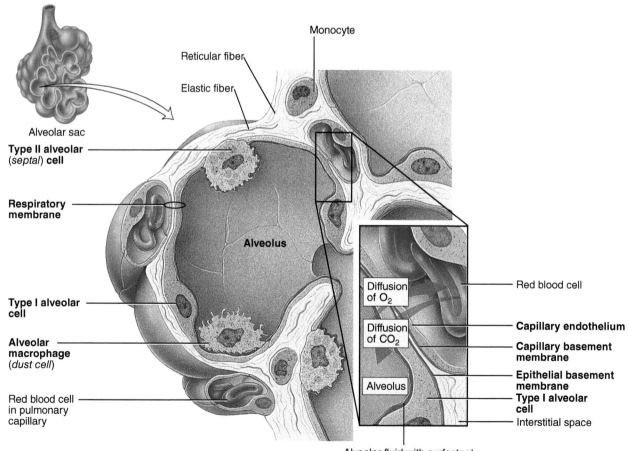

Section through an alveolus showing its cellular components

Details of respiratory membrane

FIGURE 10.4 Gas exchange within the alveoli.

Oxygen is rapidly consumed by the mitochondria during the production of energy, which is what maintains a low level of oxygen within the cell and creates the same concentration gradient as we have just discussed in the lungs (albeit in reverse). Again, this concentration gradient is what enables continuing oxygen diffusion from the blood to the cell. As glucose is metabolised by the cell in the presence of oxygen, carbon dioxide is produced and accumulates inside the cell. Capillary blood flow passing the cell has a low concentration of carbon dioxide, much lower than the concentration within the cell. This gradient allows CO_2 to move from the cell freely and rapidly through the cell membrane into the blood. When blood returns to the lung tissue, the concentration gradients favour the movement of CO_2 from the blood to the alveoli (where CO_2 levels are low) and O_2 from the highly oxygen-concentrated alveoli into the oxygen-depleted blood.

Disease Processes of the Respiratory System

Due to our constant need for oxygen, threats to the respiratory system can be life threatening. Three key respiratory presentations that are common in the prehospital environment, asthma, chronic obstructive pulmonary disorder and upper airway obstructions are discussed.

Asthma

Asthma is an incurable, but reversible, chronic airway disease causing obstruction of airflow due to a hypersensitive reaction in the airways to triggers such as dust, pollens and mites (Figure 10.5). Bronchiole smooth muscle dilates in response to increase oxygen demand, allowing a greater volume of air movement to meet the demands of exertion. In the

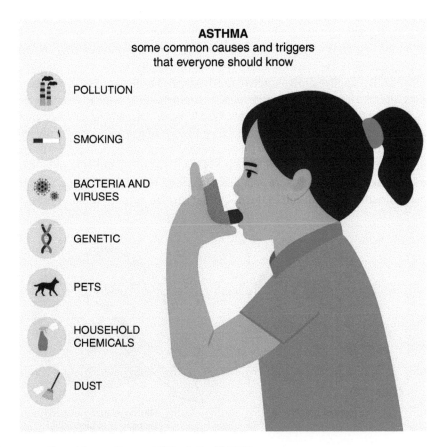

FIGURE 10.5 Common asthma triggers. Source: UC Davis Health 2023.

event that a pathogen contaminates a section of lung tissue, the bronchioles can constrict, like the fire doors of a large building, to prevent spread of the contaminant into unaffected areas. Mucus producing and secreting cells called goblet cells are spread throughout the airways. The mucus they secrete encapsulates pathogenic material, which is then expelled from the airways through action of small hairs, *cilia*, that line the airways. Without mucus, it would not be possible for a speck of dust or bacteria to be propelled out of the lungs. Bronchiole tissue, like most body tissues, can become inflamed when the immune system is activated, in an attempt to heal the body. These processes are all normal and occur in all of us.

When the airways become hypersensitive, however, they have the potential to over-respond to a trigger, which results in an exaggerated and global (large or all areas of the lungs) response. We call this state *asthma*.

Asthma is characterised by three key features:

1. Widespread airway inflammation due to the immune response.
2. Bronchoconstriction through constriction of smooth muscle.
3. Mucous oedema due to overproduction of mucus from the goblet cells.

Triggers vary between individuals; however, common causes of asthmatic episodes include dust, mites, pollens, chemicals and mould, and may be exercise induced, secondary to physical exertion.

Once exposed, the airways constrict, swell and secrete excessive quantities of mucus. This serves to narrow and obstruct the airways at the bronchioles, restricting the movement of air. The narrowing airways produce a characteristic, distorted whistling sound, which is termed *wheezing*. This occurs due to turbulence of the air as it moves in and out of the narrow airways (exactly what occurs when you purse your lips and whistle, although the sound is somewhat different).

Early in the progression of symptoms, an expiratory wheeze may be noted on exhalation, as the airways relax, narrowing further. Development of inspiratory wheeze and reduced volume are associated with worsening obstruction within the airways. Louder wheezing requires greater air movement; quiet wheezing or silence on auscultation may indicate little or no movement.

As asthma symptoms progress, mucous secretions increase and begin to clog the small bronchioles, obstructing the movement of air into or out of groups of alveoli through formation of small mucous plugs (Figure 10.6). This problem compounds the narrowing of airways, which increases airway resistance and prevents normal exhalation.

As discussed, inhalation is an active process, whereas exhalation is a largely passive process, occurring through the relaxation of respiratory muscles (as opposed to large muscle contraction). This means that the person with asthma has a greater ability to draw air into their lungs than their capacity to force air out, causing an accumulation of trapped air (gas trapping) which now stops fresh, oxygenated air from reaching the site of gas exchange. As the flow of air past the vocal cords decreases, the ability to speak is reduced from sentences to short phrases, then single words to nothing.

As the patient deteriorates, the pressure within the lungs increases to a point of hyperinflation, placing compressive pressure on the vena cava (the low-pressure vein draining blood back to the right side of the heart). As the vena cava is squeezed closed, blood flow is reduced to the point that cardiac output, so blood pressure begins to drop and

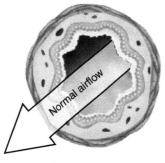
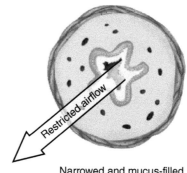

Normal bronchiole

Narrowed and mucus-filled bronchiole in bronchitis

FIGURE 10.6   Normal versus constricted bronchioles due to asthma.

hypotension begins. This raised intrathoracic pressure may also inhibit return of blood through the jugular veins, causing them to distend and become prominent on the neck; this is known as *jugular venous distention*.

The degree to which an asthma episode progresses depends on many individual, environmental and interventional features, meaning that the full sequalae are generally not present in most events; early mitigation most commonly prevents further exacerbation.

Clinical Investigations: Asthma Symptoms

Key asthma symptoms and assessments include:

- *Respiratory status signs*: anxiety or distress; difficulty speaking long sentences, tachypnoea, increased work of breathing and accessory muscle use, expiratory and or inspiratory wheeze on chest auscultation. Late signs include catatonia, bradypnea, and hypoxia (decreased oxygen saturation, SpO_2). In younger children, a dry cough may be present.
- *Perfusion status signs*: tachycardia, skin changes, and hypertension. Late signs include bradycardia and hypotension.
- *Conscious state signs*: patients should be alert and oriented initially but may decline into altered conscious states and unconsciousness as late signs.

Pharmacology

Several medications are administered in conjunction with one another to abate the symptoms of asthma. As asthma may present with varying degrees of severity, and as asthma is dynamic, meaning that symptoms can change over time, a key principle of asthma management is *escalating care* (as symptoms increase, so should your management). Local clinical guidelines must be observed in the management of episodic exacerbation of asthma; however, generally they will include the medications listed in Table 10.1.

TABLE 10.1   Medications management for asthma.

Medication	Action	Use
Salbutamol	A beta 2 agonist; it binds to beta 2 receptors (located in the smooth muscle of the bronchioles among other places), where it exerts an agonistic effect, causing bronchodilation, increasing airflow into the lungs	Delivery via PMDI with a spacer. Site of action is at the bronchioles. To escalate care, salbutamol can also be delivered via nebuliser, or intravenously in severe, life-threatening cases
Ipratropium bromide	An anticholinergic medication that works by blocking muscarinic cholinergic receptors to prevent the constriction of smooth muscles in the airways. By blocking acetylcholine, ipratropium also inhibits the secretion of mucous into the air passages	Ipratropium is generally administered by pressurised metered-dose inhaler (PMDI) or nebulised alongside salbutamol.
Corticosteroids	Steroidal medications, such as prednisolone, hydrocortisone or dexamethasone, are used to manage the inflammatory processes of airways narrowing. Corticosteroids inhibit the process of inflammation, which would otherwise cause narrowing of the airways	May be given orally or intravenously depending on the level of severity and nature of presentation
Adrenaline	Exerts beta-2 agonist effects from the bloodstream, circumventing the issue in inhaled medications of reaching the site of action through narrowed or closed airways	Adrenaline is reserved for life-threatening asthmatic events. It is administered intramuscularly or intravenously. Note: adrenaline's systemic effects, particularly on the cardiovascular system, present some unwanted adverse effects such as increased myocardial irritability in the hypoxic patient and subsequent potential for dysrhythmia

Reflective Learning Activity

People with asthma do not often use their pressurised metered dose inhaler (PMDI) properly, often omitting the use of a spacer. This means that most of the medication sprays directly on to the skin on the inside of the mouth and becomes ingested, rather than being breathed into the lungs. Next time you are on placement and encounter a patient with asthma, take some time to ask them how they are using their asthma medication and provide them with education if needed.

Medications Management: Asthma

Remember: salbutamol reverses constriction, while ipratropium bromide prevents or inhibits constriction. Long-term oral corticosteroid use is associated with several risks due to the systemic nature of its action (Ramamoorthy and Cidlowski 2016); however, corticosteroids are safe to administer in response to *acute* asthmatic events.

Clinical Investigations: History Gathering

Asthma manifests differently between individuals; history gathering must address several key criteria when assessing the patient once life-saving interventions have commenced:

- Confirm whether the patient has a medical officer diagnosis of asthma as opposed to a self-diagnosis; there may be further underlying pathologies that have not been excluded.
- Identify triggers affecting the individual and exposure to them.
- Determine the presence and content of an asthma action plan, noting that many asthmatics do not possess such a plan.
- Ascertain metered-dose inhaler usage with consideration to:
  - Whether a spacer was used; commonly incorrect technique undermines the efficacy of the medication.
  - How many doses have been administered.
  - Over what time the medication has been administered.
- Previous hospital presentations, hospital admissions and intensive care unit (ICU) stays will help to gain insight as to the potential progression of the presentation.
- Hospital presentations are a poor indicator; admission to hospital indicates a threshold or severity determined by a medical officer.
- Identify the frequency, duration of stay and last admission as an indicator of the severity of asthma.

Red and Orange Flag Alerts: Asthma

Adults

Flags for asthma assessment in adults include:

Vital sign	Red flag	Orange flag
History	Any history of ICU presentation due to asthma; frequent emergency department presentations	Frequent ambulance attendance due to asthma; any emergency department presentation due to asthma; concurrent respiratory infections
Respiratory status	Rate > 20; moderate respiratory distress; inspiratory wheeze; prolonged expiratory phase; difficultly talking; SpO_2 < 90% (note that this is a very late sign)	Mild respiratory distress; expiratory wheeze
Conscious status	Any deviation from normal (e.g. GCS score < 15)	Lethargy
Perfusion status	Heart rate > 120; blood pressure < 90; moderate hypoperfusion; cool, pale and clammy skin (denoting sympathetic activation)	Mild hypoperfusion; any skin changes

Children

- *Any* deviation from standard normal vital signs in conjunction with an asthma presentation.
- Be very suspicious of lethargy in children in the setting of asthma.
- Be aware that asthma often presents with a persistent dry cough in young children.
- Asthma symptoms can also appear in conjunction with upper respiratory tract infection, which results in a more severe presentation due to associated diminishing of respiratory capacity from the infection process.

Management

Management of asthma is based on severity of the presentation. Generally, asthma is classed in three categories, noting that symptoms may overlap or sit to one end of the range more than the other: mild/moderate, severe and life threatening.

Mild/moderate asthma refers to symptoms that are perceptible and are making breathing more difficult, but are not preventing the patient from being able to move enough air into and out of their lungs to ensure adequate oxygenation. Prehospital management in such cases generally includes salbutamol via a PMDI and spacer that resolves symptoms. Symptoms usually resolve within 5–20 minutes.

Severe asthma refers to either mild/moderate asthma which was not resolved with management after 20 minutes or symptoms that are making breathing ineffective and preventing the patient from being able to move enough air into and out of their lungs to ensure adequate oxygenation. Prehospital management in such cases generally includes repeated salbutamol and ipratropium (single dose) via nebuliser (or PMDI and spacer if nebulised medications unavailable). Fast-acting corticosteroids, such as dexamethasone, should also be administered orally or intravenously. Symptoms generally resolve or begin to improve after 5–20 minutes.

Life-threatening asthma refers to either severe asthma that was not improved with management to an acceptable level or symptoms that are causing ineffective breathing and oxygenation, which will result in cessation of breathing. Prehospital management generally includes severe management and intramuscular or intravenous adrenaline administration.

Chronic Obstructive Pulmonary Disease

Chronic obstructive pulmonary disease (COPD) refers to a group of chronic, irreversible and incurable diseases which limit the movement of air through the lungs. Beneath the umbrella term of COPD sits emphysema, chronic bronchitis and chronic asthma. The primary cause of COPD is tobacco smoking (World Health Organization 2023), followed by inhalation of second-hand smoke, environmental pollution and industrial chemicals, and finally genetics and the pre-existence of asthma or other respiratory pathologies also contribute to a lesser degree. COPD is more prevalent in indigenous and low socioeconomic groups within a population (Cooksley et al. 2015).

Chronic bronchitis refers to a productive cough occurring more than three months within a span of two years (Widysanto and Mathew 2022). The condition involves widespread inflammation of the bronchi, excessive mucus production and an associated destruction of cilia, which results in reduced capacity for mucociliary clearance. The net result is narrowed and obstructed airways, limiting airflow.

The key symptom is a chronic, productive cough with increasing dyspnoea as the disease process progresses. Narrowed, inflamed airways give rise to wheezing and crackling airflow and a prolonged expiratory phase of ventilation (Figure 10.7).

Emphysema refers to a combination of the loss of alveolar elasticity, breakdown of the alveoli and widespread gas trapping, all contributing to shortness of breath, which is exacerbated upon exertion. Emphysema is a condition that is primarily associated with reduced overall lung tissue, rather than reduced availability of existing lung tissue as is found in chronic bronchitis and asthma. Dyspnoea is the key symptom of emphysema and is accompanied by a compensatory increased respiratory rate and minute ventilation (total volume of inhaled air per minute). Breakdown of the functional tissue of the lungs results in air-filled spaces (bullae), which may lead to pneumothorax.

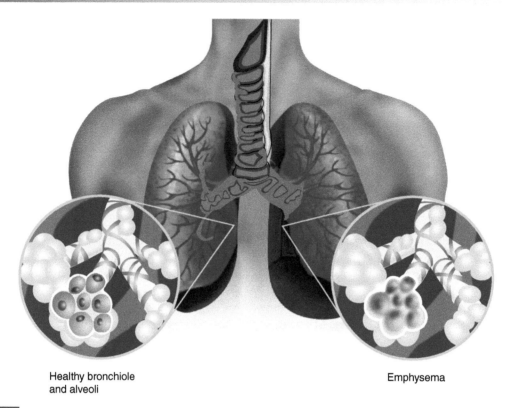

Healthy bronchiole
and alveoli

Emphysema

FIGURE 10.7   Emphysema.

Clinical Investigations: History Gathering

COPD manifests differently between individuals; history gathering must address several key criteria when assessing the patient once life-saving interventions have commenced.

- Confirm whether the patient has a diagnosis of COPD, as opposed to a self-diagnosis; there may be further underlying pathologies that have not been excluded.
- Identify triggers affecting the individual and exposure to them, common exacerbation triggers include smoking, increased exertion, stress and concurrent respiratory infections.
- Previous ambulance or hospital presentations, hospital admissions and ICU stays will help to gain insight as to the potential progression of the presentation.

Red and Orange Flag Alerts: Chronic Obstructive Pulmonary Disease

Flags for COPD assessment in adults (children do not usually get COPD except in incredibly rare circumstances) are the same to those for asthma. Note, however, that patients with COPD are chronically hypoxaemic and will generally tolerate an SpO_2 of 88–92%.

Management

As is the case with all chronic disease, management addresses both the chronic, day-to-day disease symptoms and acute exacerbations. For all exacerbations of COPD, a combination of short- and long-lasting bronchodilators (usually salbutamol and ipratropium) and corticosteroids is provided. Oxygen therapy is also indicated, titrating to an SpO_2 of 88–92%.

Non-pharmacological management of COPD is a critical adjunct to medications (Safka and McIvor 2015). These include avoidance of the exposure, namely cessation of tobacco smoking and pulmonary rehabilitation. Pulmonary rehabilitation is a multifaceted process facilitated by the patient's general practitioner (GP), which begins with respiratory assessment and stress testing to determine lung function. Education is provided to patients and support persons in the management of chronic respiratory disease. Psychological support is provided for the potential associated symptoms of the disease, such as depression and anxiety that may accompany chronic illness. Respiratory muscle exercise and improvement in general cardiopulmonary fitness improve ventilatory efficacy and respiration, easing dyspnoea associated with activities of daily life and improving quality of life; general fitness is supported through counselling in appropriate nutrition. At the conclusion of the programme, which is generally several months, lung function testing is repeated to assess efficacy of the rehabilitation process. It is important that prehospital practitioners revisit care plans with patients and work with them to encourage compliance with prevention strategies to prevent future call outs.

Snapshot 10.1

Scenario

You are examining a 40 year old female patient who is in respiratory distress after walking to the shops, which are approximately 500 metres from her house. Your patient is presenting with tachypnoea (respiratory rate 22 breaths/minute), an SpO_2 of 88% and an audible expiratory wheeze. She is afebrile and her GCS score is 15. Your patient is a pack a day smoker and has been for 25 years. The patient is regularly short of breath post exertion, but does not go to a GP or the emergency department as she does not trust doctors.

Your Diagnosis?

Before you read on, what do you think is the most likely cause of this patient's respiratory distress? What aspects of her presentation lead you to that conclusion?

Differential Diagnosis

This patient could be presenting with asthma, COPD, a simple chest infection or even something less common like a pulmonary embolism. This patient is relatively young, which makes COPD less likely, as this condition needs time to develop. However, she has been a pack a day smoker for 25 years, and that can certainly be sufficient time to destroy enough lung tissue to cause COPD. The onset of shortness of breath with associated wheezing post exertion can be present in both asthma and COPD, but walking for 500 m is a very short distance to induce exercise-related asthma (this is also far more common in children than adults). Her SpO_2 of 88% is quite telling. Asthma is unlikely to lead to a drop in oxygen saturations, except as a late sign, as the issue with asthma is not getting air into the lungs, it is getting air out of the lungs. Once gas trapping associated with asthma results in reduced airflow, SpO_2 can certainly drop, but this would most probably be associated with an altered conscious state and severe respiratory distress. Far more likely is that this patient has a reduced lung density because of her smoking, which has resulted in a very low exercise capacity before her respiratory system can no longer meet her body's oxygenation demands. Her lack of healthcare means that she would be unlikely to be managing her condition well, and therefore even a 500-metre walk is enough to cause an exacerbation of her COPD.

Acute Pulmonary Oedema

Acute pulmonary oedema (APO) refers to the rapid accumulation of fluid in the lungs, in particular in the alveoli, leading to impaired gas exchange and respiratory distress. The most common cause of acute pulmonary oedema is left ventricular heart failure, specifically systolic dysfunction. In this condition, the left ventricle is unable to pump blood forwards adequately, leading to an increase in left atrial pressure. This elevated pressure is transmitted backwards through the pulmonary veins into the pulmonary capillaries, raising the hydrostatic pressure within these vessels. Increased hydrostatic pressure in the pulmonary capillaries forces fluid out of the capillary walls and into the alveoli and interstitial spaces. This fluid accumulation in the alveoli impairs gas exchange by washing out the surfactant lining of the alveoli, meaning that the alveoli close during expiration, thus preventing gas exchange in this phase.

In addition to heart failure, other factors can contribute to the development of APO. These include myocardial infarction (heart attack), which can lead to ventricular dysfunction and increased pulmonary venous pressure. Valvular heart diseases, such as aortic or mitral valve stenosis or regurgitation, can also disrupt the normal flow of blood and result in elevated pulmonary pressures.

Non-cardiac causes of APO include kidney failure, where fluid overload can overload the circulation and increase capillary hydrostatic pressure. Acute respiratory distress syndrome and severe lung infections can also damage the capillary walls and increase their permeability, allowing fluid to leak into the alveoli.

The hallmark symptom of APO is severe shortness of breath, accompanied by a sensation of suffocation and a feeling of impending doom. Other common signs and symptoms include rapid and laboured breathing, coughing with frothy pink or blood-tinged sputum, wheezing and cyanosis (blue-purple, grey-green or pale white discoloration of the skin and mucous membranes). The patient may also exhibit anxiety, restlessness and confusion due to inadequate oxygen supply to the brain.

Pharmacology

The key medication used in the treatment of APO is glyceryl trinitrate (GTN). GTN is a prodrug that is converted to nitric oxide within the smooth muscle cells. Nitric oxide activates the enzyme guanylate cyclase, leading to the formation of cyclic guanosine monophosphate (cGMP). Increased levels of cGMP result in smooth muscle relaxation, leading to vasodilation.

In the context of APO, the venous vasodilatory effects of GTN reduce the volume of blood returning to the heart (preload) and decrease the pressure in the pulmonary vasculature. This reduces the hydrostatic pressure within the pulmonary capillaries, alleviating fluid accumulation and pulmonary congestion.

Medications Management: Glyceryl trinitrate

GTN is a potent vasodilator that acts primarily on the venous system, although it also has some arterial vasodilatory effects. GTN can be administered via various routes, including sublingual tablets, transdermal patches or intravenous infusion. When given sublingually, GTN is rapidly absorbed through the oral mucosa and enters the systemic circulation. It has a short half-life of a few minutes, requiring frequent administration to maintain therapeutic levels.

Management

The management of APO focuses on improving oxygenation, relieving symptoms and addressing the underlying cause. Immediate interventions may include upright positioning to facilitate breathing and administering supplemental oxygen. In the setting of cardiogenic APO, vasodilators such as GTN can help to decrease preload and afterload on the heart, which reduces pressure in the pulmonary circuit and reduces fluid accumulation in the lungs.

For more severe cases, continuous positive airway pressure (CPAP) can be used to deliver a continuous flow of positive pressure to the patient's airways throughout the respiratory cycle, which helps to prevent fluid from entering the alveoli. This also serves to keep the alveoli open during expiration, preventing alveolar collapse due to surfactant washout. CPAP is typically applied using a mask, allowing the patient to breathe spontaneously.

Upper Airway Obstruction

Upper airway obstruction refers to any narrowing or occlusion (partial or complete) that leads to a compromise in ventilation. It may arise as a result of foreign body (airway) obstruction (FBAO), relaxation of the tongue, or be due to swelling of the airway structures which causes a reduction in lumen size. Pathologies such as anaphylaxis, croup, airway burns, epiglottitis and related events, in addition to traumatic injury, may narrow the airway to a point of restricted airflow and may completely close the airway.

Foreign Body Airway Obstruction

Foreign body airway obstruction (FBAO) may present an immediately life-threatening situation. FBAO may present as either *complete*, in which no air movement can occur, or *partial*, in which some amount of air may pass the obstruction. The underlying pathology will determine the required management; however, partial obstruction may progress as the airway swells and spasms, or as the object moves or conforms to the shape of the airway.

Red Flag: Paediatric Concerns

Common causes of FBAO in paediatrics includes items such as batteries, balloons, marbles, coins and paper; however, almost 60% of all cases are food. Difficulty swallowing associated with neurological impairment carries a higher risk of airway comprise through obstruction (Dodson and Cook 2023).

Partial Foreign Body Airway Obstruction

Partial FBAO is likely to present with gasping, noisy breathing, coughing and panic. A stridor may be present, which is not the same as a wheeze and sounds more like a high-pitched whistle. In the out-of-hospital context, an incomplete obstruction caused by a foreign body is best managed by reassuring the patient and encouraging them to slow their breathing and to cough. Helping the patient to position themselves so that their head and shoulders are forward may use gravity to expel the obstruction if coughed upwards. Attempting other interventions may result in the obstruction turning from partial to complete, so must not be performed.

Complete Foreign Body Airway Obstruction

In complete obstruction, the patient will likely clutch their throat (the universal choking sign) and will present with extreme distress. Although the respiratory muscles may be working, there will be no air movement or associated sound. As the respiratory muscles reduce intrathoracic pressure against an occluded airway, there may be tracheal tugging or intercostal recession and, as the patient becomes hypoxic, changes in skin colour, cyanosis and altered level of consciousness may ensue.

Management of a complete obstruction requires up to five sharp back blows with the hand in the middle of the back between the shoulder blades. If five back blows do not resolve the obstruction, then five chest thrusts should be administered similar to chest compressions but sharper. The intent is that following each back blow or chest thrust, the patient is rapidly reassessed to ascertain any success in partially or fully resolving the obstruction. Back blows and chest thrusts should alternate (five then five) until the obstruction is cleared or until the patient becomes unresponsive, at which time you would enter into a cardiac arrest protocol. Ideally, the patient will be positioned with their upper airway facing downwards, so that gravity can assist. Should the obstruction partially resolve, then management must be as for partial FBAO above.

213

Relaxation of the Tongue

The tongue is a voluntarily controlled muscle attached to the mouth floor, meaning that an obtunded patient's tongue may become relaxed as tone decreases. Where a patient is positioned semi-recumbent or supine, relaxation of the tongue may result in obstruction to the airway (Figure 10.8). Partial obstruction causes snoring respirations and may produce gasping or choking, which would normally rouse a patient. In patients who are obtunded due to injury, medical event or pharmacology, an oropharyngeal airway (or superior airway) and manual airway manoeuvres should be initiated.

Trauma

Traumatic injury may compromise the airway through several mechanisms: swelling, structural damage, bleeding and loss of neural control and muscle tone. Airway compromise may arise as an isolated injury or in the setting of polytrauma. These cases are further complicated by concurrent spinal management, haemodynamic instability and problems sealing the mask to the traumatised face. Jaw thrust is the mainstay of immediate management; care must be taken to exclude basal skull injury where a nasopharyngeal airway is considered; intubation or surgical airway may be warranted.

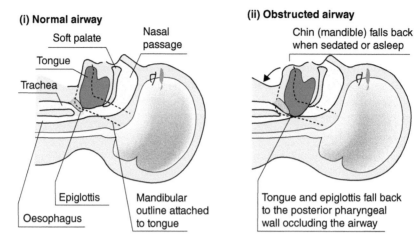

FIGURE 10.8   Obstruction of the airway caused by relaxation of the tongue.

Medical Events

Medical events such as anaphylaxis, croup and epiglottitis may result in swelling of the airways and associated structures. Tissue inflammation and oedema causing the airway walls to swell results in narrowing of the lumen and reduced airflow. Management of the underlying medical event may involve the administration of intramuscular or intravenous adrenaline in the setting of anaphylaxis or nebulised adrenaline and steroidal medications, in cases of severe croup or epiglottitis.

Snapshot 10.2

Pre-arrival Information

You are dispatched to a residential address for a 45-year-old man.

On Arrival with the Patient

On arrival, you find the patient sitting in a chair, visibly distressed and struggling to breathe. He is sweating profusely and keeps saying 'cannot breathe' every few moments. He smells of cigarette smoke.

Patient Assessment

You perform a quick assessment and find:

- Respiratory rate 28 breaths/minute. He is using accessory muscles to breathe, and you can hear audible inspiratory and expiratory wheezing. His SpO$_2$ is 94%.
- Heart rate 130 beats/minute and blood pressure 140/90 mmHg.
- He will not answer any questions due to his shortness of breath but makes purposeful movements when asked.
- Electrocardiogram (ECG): normal sinus rhythm
- Blood Glucose level 4.2 mmol/l
- Temperature 36.9°C.

   The patient is clutching a salbutamol inhaler, with no spacer, and you note that it is both expired and empty. You ask him if he has a history of COPD and he shakes his head and says the word 'asthma', followed by 'cannot breathe' again.

Intervention

Given this assessment, you determine that the patient is in severe respiratory distress due to an acute exacerbation of asthma. You request intensive-care paramedic backup and begin your treatment.

   The patient is well positioned, so you administer salbutamol and ipratropium bromide through a nebuliser mask. You attempt to administer a corticosteroid orally, but the patient is still in too much distress to take the medication, so you administer an intravenous dose.

After five minutes of this treatment, the patient is showing signs of exhaustion. His respiratory rate, heart rate and blood pressure are all dropping. His SpO_2 is now 90% and he is beginning to become drowsy and hard to rouse. You therefore administer adrenaline intramuscularly.

Five minutes later, the patient's breathing begins to settle down. He is still drowsy, but the audible wheeze has lessened and his SpO_2 has risen to 92%. You provide an additional dose of salbutamol, but no additional doses of ipratropium or dexamethasone, as you have given the maximum dose already. Five minutes after this, the patient is able to breathe relatively easily, and his conscious state has returned to normal. You transport the patient to hospital with the intensive-care paramedic, monitoring his respiratory status to see if he requires additional doses of salbutamol.

Take Home Points

- The respiratory system is responsible for ventilation and respiration, so that the body can deliver oxygen to the tissues and maintain homeostasis.
- Asthma is an incurable but reversible chronic airway disease, causing obstruction of airflow due to a hypersensitive reaction, and is characterised by widespread airway inflammation, bronchoconstriction and excessive mucous oedema. Asthma is generally treated with bronchodilators, such as salbutamol and ipratropium, corticosteroids and, in severe cases, adrenalin.
- COPD refers to a group (emphysema, chronic bronchitis and chronic asthma) of chronic, irreversible and incurable diseases that which limit the movement of air through the lungs. The key difference between COPD and asthma is that, in COPD, lung tissue is destroyed, often due to smoking. Treatment is the same as for asthma.
- APO refers to the rapid accumulation of fluid in the lungs, in particular in the alveoli, leading to impaired gas exchange and respiratory distress. Treatment seeks to reduce the pressure in the pulmonary blood vessels, using nitrates and providing CPAP to maintain pressure in the alveoli and prevent closure.
- Upper airway obstruction refers to any narrowing or occlusion (partial or complete) which leads to a compromise in ventilation. Foreign body removal treatment focuses on removing the obstruction, while obstructions due to swelling following other disease processes require reversal of the root cause.

Summary

215

The respiratory system is responsible for ensuring that the cardiovascular system is able to provide oxygenated blood to the tissues, and for excreting the key metabolic waste of carbon dioxide. The respiratory system achieves this through facilitation of ventilation and respiration. Several conditions can prevent the respiratory system from performing its function; for example, asthma reduces the ability to easily draw air into and expel out of the lungs; COPD reduces the lung tissue available for gas change; APO results in fluid accumulation in the lungs, preventing gas exchange; and upper airway obstructions block air from entering the system. Rapid identification and treatment of these conditions requires the capacity to identify and manage symptoms using a range of pharmacology and non-pharmacological options.

References

Brinkman, J.E., Toro, F., and Sharma, S. (2023). *Physiology, Respiratory Drive*. Treasure Island, FL: StatPearls Publishing https://www.ncbi.nlm.nih.gov/books/NBK482414.

Cooksley, N.A., Atkinson, D., Marks, G.B. et al. (2015). Prevalence of airflow obstruction and reduced forced vital capacity in an aboriginal Australian population: the cross-sectional BOLD study. *Respirology* 20 (5): 766–774. https://doi.org/10.1111/resp.12482.

Delgado, B.J. and Bajaj, T. (2022). *Phyiology, Lung Capacity*. Treasure Island, FL: StatPearls Publishing https://www.ncbi.nlm.nih.gov/books/NBK541029.

Dezube, R. (2023). Exchanging oxygen and carbon dioxide. In: *MSD Manual: Consumer Version*. Rahway, NJ: Merck & Co. Inc. https://www.msdmanuals.com/en-au/home/lung-and-airway-disorders/biology-of-the-lungs-and-airways/exchanging-oxygen-and-carbon-dioxide.

Dodson, H. and Cook, J. (2023). *Foreign Body Airway Obstruction*. Treasure Island, FL: StatPearls Publishing https://www.ncbi.nlm.nih.gov/books/NBK553186.

Ramamoorthy, S. and Cidlowski, J.A. (2016). Corticosteroids. *Rheumatic Disease Clinics of North America* 42 (1): 15–31. https://doi.org/10.1016/j.rdc.2015.08.002.

Safka, K.A. and McIvor, R.A. (2015). Non-pharmacological management of chronic obstructive pulmonary disease. *The Ulster Medical Journal* 84 (1): 13–21.

UC Davis Health. (2023). *Asthma in Children and Teens*. Sacramento, CA: UC Davis Health Children's Hospital. https://health.ucdavis.edu/children/patient-education/asthma-children-teens/asthma-triggers (accessed 5 October 2023).

Widysanto, A. and Mathew, G. (2022). *Chronic Bronchitis*. Treasure Island, FL: StatPearls Publishing https://www.ncbi.nlm.nih.gov/books/NBK482437.

World Health Organization. (2023). *Chronic obstructive pulmonary disease (COPD)*. https://www.who.int/news-room/fact-sheets/detail/chronic-obstructive-pulmonary-disease-(copd)#:~:text=Smoking%20and%20air%20pollution%20are,gets%20vaccines%20to%20prevent%20infections. (accessed 5 October 2023).

Further Reading

Davies, A. and Moores, C. (2014). *The Respiratory System: Basic Science and Clinical Conditions*. Burlington, MA: Elsevier Health Sciences.

Gregory, P. and Ward, A. (2018). *Sanders' Paramedic Textbook*, 5e. St Louis, MO: Mosby.

Peate, I. (ed.) *Fundamentals of Applied Anatomy and Pathophysiology. An Essential Guide for Nursing and Healthcare Students*, 4e. Chichester: Wiley.

Peate, I. and Evans, S. (ed.) (2020). *Fundamentals of Anatomy and Physiology for Nursing and Healthcare Students*, 3e. Chichester: Wiley.

West, J.B. and Luks, A.M. (2020). *West's Respiratory Physiology*. Philadelphia, PA: Lippincott Williams & Wilkins.

Online Resources

Biology Forums. *Asthma*. https://biology-forums.com/index.php?action=gallery;sa=view;id=10051.

Nickson, C. (2020). Spirometry. *Life in the Fast Lane* 3 November. https://litfl.com/spirometry (accessed 5 October 2023).

Northshore University Health System. (2022). Spacer for metered dose inhaler. *Health Encyclopedia* 13 November. https://www.northshore.org/healthresources/encyclopedia/encyclopedia.aspx?DocumentHwid=aa126687.

Glossary

Asthma	An incurable, but reversible, chronic airway disease causing obstruction of airflow due to a hypersensitive reaction in the airways.
Acute pulmonary oedema (APO)	The rapid accumulation of fluid in the lungs, in particular in the alveoli, leading to impaired gas exchange and respiratory distress.
Chronic obstructive pulmonary disease (COPD)	A group of chronic, irreversible and incurable diseases which limit the movement of air through the lungs, including emphysema, chronic bronchitis and chronic asthma.

Continuous positive airway pressure (CPAP)	Delivery of oxygen in a continuous flow of positive pressure to the patient's airways throughout the respiratory cycle
Foreign body airway obstruction (FBAO)	Any occlusion of the airway due to a foreign body, relaxation of the tongue or swelling of the airway structures.
Gas trapping	An accumulation of trapped air in the alveoli due to bronchoconstriction and mucous plugs.
Lower respiratory tract	The trachea, primary bronchi, bronchioles and alveoli (the elements of the system within the thorax).
Mucous plugs	A blockage of the small airways due to excessive mucous secretion.
Respiration	The process of gas exchange occurring in the alveoli.
Respiratory tract	The group of airway structures which warm, humidify, filter and conduct air from the atmosphere to the alveoli.
Upper airway obstruction	Any narrowing or occlusion of the airways (partial or complete) which leads to a compromise in ventilation.
Upper respiratory tract	The nasal cavity, larynx and pharynx (those elements above the thorax).
Ventilation	The mechanical act of drawing air in and out of the lungs, includes inhaling and exhaling.

Multiple Choice Questions

1. What is the pharynx more generally known as?
   a. The mouth
   b. The throat
   c. The vocal chords
   d. The lungs

2. Surfactant is used in the alveoli for what purpose?
   a. To prevent them collapsing on expiration
   b. To prevent them collapsing on inspiration
   c. To capture pathogens and remove them from the respiratory system
   d. To secrete mucous

3. The mechanical act of drawing air in and out of the lungs is known as what?
   a. Perfusion
   b. Homeostasis
   c. Respiration
   d. Ventilation

4. Which of these is NOT a characteristic of asthma?
   a. widespread airway inflammation
   b. Bronchoconstriction
   c. Over production of mucus from the goblet cells
   d. Destruction of lung tissue

5. Emphysema is characterised by what?
   a. Fluid build up in the lungs
   b. Smooth muscle constriction in the lungs
   c. Reduced lung tissue
   d. A blockage of the lower airways

6. In which of the following conditions is wheezing NOT present as a symptom?
   a. Asthma
   b. COPD
   c. APO
   d. Partial upper airway obstruction due to a foreign body

7. Which medication reduces preload?
   a. Salbutamol
   b. Adrenalin
   c. GTN
   d. CPAP

8. Which medication blocks muscarinic cholinergic receptors?
   a. Ipratropium
   b. Salbutamol
   c. Dexamethasone
   d. GTN

9. Which of the following is a cardiogenic cause of APO?
   a. Kidney failure
   b. AMI
   c. Acute respiratory distress syndrome
   d. Severe lung infections

10. First-line treatment for complete upper airway obstructions is what?
    a. Chest thrusts
    b. Encouraging the patient to cough
    c. Back blows
    d. Administering adrenaline

CHAPTER 11

The Gastrointestinal System and Associated Disorders

Ian Peate and Neil Coleman

AIM

This chapter aims to introduce the reader to the gastrointestinal system and its functions.

LEARNING OUTCOMES

After completing this chapter, you will be able to:

- Identify the organs of the gastrointestinal system.
- Explain how food moves from the mouth through the gastrointestinal system.
- Describe the structures of the gastrointestinal system.
- Discuss the role of the paramedic when responding to people who have gastrointestinal disorders.

Test Your Prior Knowledge
1. When food enters the mouth, approximately how far must it travel before excretion will occur?
2. Where and how are the major nutrients used in the body?
3. Describe common reasons why a patient might experience diarrhoea?
4. Why might pain in the lower right quadrant of the abdomen indicate a potentially serious condition?

Fundamentals of Applied Pathophysiology for Paramedics, First Edition. Edited by Ian Peate and Simon Sawyer.
© 2024 John Wiley & Sons Ltd. Published 2024 by John Wiley & Sons Ltd.

Introduction

The gastrointestinal (GI) system is often interchangeably referred to as the digestive tract or the alimentary canal (Figure 11.1). The track from mouth to anus is approximately 8 m long. This system is responsible for the intake of raw materials (from the mouth), the absorption of nutrients from food and fluids and elimination of waste material from the body. This process is broken down into six stages:

1. Ingestion
2. Propulsion
3. Digestion
4. Absorption
5. Assimilation
6. Elimination.

The body moves food and fluids through the gastrointestinal system, taking what nutrients it can from it, and removing what is left. Table 11.1 details these six stages.

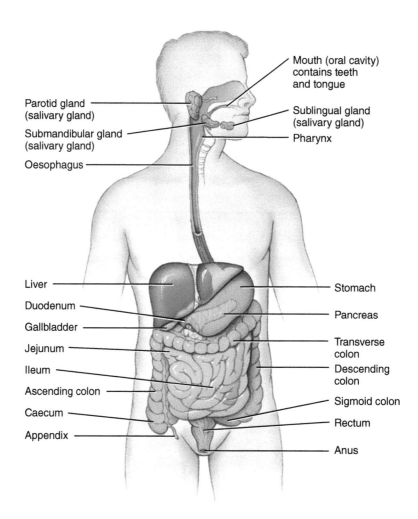

Mouth (oral cavity) contains teeth and tongue

Parotid gland (salivary gland)

Submandibular gland (salivary gland)

Oesophagus

Sublingual gland (salivary gland)

Pharynx

Liver

Duodenum

Gallbladder

Jejunum

Ileum

Ascending colon

Caecum

Appendix

Stomach

Pancreas

Transverse colon

Descending colon

Sigmoid colon

Rectum

Anus

FIGURE 11.1   The gastrointestinal system. Source: Peate and Evans (2020)/John Wiley & Sons.

TABLE 11.1 The stages of digestion.

Stage	Description
Ingestion	Eating and drinking; the process by which raw materials are introduced to the digestive system
Propulsion	Movement of food through the digestive system, facilitated by muscular contractions such as peristalsis
Digestion	The breaking down of food within the system; this commences with chewing (mastication). As the food moves down the tract, a chemical process takes place that further breaks the food down
Absorption	The nutrients from the digestive process are now 'absorbed' into the blood stream
Assimilation	The use of absorbed nutrients by the cells and integration into the body's tissues and organs
Elimination	Materials that have been eaten but cannot be digested and absorbed are passed out of the body as waste (faeces)

Components of the Gastrointestinal System

The Mouth

The mouth is where ingestion takes place but also where digestion begins. Food in its solid form starts to break down from a combination of mastication and the release of saliva into the mouth. The saliva contains an enzyme called amylase or salivary amylase. Saliva is released into the mouth from three paired primary salivary glands, which are located under at the floor of the mouth (sublingual glands), in the cheeks (parotid glands) and under the angle of the jaw (submandibular glands; Figure 11.2).

Mechanical digestion refers to chewing and ripping of the food by the teeth to make the object smaller and therefore easier to swallow. Chemical digestion refers to the use of amylase to break down the food. Both take place before the food has even left the mouth. As an additional benefit, reducing the size of the food particles increases the surface area of each particle, thus making chemical digestion easier.

Pharynx

The pharynx connects the mouth to the oesophagus. When mastication is complete, food is pushed backwards towards the pharynx. This is achieved by a reflex action that takes places in the wall of the oropharynx, and the process is coordinated by the swallowing centre of the brain, which is located in the medulla. The chewed food (referred to now as a bolus) is prevented from being aspirated by an involuntary process where the soft palate rises up and closes off the nasopharynx while the larynx lifts up and forwards Additionally, the epiglottis occludes the opening to the trachea so that the bolus cannot enter the airway (Figure 11.3).

Oesophagus

Located posteriorly to the trachea, the oesophagus is the muscular tube running from the pharynx to the stomach. Once the bolus is in the pharynx, the oesophagus is stimulated to commence the process of peristalsis. Peristalsis is a rhythmic muscular contraction and relaxation of muscles causing a wave life movement; in this case, the action forces the food downwards towards the opening to the stomach (Figure 11.4).

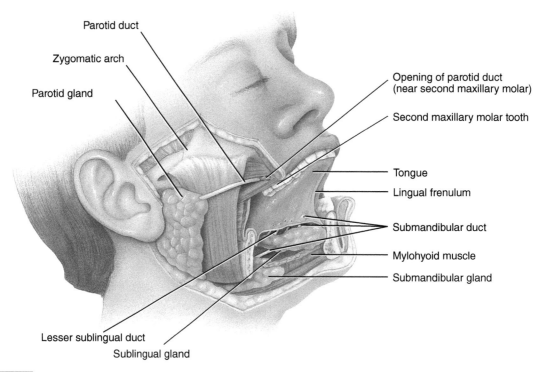

FIGURE 11.2 The salivary glands. Source: Peate and Evans (2020)/John Wiley & Sons.

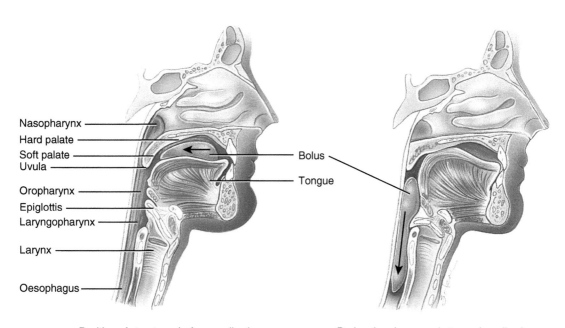

Position of structures before swallowing   During the pharyngeal stage of swallowing

FIGURE 11.3 Swallowing. Source: Peate and Evans (2020)/John Wiley & Sons.

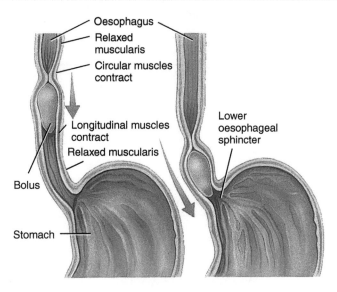

Anterior view of frontal sections of peristalsis in oesophagus

FIGURE 11.4 Peristalsis. Source: Peate and Evans (2020)/John Wiley & Sons.

At the bottom of the oesophagus is the lower oesophageal sphincter, the muscle which guards the opening to the stomach. Just prior to peristalsis, this sphincter relaxes and opens to allow the bolus to enter the stomach. It closes again once the bolus has passed into the stomach to prevent regurgitation of gastric content into the oesophagus.

Stomach

The stomach begins at the lower oesophageal sphincter and ends at the pyloric sphincter (Figure 11.5). The stomach churns food and breaks it down further into a milky material known as chyme. Gastric juices assist in the process. They are released by the walls of the stomach, which contains millions of glands (Figure 11.6).

Small Intestine

The small intestine is composed of three parts (Figure 11.7):

1. *The duodenum* is approximately 25 cm long and 5 cm wide. It commences at the pyloric sphincter and continues into the jejunum.
2. *The jejunum* is the middle section of the small intestine and is approximately 2 m long.
3. *The ilium* is the 'end' section of the small intestine but is also the longest, at approximately 3 m long.

By the time that the chyme reaches the small intestine, digestion is complete, and the majority of absorption is also complete. In the small intestine, the pancreas releases pancreatic amylase via a duct and this serves to make the perfect pH in the small intestine for several processes:

- Digestion of proteins: converts proteins to amino acids.
- Digestion of carbohydrates: converts all digestible starches that have not already been digested by salivary amylase into glucose, fructose or galactose.
- Digestion of fats: converts fats to fatty acids and glycerol.

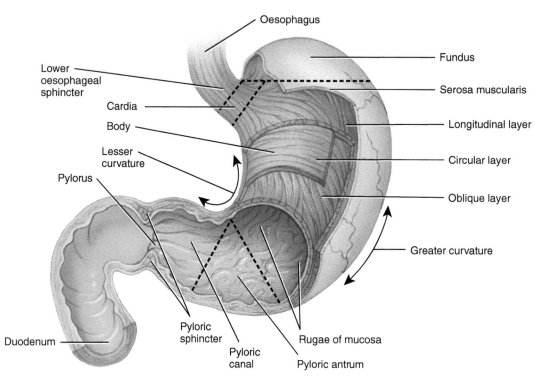

Anterior view of regions of stomach

FIGURE 11.5 The stomach. Source: Peate and Evans (2020)/John Wiley & Sons.

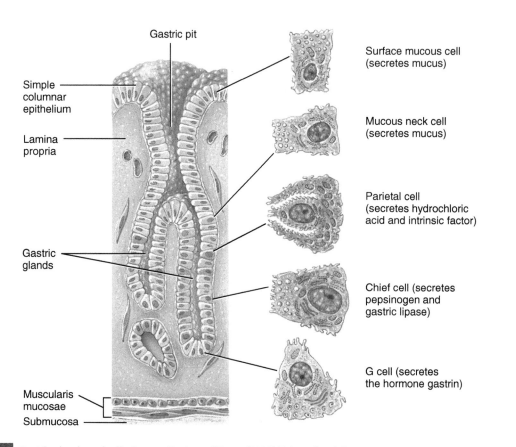

FIGURE 11.6 Gastric glands and cells. Source: Peate and Evans (2020)/John Wiley & Sons.

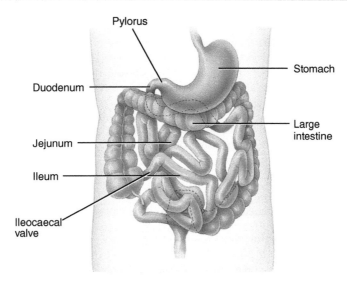

Pylorus

Stomach

Duodenum

Large
intestine

Jejunum

Ileum

Ileocaecal
valve

FIGURE 11.7 The small intestine. Source: Peate and Evans (2020)/John Wiley & Sons.

Large Intestine

The large intestine is divided into three parts: the ascending colon, which begins at the caecum, the transverse colon and the descending colon. This is the final part of the gastrointestinal system. Content can remain here for 10 hours to several days. The large intestine is actively involved in the reabsorption of water from the remnants of food, and what is left is known as faeces. Faeces are stored in the rectum until ejected from the system via the anal canal.

Rectum

The rectum is continuous with the descending colon. It is from here that the faeces are stored and then expelled via the anus and the process of elimination is completed.

Clinical Investigations: Gastrointestinal Disorders

GI emergencies are commonly precipitated by lifestyle, and these factors can indicate what may be the underlying issues. Excessive alcohol consumption, excessive smoking and increased stress are all common causes of GI presentations at hospital (Haber and Kortt 2021). However, it is important to note that a comprehensive assessment of the patient is required before making a field diagnosis, as many GI disturbances can be indicative of, or associated with, other conditions.

The assessment of the patient with a gastrointestinal disorder will not differ from the assessment of any other patient; however, there is scope within assessment protocols to expand history taking with a patient whose primary complaint appears to be GI in nature.

The paramedic's first concern should be for their own safety, but once this is ascertained, perusing the scene to attempt to establish whether the complaint is mechanical or non-mechanical should be prioritised. Did the patient fall and now has bruising to the abdomen or was the pain acute in nature?

The 'OPQRST' evaluation of the person with GI disorder can be particularly telling. This should be completed after a SAMPLE history has been taken and should be used as an additional tool to help reach a working diagnosis. Some key points of this assessment include:

- **Onset**: in a GI complaint, acute pain is often associated with perforation of an organ whereas chronic pain is more commonly associated with obstructions.
- **Provocation or palliation**: if walking relieves the pain, consider a GI or urinary root cause, such as a renal stone (renal calculi) lodged in the renal pelvis or obstruction of the gallbladder caused by cholelithiasis (gallbladder stones). If moving the knees towards the abdomen relieves pain, consideration should be given to peritoneal inflammation, which is commonly GI in nature.

- **Quality**: dull pain usually equates to obstruction; sharp pain may indicate renal calculi, especially if localised to one side. You can read more about this in Chapter 9.
- **Radiation**: pain referred to the shoulder or neck is often linked to the diaphragm. This referred pain is common in cholecystitis.
- **Severity**: severity of pain commonly increases as the condition progresses.
- **Time**: generally, abdominal pain in excess of six hours is considered to be an emergency, although exact timings vary with jurisdictional norms.

Associated symptoms should also be assessed. If the patient has vomited, what colour was the vomit? What did it look like? Was it an isolated or repeated vomiting spell? This can give valuable clues as to where the issue may lie.

In an out-of-hospital environment, patient presentations that involve the GI tract can be divided into two broad categories:

- Upper GI – which consists of the mouth, pharynx, oesophagus, stomach and duodenum.
- Lower GI – which consists of the small and large intestines and the anus.

The assessment and management of upper and lower gastrointestinal problems in the prehospital care setting can range from mild discomfort to serious emergencies. Depending on the severity and specific diagnosis, the patient may require urgent transport to hospital for further evaluation, management and continuing care (Greaves and Porter 2021).

Table 11.2 provides a list of common gastrointestinal conditions that the paramedic may encounter in the out-of-hospital care setting.

TABLE 11.2   Common gastrointestinal conditions.

Condition	Discussion	Common management
Gastroenteritis	The inflammation of the stomach and intestines, often caused by viral or bacterial infections. It may lead to symptoms such as diarrhoea, vomiting, abdominal pain and dehydration	Antiemetics to reduce vomiting; analgesics for pain relief; fluid for dehydration
Gastric ulcers	Open sores developing on the lining of the stomach. They can cause symptoms such as abdominal pain, nausea, vomiting (sometimes with blood) and melaena	Analgesics for pain relief
Gallstones	Cholelithiasis; hardened deposits that form in the gallbladder. They may result in severe abdominal pain, typically in the upper right quadrant, together with nausea and vomiting	Analgesics for pain relief
Appendicitis	Inflammation of the appendix, known as appendicitis, is a common surgical emergency. It causes severe abdominal pain, usually starting around the navel and moving to the lower right side (Figure 11.9), together with pyrexia and nausea	Analgesics for pain relief
Bowel obstruction	An obstruction in the intestines, preventing the passage of faeces. It leads to symptoms that include severe abdominal pain, bloating, constipation and vomiting	Antiemetics to reduce vomiting; analgesics for pain relief
Gastrointestinal bleeding	Haemorrhage can occur in any part of the gastrointestinal tract; it can range from mild to life-threatening. It may present with symptoms such as haematemesis or haematochezia, melaena and abdominal pain	Analgesics for pain relief

Conditions of the Upper Gastrointestinal Tract

Upper Gastrointestinal Haemorrhage

Upper GI haemorrhages are common and account for a significant number of hospital admissions annually. It should be noted that locating the exact cause of a haemorrhage in an out-of-hospital environment is often challenging. Overall, the majority of gastrointestinal haemorrhages will be caused by erosion of the gastric mucosa. Many patients may present with nausea and vomiting, as blood severely irritates the GI system. In addition, the patient may have experienced haematemesis (bloody vomitus) or melaena (bloody stool). For melaena to be present, there must have been blood present in the GI tract for at least five to eight hours.

Orange Flag Alert: Homelessness

Homeless people are at relatively high risk for a broad range of acute and chronic illnesses. Precise data on the prevalence of specific illnesses among homeless people compared with those among people with settled homes are difficult to obtain. Homeless people have many risk factors for dyspepsia (indigestion), but little information is available on gastrointestinal symptoms in this population. The presence of upper stomach pain is most strongly associated with a history of gastrointestinal disease. Chronic homelessness is characterised by a trimorbidity: homeless people are more likely to experience poor mental ill health, poor physical health and to engage in substance use. Additionally, homeless people have much higher barriers to accessing the health services they need (Snellaert 2018).

227

Peptic Ulcer Disease

An ulcer is a sore, while a peptic ulcer is a sore that forms in the stomach or oesophagus. Peptic ulcers formed in the stomach will also sometimes be referred to as gastric ulcers. Peptic ulcer disease accounts for a significant amount of upper GI bleeds. This number is estimated to be in the region of 50% of all upper GI bleeds. Figure 11.8 shows common sites for peptic ulcers.

Common complaints from patients with peptic ulcers may include:

- Dull pain in the abdomen (dull burning pain is the often stated as a symptom).
- Unexplained weight loss.

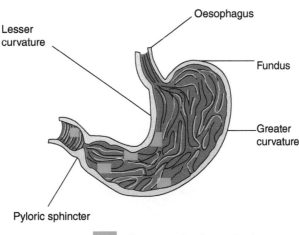

Commom sites for peptic ulcer

FIGURE 11.8 Common sites for peptic ulcer. Source: Peate and Evans (2020)/John Wiley & Sons.

- Indigestion or gastric reflux.
- Change in colour of the stool.

Red Flag Alert: Chronic Abdominal Pain

- Abdominal pain that is chronic and in excess of six hours should be considered an emergency.

Medications Management: Proton Pump Inhibitors

Proton pump inhibitors work by inhibiting gastric hydrogen potassium ATPase (H^+K^+ ATPase; the proton pump) in the stomach. It may be important for paramedics to consider if patients are indeed compliant with their prescribed proton pump inhibitor medication. Examples of proton pump inhibitors include omeprazole, lansoprazole, pantoprazole, rabeprazole, esomeprazole and dexlansoprazole.

Treatment is often based around medications aimed at reducing gastric acid reflux (a group of medications called proton pump inhibitors), and antacids to reduce indigestion such as symptoms (by neutralising gastric acid). The patient may also be prescribed histamine blockers which also act to reduce gastric acid by blocking H2 receptor sites.

Reflective Learning Activity

Choose three proton pump inhibitors and make notes on them. Include the dose, route of administration, adverse effects and contraindications.

Medications Management: Non-steroidal Anti-inflammatory Drugs

Non-steroidal anti-inflammatory drugs (NSAIDs) can damage the gastroduodenal mucosa. They can reduce the positive barrier properties of the mucus, suppress gastric prostaglandin synthesis and interfere with the natural repair of mucosal injury.

Treatment for peptic ulcers not linked to *Helicobacter pylori* does not need an antibiotic. An H2-receptor antagonist such as ranitidine, cimetidine or famotidine is usually sufficient to promote healing of the ulcer. H2-receptor antagonists are often given prophylactically to prevent gastrointestinal complications.

Gastritis

Gastritis is an inflammation of the mucosa of the stomach. It is commonly caused by the same process that will cause peptic ulcers. Treatment is similar to that of peptic ulcer disease, and patients may also be advised to avoid spicy foods or foods that cause further irritation.

Medications are often antacids; however, if on examination and testing the clinician feels that the condition is being caused by *H. pylori* bacteria, the patient will most like be on, or have recently completed a course of prescribed antibiotics (this also applies to peptic ulcer disease).

Medicine Management: Antacids

Antacids are not usually prescribed for gastric ulcer, nor are they encouraged, as they only manage the symptoms. Antacids do not eradicate the ulcer; however, they can be given for symptom management.

Variceal Rupture

Varices are veins that are dilated beyond what is normal. Variceal bleeding refers to bleeding that occurs in the GI tract. A rupture of an oesophageal varix will cause copious bleeding and is a life-threatening emergency. Signs and symptoms will be similar to those seen in a patient who is in hypovolaemic shock (Chapter 5), as the patient may be losing a significant amount of blood. Your primary concern will be airway management if the bleed is occurring in the oesophagus, as there is a higher chance of respiratory compromise and ultimately respiratory arrest.

Mallory–Weiss Tears

Mallory–Weiss tears are oesophageal lacerations most commonly secondary to bouts of significant vomiting. These tears are most commonly in the lower oesophageal tract (although they can also occur in the upper oesophagus), and patients may complain of abdominal pain, haematemesis and/or melaena.

In an out-of-hospital environment, there is little that can be done for this condition other than analgesia. The patient should be transferred or referred to an appropriate care provider. Many of these tears will self-heal, usually within approximately eight days. If the symptoms persist, hospital-based treatments are required.

Oesophagitis

Commonly caused by the reflux of gastric acid, oesophagus is inflammation of the oesophagus. Patients may present with chest pain, indigestion symptoms and dysphagia (difficulty swallowing). Assessment of these patients should not focus on GI suspicions, as many of these symptoms may also be common in other conditions. In an out-of-hospital setting, treatment is based on patient comfort and treating the presenting symptoms.

Duodenitis

As the name suggests, duodenitis is inflammation of the lining of the duodenum. This condition commonly presents with gastritis and, when this occurs, it is referred to as gastroduodenitis. Symptoms are similar to gastritis.

Conditions of the Lower Gastrointestinal Tract

Lower Gastrointestinal Tract Bleeds

Lower GI bleeds tend to be chronic in nature and are often associated with the process of ageing.

Haemorrhoids

Haemorrhoids are swollen veins that occur in the anus, often in groups or masses. The cause of most haemorrhoids is idiopathic (of unknown cause). Of the known causes, portal hypertension, pregnancy and lifting heavy objects are common. People who have low-fibre diets are more prone to this condition, as with other conditions of the lower GI tract. Morbidity from haemorrhoids is low, but care should be taken with patients who are alcohol dependent, as there may also be cirrhosis of the liver.

Symptoms would commonly be bright red bleeding and/or pain when defaecating. While the majority of these patients will require only support and transport, there should always be an awareness of the possibility of significant bleeding due to this condition.

Red Flag Alert: Gastrointestinal Bleeding

Gastrointestinal bleeding can be obscure or occult (not visible externally). There is a high risk of occult bleeding in the gastrointestinal tract, which may delay identification and management, thus impacting prognosis.

Snapshot 11.1

Pre-arrival Information

You are responding to a 33 year old woman who is complaining of lower left quadrant pain. The pain was acute in nature, and onset two days ago. The patient states that it is becoming progressively worse.

On Arrival with the Patient

The patient is significantly overweight and informs you that her diet is based largely on takeaway and convenience foods of low nutritional quality.

History

Her medical history reveals no medical conditions of note; however, the patient says that her bowel movements for the have been reduced for the past two days.

Reflective Learning Activity

Outline your differential diagnosis for the patient in Snapshot 11.1. What is the most likely cause of this condition? What is your treatment protocol for this patient?

Crohn's Disease

Crohn's disease, is an idiopathic inflammatory bowel disease. It is a chronic, relapsing, non-infectious inflammatory disease of the gastrointestinal tract (National Institute for Health and Care Excellence 2020a). It is one of two idiopathic bowel diseases, the other being ulcerative colitis. The disease has a strong genetic connection and is more common in white females than any other ethnic group. Crohn's can occur in both the upper and lower GI tract, and approximately 35% of cases will include the small intestine. A clinical definition of Crohn's disease is 'inflammation of part of the digestive tract'.

Symptoms of Crohn's can vary. Some patients will complain of diarrhoea, abdominal pain, reduced appetite and/or unexplained weight loss. Symptoms, however, may vary depending on what part of the digestive tract is affected. Significant bleeding with Crohn's is uncommon, so out-of-hospital treatment is usually supportive.

Orange Flag Alert: Pregnancy

In female patients post puberty, pregnancy must be ruled out as the cause of abdominal pain.

Ulcerative Colitis

Ulcerative Colitis is the other idiopathic bowel disease. This disease leads to a continuous length of ulcers in the colon. Clinically defining ulcerative colitis in the out-of-hospital environment may be challenging, as it will often present similar in nature to many other lower GI tract presentations.

Treatment is based on the presentation of the patient. The presence of melaena may indicate significant internal bleeding, so the paramedic should be aware for the possibility of hypovolaemic shock. Patients should be transported to hospital for diagnostic testing, with the use of antiemetics (medications that offset nausea and vomiting) if appropriate.

Diverticulitis

Diverticula are small pouches that form in the intestine. Diverticulitis is an inflammation of the diverticula, which is usually caused by an infection. This is a relatively common condition, with estimates from some countries putting the prevalence at approximately 50% in the population over 60 years of age.

The condition can lead to even further complications, such as larger perforations of the colon and bleeding. Common presentations would include abdominal tenderness on examination, low grade pyrexia and a 'colicky' pain.

In the absence of significant haemorrhage, treatment is largely supportive in the out-of-hospital setting. A high-fibre diet is often recommended for patients diagnosed with diverticulitis.

Orange Flag Alert: Constipation

Any information that the paramedic provides about constipation and its management, including laxative treatment, should be accessible to the patient and their carers.

Bowel Obstruction

Most bowel obstructions are secondary to adhesions as a result of previous surgery (Greaves and Porter 2021). It is most common for obstruction to occur in the small intestine. Any number of causes may lead to an obstruction, although hernia is a common cause. Patients may present with a distended abdomen, but the absence of a distended abdomen should not exclude an obstruction from a differential diagnosis. The paramedic should also observe the abdomen for scars that could indicate previous surgery. Specifically, care should be taken with this patient, as this condition can lead to strangulation of other organs and significant internal bleeding. Pain is often diffuse in nature and the patient may have difficulty identifying the exact location of the pain. Greaves and Porte (2021) identify the following presenting features of bowel obstruction:

- Abdominal pain
- Nausea and vomiting (this may not occur where this distal small bowel and large bowl obstruction)
- Distended abdomen
- Abdominal tenderness
- Constipation
- Abdominal scars, which could indicate previous surgery.

The Acute Abdomen

The clinical presentation of an acute abdomen involves a broad spectrum of disease. The patient can be very unwell or they may deteriorate rapidly and often require early input from a hospital intensive care team. The abdominal cavity itself hosts vast potential for catastrophe, predominantly through haemorrhage, sepsis or ischaemia

(Buczacki and Davies 2018). The prompt assessment of patients reporting or illustrating signs of an acute onset of abdominal symptoms is key in determining an early diagnosis. Diagnosis is facilitated by a systematic approach to history taking, clinical examination, imaging and laboratory results. The need for early detection of abnormal abdominal pathology is further added to by the associated increase in mortality and prevalence of multiorgan failure that is faced by those who need critical care admission (Riley et al. 2023).

In the out-of-hospital setting, managing a patient with an acute abdomen requires the paramedic to undertake prompt and thorough assessment, stabilise the patient and instigate appropriate interventions according to local policy and procedure. Steps for managing an acute abdomen usually include the following:

1. Undertake an initial assessment of the patient's condition, with a focus on a systematic ABCDE approach. First address any immediate life-threatening issues.

2. Generate information about the individual's medical history and any previous surgery, and determine their current symptoms. Ask about the onset, location, severity and character of the abdominal pain and associated symptoms, such as nausea, vomiting or changes in bowel movements.

3. Assess vital signs including heart rate, blood pressure, respiratory rate and oxygen saturation. Monitor the patient's vital signs continuously and reassess as the patient's condition dictates.

4. Perform a secondary survey, examining the patient's abdomen and assessing quadrants for tenderness, distention or other indications of disease.

5. Administer appropriate pain relief measures, adhering to local protocols and guidelines. This could involve the administration of non-opioid analgesics such as paracetamol or NSAIDs. Avoid opioids unless it is necessary, due to their potential adverse effects and the risk of masking symptoms.

6. If the patient shows signs of hypovolaemia or dehydration, provide fluid resuscitation following local protocols to restore and maintain adequate circulation.

7. Arrange for timely transport to the hospital. An acute abdomen will often require surgical evaluation and management. Contact the receiving hospital, informing them about the patient's condition and the suspected diagnosis. This will enable the receiving hospital to prepare for the patient's arrival.

8. Offer emotional support and reassurance to the patient (and if appropriate their family); explain the actions that are being taken and the reasons behind them. Maintain a calm and empathetic approach, alleviating anxiety and stress.

9. Document and communicate your actions.

Care for a patient with an acute abdomen in an out-of-hospital setting requires clinical judgement and may vary depending on the specific cause. Abdominal pain can have several underlying aetiologies (e.g. appendicitis, gallstones, bowel obstruction or perforation) and each will require specific interventions and treatment.

Accessory Organs

While not technically classed as part of the GI tract, there are some accessory organs of the GI tract:

- Appendix
- Liver
- Gall bladder
- Pancreas.

Accessory organs may also give rise to some conditions that the paramedic will also need to consider.

Acute Appendicitis

Appendicitis is an inflammation of the appendix. There are no risk factors that predispose a certain group to this condition, and it is a relatively common emergency. It is more common in young adults and teenagers. The purpose of the appendix is not known, but if it ruptures it can lead to peritonitis as a result of emptying its contents into the peritoneal cavity.

Paramedics play a crucial role in the management of acute appendicitis, primarily in the out-of-hospital setting. While the definitive treatment for acute appendicitis is surgical intervention, paramedics focus on undertaking an initial assessment, administration of analgesia and prompt transport to the appropriate hospital.

It should be noted that a definitive diagnosis and the treatment of acute appendicitis can only be made by a physician in a hospital setting. The paramedic's role is to recognise the signs and symptoms, offer supportive care and arrange for timely transport for definitive management.

Right-sided lower abdominal pain is common, and an accepted test is palpation of McBurney's point (Figures 11.9 and 11.10).

Clinical Investigations: Examination

Performing an abdominal examination is an intimate examination. It is an important skill that is used to assess a patient's abdomen for any signs of potential problems. Consider the following when performing an abdominal examination:

- Introduce yourself to the patient and explain the examination you will be performing. Obtain the patient's consent and ensure comfort and privacy. Determine whether a chaperone is required.
- Decontaminate your hands.
- Ask the patient to lie flat on their back, offering support if needed. The patient's knees should be slightly bent, helping to relax the abdominal muscles.
- Start by inspecting the patient's abdomen visually, noting any abnormalities such as scars, rashes, distension or discoloration.
- Palpate the abdomen. Palpation involves using your hands to feel different areas of the abdomen to assess for tenderness, masses or organ enlargement (organomegaly). Only trained and competent staff should undertake palpation. Follow these steps:
  - *Light palpation*: start by gently pressing all over the abdomen in a systematic manner, use gentle, circular movements. This can help to identify any superficial tenderness or areas of discomfort.
  - *Deep palpation*: with the patient's permission and if there is no significant tenderness, proceed to deep palpation. Apply more pressure, using your fingertips or the palm of your hand; press down slowly and evenly. Assess for masses, organ enlargement or deep tenderness. At all times, observe the patient for signs of pain or discomfort.
  - *Palpate specific organs*: assess individual organs, such as the liver, spleen and kidneys. To palpate the liver, place your left hand under the patient's back at the 11th and 12th ribs, and press your right hand into the abdomen just below the right ribcage. Request the patient to take a deep breath. If there is enlargement (hepatomegaly), you may feel it move downward. Repeat the process to assess the spleen and kidneys.
- Auscultation requires the use of a stethoscope. Listen for bowel sounds over different quadrants of the abdomen. Begin in the right lower quadrant and move clockwise (Figure 11.10). Normal bowel sounds are high-pitched and gurgling. Absence or abnormal sounds may indicate an obstruction or other gastrointestinal issues. It should be noted that, in some jurisdictions, auscultation of the abdomen is not a standard or primary part of the abdominal examination. While auscultation is commonly used to assess lung sounds and heart sounds, it is not normally relied upon for evaluating the abdomen.
- Additional assessments: depending on the patient's symptoms and findings, there may be a need to perform additional assessments such as checking for rebound tenderness (pressing down slowly and releasing quickly to assess for pain), assessing for hernias or examining the inguinal area.
- Documentation: record findings accurately and thoroughly in the patient's medical records, including any abnormal findings, tenderness, masses or other pertinent details.
- Decontaminate your hands as per local policy.

Examination of the abdomen requires practice and experience to become proficient. If you encounter any concerning or complex findings during the examination, you must consult a more senior colleague or refer the patient for further evaluation and management of their condition.

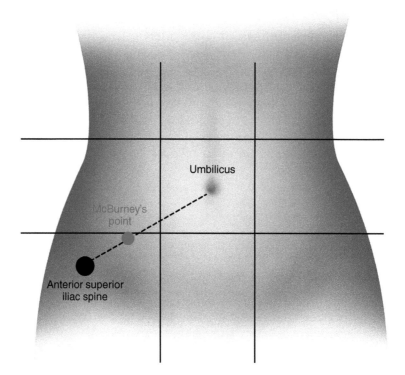

FIGURE 11.9   Mc Burney's point. Source: Peate and Evans (2020)/John Wiley & Sons.

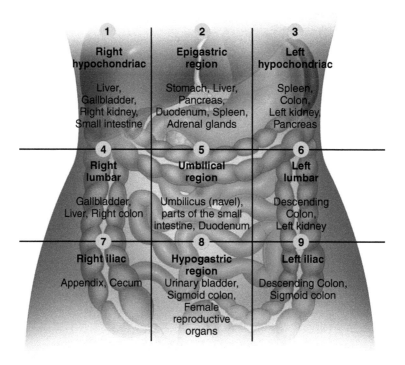

FIGURE 11.10   The abdominal quadrants.

Having a chaperone with a paramedic during medical procedures or examination is important for several reasons. It ensures patient safety by providing additional support and monitoring. Collaboration between the paramedic and chaperone can improve teamwork and coordination. The chaperone may assist with physical tasks and provides emotional support to patients. They also act as a witness for documentation and can help to manage risks associated with procedures.

Cholecystitis

Cholecystitis refers to inflammation of the gall bladder. An inflamed gall bladder will often cause upper right quadrant pain, which may radiate to the right shoulder (Figure 11.10). Most gallstones (the main cause of the inflammation) are caused by cholesterol. Pain will often present after a meal that is high in fat. A positive McBurney's sign (Figure 11.9) tenderness under the right costal arch, may lend to a diagnosis of cholecystitis. Patients will often feel nauseous and will vomit. Out-of-hospital treatment is largely supportive.

Reflective Learning Activity

Reflect on the role of the paramedic and think about how you could help and support a person for whom you are caring who has nausea and vomiting. What actions can you take to provide high-quality effective care?

In the organisation(s) where you undertake clinical practice is there a nausea and vomiting protocol in place? If so, where is it located? Write notes on the key points contained in the protocol.

Pancreatitis

The pancreas is an accessory organ of the digestive system and when it becomes inflamed the condition is referred to as pancreatitis. Pancreatitis can be acute or chronic. Pancreatitis predominantly affects those aged 50–60 years (McErlean 2021).

Risk factors include alcoholism, peptic ulcer disease, trauma affecting the abdomen, hyperlipidaemia, some medications (e.g. some diuretics) and genetic factors. Heavy drinking is the single most important risk factor for chronic pancreatitis, and is responsible for 70–80% of cases in western Europe (National Institute for Health and Care Excellence 2020b).

As pancreatitis progresses, it can lead to sepsis and shock and, as a result, mortality is relatively high. Out-of-hospital treatment is largely supportive.

Snapshot 11.2

You are presented with a 57 year old man, Mr Krish, who has a history of alcohol dependency. He appears to have jaundiced skin and has yellowing of the sclera. The patient complains of feeling unwell. His malaise has become progressively worse over the previous three months. He is still actively drinking up to 14 units per day.

Reflective Learning Activity

Outline your differential diagnosis for the patient in Snapshot 11.2. State any medications that may be ineffective in this patient. What other questions in relation to history would you ask this patient?

Hepatitis

Hepatitis refers to damage to the liver cells associated with inflammation. Hepatitis has many subdivisions: hepatitis A, B, C, D and E. Owing to the large number of causes of hepatitis, mortality is high. Hepatitis A is spread by the oral–faecal route. Hepatitis B is a bloodborne pathogen. Hepatitis C is also bloodborne and is the most common form of hepatitis post blood transfusion. Hepatitis D can only be contracted if the patient is already hepatitis B positive, as hepatitis D is dormant until activated by hepatitis B. Finally, hepatitis E is waterborne and is most prevalent in lower socioeconomic groups. With many of these conditions, out-of-hospital care is supportive in nature.

Manging hepatitis in an out-of-hospital care setting involves ensuring the safety of both the patient and the paramedic. General guidelines for managing a patient with suspected or known hepatitis include the following:

- Wear appropriate personal protective equipment, which may include gloves, face masks, goggles and disposable gowns, to minimise the risk of exposure to blood or body fluids, particularly during procedures such as intravenous insertion or airway inspection.
- Carry out a thorough assessment of the patient's condition, including vital signs, level of consciousness and symptoms. Monitor the patient closely for any indication of deterioration.
- Adhere to standard infection control precautions, with the aim of preventing the transmission of hepatitis. This will include correct hand hygiene, safe disposal of contaminated materials and disinfection of equipment.
- Offer supportive care as needed. This could include managing pain and providing fluids to maintain hydration, as well as ensuring a comfortable environment for the patient.
- Avoid blood contact, taking precautions to prevent direct contact with the patient's blood or their body fluids. If there is a need to provide first aid or to perform any procedures that may involve exposure to blood, adhere to local guidelines and protocols.
- Communicate the patient's condition and suspected or known hepatitis to the receiving hospital. They may provide guidance on further management and any specific precautions needed.
- Ensure that all actions are documented.

The management of hepatitis can vary depending on the type and severity of the infection. These are general guidelines that can help to minimise the risk of transmission and provide supportive care until the patient can receive appropriate medical treatment in a healthcare facility.

It is essential that the paramedic adheres to their organisation's specific protocols and guidelines for managing infectious diseases, including hepatitis.

Take Home Points

- The gastrointestinal system is complex and often difficult to assess in an out-of-hospital environment.
- Pregnancy must be ruled out with all female patients post puberty who present with any GI complaints.
- In an out-of-hospital setting, complications of the GI system can rarely be resolved and care is often based on pain and symptom management.
- Caution should be exercised with patients who are insistent that they just have 'indigestion'. This is often a comment from patients who are experiencing cardiac issues, especially myocardial infarction.
- You are not expected to have the answer to every GI presentation. A solid assessment and logical and timely care, within the remit of your service provider, are key tenets in the care of these patients.

Summary

The GI tract will present many challenges to you as a paramedic during your career. Many of the conditions that affect both the upper and lower GI tract will either share the same symptoms or have symptoms that are similar. A high index of suspicion must be maintained in relation to the possibility of blood loss. You should always consider the patient's vital signs and the responses you receive to your assessment questions as key identifiers of potentially serious underlying issues.

References

Buczacki, S.J. and Davies, J. (2018). The acute abdomen in the cardiac intensive care unit. In: *Core Topics in Cardiothoracic Critical Care* (ed. K. Valchanov, N. Jones, and C.W. Hogue), 294–300. Cambridge: Cambridge University Press.

Greaves, I. and Porter, K.M. (2021). *Oxford Handbook of Pre-hospital*, 2e. Oxford: Oxford University Press.

Haber, P.S. and Kortt, N.C. (2021). Alcohol use disorder and the gut. *Addiction* 116 (3): 658–667.

McErlean, L. (2021). The gastrointestinal system and associated disorders. In: *Fundamental of Applied Pathophysiology*, 4e, vol. 13 (ed. I. Peate), 361–397. Oxford, CH: Wiley.

National Institute for Health and Care Excellence. (2020a) Crohn's Disease: What is it? Clinical Knowledge Summaries. https://cks.nice.org.uk/topics/crohns-disease/background-information/definition (accessed 7 October 2023).

National Institute for Health and Care Excellence. (2020b) *Pancreatitis*. NICE Guideline NG 104. London: National Institute for Health and Care Excellence. https://www.nice.org.uk/guidance/ng104 (accessed 7 October 2023).

Riley, A., Box, J., and Aherne, A. (2023). Gastrointestinal critical care. In: *Fundamental of Critical Care*, vol. 22 (ed. I. Peate and B.,.B. Hill), 313–329. Oxford, CH: Wiley.

Snellaert, S. (2018). There is no excuse for homelessness in Britain in 2018. *British Medical Journal* 360: https://doi.org/10.1136/bmj.k902.

Further Reading

Peate, I. (2021) (4th Ed) (Ed) "Fundamentals of Applied Pathophysiology" Wiley Oxford.

Peate, I., Evans. S. and Clegg, L. (2022) (Eds) "Fundamentals of Pharmacology for Paramedics" Wiley Oxford.

237

Online Resources

British Liver Trust (resources for those working in primary care): https://britishlivertrust.org.uk/health-professionals/primary-care-resources.

Crohn's & Colitis UK: http://crohnsandcolitis.org.uk.

National Institute for Health and Care Excellence (digestive tract conditions guidance): www.nice.org.uk/guidance/conditions-and-diseases/digestive-tract-conditions.

Glossary

Amino acids	Organic compounds that serve as the building blocks of proteins.
Cholelithiasis	Gallbladder stones.
Chyme	The partially digested, semi-liquid mixture of food and digestive juices that is produced in the stomach.
Contraindication	A specific circumstance or condition that makes a particular treatment, procedure or medication potentially harmful or unsuitable for an individual.
Haematemesis	Blood in vomit.
Haematochezia	Blood in stool.
Haemorrhage	Bleeding.
Hernia	A condition where an organ or fatty tissue protrudes through a weak spot or opening in the surrounding muscle or connective tissue.
Melaena	The passage of dark, tarry stools.
Nausea	A sensation or feeling of discomfort in the stomach, often accompanied by a strong urge to vomit.
Pancreatic amylase	An enzyme produced by the pancreas, specifically in the acinar cells of the pancreas.

Multiple Choice Questions

1. What is the longest part of the small intestine?
   a. Ileum
   b. Duodenum
   c. Jejunum
   d. Colon

2. The alimentary canal is approximately how wide?
   a. 4 cm
   b. 5 cm
   c. 9 cm
   d. 10 cm

3. Acute severe abdominal pain is usually associated with what?
   a. Pregnancy
   b. Blockages
   c. Perforations
   d. Gastric reflux

4. Cholecystitis will commonly refer pain to where?
   a. The right leg
   b. The lower abdomen
   c. The right chest wall
   d. The shoulders and neck

5. Digestion begins where?
   a. The stomach
   b. The mouth
   c. The small intestine
   d. The large intestine

6. Digestion is complete by the time the bolus reaches where?
   a. Ascending colon
   b. Transverse colon
   c. Descending colon
   d. Sigmoid colon

7. Diverticulitis is often associated with pain where in the body?
   a. Right-sided abdominal pain
   b. Upper abdominal pain
   c. Left-sided abdominal pain
   d. Chest pain

8. Which of the following is NOT considered part of the upper GI tract?
   a. Mouth
   b. Oesophagus
   c. Stomach
   d. Rectum

9. A Mallory–Weiss tear is usually associated with what symptom?
    a. Vomiting
    b. Fever
    c. Nausea
    d. Defaecation

10. Cholecystitis is inflammation of which organ?
    a. The liver
    b. The kidneys
    c. The gallbladder
    d. The pancreas

CHAPTER 12

The Endocrine System and Associated Disorders

Sadie Diamond-Fox and Alexandra Gatehouse

AIM

The aim of this chapter is to provide the reader with an introduction to the physiological, pathological, assessment and evidence-based management considerations pertaining to the endocrine system.

LEARNING OBJECTIVES

After completing this chapter, you will be able to:

- Gain an understanding of the physiology of the endocrine system and the associated common disorders.
- Discuss the different types of endocrine glands and tissues, their related hormones and action.
- Appreciate the control of hormones and the role of homeostasis and feedback mechanisms within the endocrine system.
- Consider the clinical examination findings and features of common endocrine conditions.
- Understand the causes, identification and management of specific endocrine disorders.

Test Your Prior Knowledge

1. Describe the principal functions of the endocrine system and its main components.
2. Name four common endocrine conditions.
3. Differentiate between neural, hormonal and humoral endocrine responses.
4. Based upon current evidence, critically discuss the management of the various endocrine emergencies.
5. Discuss the importance of the biochemical tests used to identify endocrine disorders.

Fundamentals of Applied Pathophysiology for Paramedics, First Edition. Edited by Ian Peate and Simon Sawyer.
© 2024 John Wiley & Sons Ltd. Published 2024 by John Wiley & Sons Ltd.

Introduction

The endocrine system is one of the body's major control processes that regulates water, electrolytes, nutrients and digestion, in addition to growth development, reproduction and stress adaptation. It plays a crucial role in homeostasis through regulation of hormones and is inextricably linked with the central nervous and immune systems (see Chapters 3 and 6). The endocrine system comprises both primary and secondary endocrine glands, each releasing specific hormones that affect target tissues (Figure 12.1).

It is essential to have an understanding of the anatomy and physiology of the endocrine system to be able to recognise and appreciate the pathophysiology of specific endocrine disorders. Diabetes mellitus and thyroid disease are the most common endocrine conditions. Other less common conditions include Addison's disease, Cushing syndrome, hypopituitarism and acromegaly.

Physiology of the Endocrine System

The central endocrine glands include the hypothalamus, the pituitary gland and the pineal gland while the principal peripheral glands include the thyroid, parathyroids, adrenal, pancreas, ovaries and testes. The hypothalamus directly controls the pituitary gland, resulting in regulation of the major physiological processes including reproduction, stress, metabolism, lactation and growth. Endocrine glands release hormones which exert their effects at distant target cells, regulating slower physiological processes that require longer duration and sustainability. Knowledge and understanding of endocrine glands, hormones and their action is vital in recognition of endocrine pathology (Table 12.1).

Hormones

Classification of hormones is based upon structure, including amino acids, peptides, polypeptides and proteins or steroids. Protein and polypeptide hormones tend to be synthesised and stored intracellularly then released upon cell activation. Steroid and thyroid hormones are lipid soluble and therefore unable to be stored, so they are secreted on synthesis. Transport of hormones within the circulation is either free or bound to plasma proteins. Bound hormones are protected from metabolic degradation but unable to exert their effects at the site of action until released. However, falling plasma levels result in unbinding from these proteins, maintaining a steady state of free circulating hormone.

Hormones released from endocrine glands act as chemical messengers, exerting their effects on specific receptors, which results in the activation of secondary messenger mechanisms or intracellular modulation of synthesis of proteins or enzymes. Tissues with specific receptor sites will be activated by free-circulating hormones, potentially resulting in simultaneous stimulation of multiple organs and physiological processes.

Hormones are either directly secreted into the blood, exerting effects at distant sites of action, or have a 'paracrine' effect upon nearby cells or 'autocrine' effect on the cells by which they are produced (Figure 12.2). Neurosecretory neurons release neurohormones from the axon terminals into the blood, where they exert their effects on target cells and are considered to be part of the endocrine system. Neurotransmitters are released from axon terminals, diffuse across the narrow synaptic cleft to an adjacent neuron (Figure 12.2).

Medications Management: Aspirin

Aspirin is associated with displacement of thyroid hormone from thyroid-binding globulin, leading to an excess of circulating thyroid hormone. There is therefore an increased risk of thyroid storm.

Secreting tissue		Main hormone(s)	Main target tissue(s)	Discussed in chapter
Glands				
Anterior pituitary (P)		Adrenocorticotrophic hormone (ACTH)	Adrenal cortex (M)	52
		Growth hormone (GH)	Liver, bones, muscle (G)	50
		Follicle-stimulating hormone (FSH)	Gonads (R)	
		Luteinizing hormone (LH)	Gonads (R)	53
		Prolactin	Mammary glands (R)	56
		Thyroid-stimulating hormone (TSH)	Thyroid gland (G, M)	48
Intermediate pituitary (P)		Melanotrophin-stimulating hormone (MSH)	Melanocytes (H)	47
Posterior pituitary (P)		Antidiuretic hormone (ADH)	Kidney (H)	38
		Oxytocin	Mammary glands	56
			Uterus (R)	55
Pineal (A)		Melatonin	Hypothalamus (H)	
Thyroid (A)		Thyroxine (T4)	Most tissues (G, M)	49
		Tri-iodothyronine (T3)	Most tissues (G, M)	
		Calcitonin	Bones, gut (H)	51
Parathyroid (P)		Parathyroid hormone (PTH)	Bones, gut (H)	51
Pancreas (P)		Insulin	Liver, muscle, adipose tissue (G, M, H)	46
		Glucagon		
Adrenal cortex (S)		Corticosteroids (including cortisol)	Multiple (G, M)	52
		Aldosterone	Kidney (H)	38 and 52
Adrenal medulla (A)		Adrenaline (epinephrine)	Multiple (H, M)	52
		Noradrenaline (norepinephrine)	Multiple (H, M)	
Gonads: male (S)		Testosterone	Testes (R)	53
Gonads: female (S)		Oestradiol	Ovaries, uterus (R)	53 and 55
		Progesterone	Ovaries, uterus (R)	
		Human chorionic gonadotrophin (hCG)	Uterus (R)	55
Placenta (P, S)		Oestradiol	Ovaries, uterus (R)	
		Progesterone	Ovaries, uterus (R)	
Non-glands				
Brain (P, A)		Hypothalamic-releasing hormones	Anterior pituitary gland (H, R, M)	47
		Growth factors	Various (M)	
Heart (P)		Atrial natriuretic peptide (ANP)	Kidney	38
Kidney (P, S)		Erythropoietin (EPO)	Bone marrow (M)	9
		1,25-Dihydroxycholecalciferol	Gut, kidney (H)	51
		Renin	Plasma proteins (H)	38
Liver (P)		Insulin-like growth factor-1 (IGF-1)	Various (M)	50
Adipose tissue (P)		Leptin	Hypothalamus (M)	47
Gastrointestinal tract (P, A)		Gastrin	Gut (H, M)	40–44
		Secretin		
		Cholecystokinin (CCK)		
		Vasoactive intestinal polypeptide (VIP)		
		Gastrin-releasing peptide (GRP)		
Immune cells (P)		Cytokines	Hypothalamus (H, M)	11
Platelets (P)		Growth factors	Various (G)	49
Various sites (P)		Growth factors	Various (G)	49
		Neurotrophins	Neurones (G)	

Molecules: A, modified amino acid; P, peptide/protein; S, steroids/sterols.
Functions: H, homeostasis; R, reproduction; G, growth and development; M, metabolism.

FIGURE 12.1 Tissues involved in endocrine control systems. The top half of the table shows the products of classical glandular tissue; the bottom half lists some of the other organs that release hormones. Source: Ward and Linden (2017)/John Wiley & Sons.

242

TABLE 12.1 Endocrine glands and tissues, hormones and action.

Endocrine gland or tissue	Hormone	Hormone action
Gland		
Hypothalamus	Corticotropin-releasing hormone	Exert effects upon pituitary gland hormone release
	Thyrotropin-releasing hormone	
	Growth hormone-releasing hormone	
	Gonadotropin-releasing hormone	
	Somatostatin	Inhibits thyroid-stimulating hormone and growth hormone
Anterior pituitary	Growth hormone	Stimulates growth of bone and soft tissue
	Adrenocorticotropic-hormone	Stimulates cortisol release
	Thyroid-stimulating hormone	Stimulates T_3 and T_4 release
	Follicle-stimulating hormone	Female: ovulation, ovarian follicle growth; male: sperm production
	Luteinising hormone	Female: stimulates ovulation, estrogen and progesterone release Male: stimulates testosterone release
	Prolactin	Female: breast development and milk production
Posterior pituitary	Antidiuretic hormone	Increases renal reabsorption of water, arteriole constriction
	Oxytocin	Increases uterine contraction
Parathyroid	Parathyroid hormone	Regulation of serum calcium and phosphate, activation of vitamin D
Thyroid	Follicular cells – tri-iodothyronine (T_3), tetraiodothyronine (T_4)	Increase metabolic rate and bone or protein turnover
	C cells – calcitonin	Reduces calcium and phosphate serum levels
Adrenal	Cortex – aldosterone (mineralocorticoid)	Increases reabsorption of sodium and secretion of potassium
	Cortisol (glucocorticoid)	Regulation of blood glucose, metabolism and stress adaptation
	Androgens	Converted to progesterone and testosterone
	Medulla – adrenaline/epinephrine	Neurotransmitters within the sympathetic nervous system
	Noradrenaline/norepinephrine	
Pancreas	Insulin	Decreases blood glucose
	Glucagon	Increases blood glucose
	Somatostatin	Delays intestinal digestion and absorption of glucose
Ovaries	Estrogen	Development of female secondary sex characteristics and sex organs
	Progesterone	Menstrual cycle
Testes	Testosterone	Development of male secondary sex characteristics and sex organs, stimulates sperm production

TABLE 12.1   (*Continued*)

Endocrine gland or tissue	Hormone	Hormone action
Thymus	Thymosin	Proliferation and enhancement of T lymphocyte function
Organ		
Heart	Atrial natriuretic peptide	Inhibition of renal tubule absorption of sodium, systemic vasodilatation, inhibition of renin
	Brain natriuretic peptide	
Stomach	Gastrin	Secretion of hydrochloric acid, gastric mucosal growth
Duodenum and small intestine	Secretin	Control secretion of gastric enzymes for digestion and gut motility
	Gastric inhibitory peptide	
	Cholecystokinin	
	Vasoactive intestinal peptide	
	Motilin	
Kidneys	Renin	Regulation of blood pressure
	Vitamin D	Absorption of calcium from the intestines

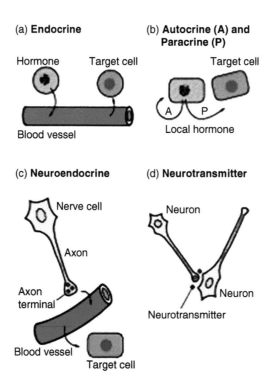

FIGURE 12.2   Types of hormone signalling. Source: Holt and Hanley (2011)/John Wiley & Sons.

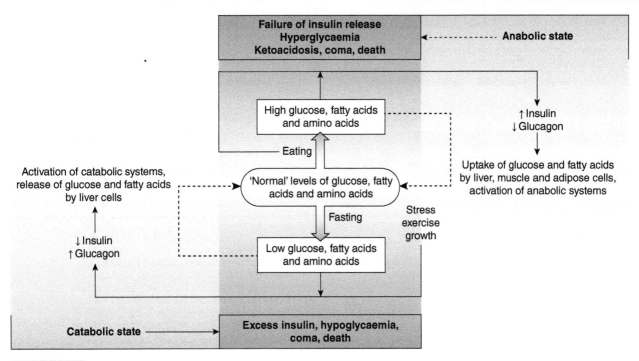

Control of Hormones

The initial stimulus to cause an endocrine response may be hormonal, neural or humoral. The hormonal response occurs when the initial stimulus is a hormone, where the rate of secretion fluctuates and tends to be rhythmical. The hypothalamus secretes hormones that regulate the pituitary gland. Stimulation of a nerve may cause a neural response, an example of which is sympathetic nerve stimulation of the adrenals, which results in the release of adrenaline and noradrenaline. Alternatively, some hormones are regulated by the substance that they control. The humoral response, the release of insulin or glucagon, is under the control of blood glucose levels (Figure 12.3), aldosterone is regulated by plasma sodium and potassium concentration, and parathyroid hormone by falling levels of plasma calcium.

The circulating blood concentration of a hormone is proportional to its effects. Control mechanisms are necessary to maintain and regulate homeostasis. The amount of hormone available to exert its effects is dependent upon one or all of the following:

- The central nervous system.
- Other endocrine glands.
- The rate of metabolic inactivation or activation.
- The rate of urinary excretion.
- Plasma protein binding.

The general mechanisms for regulation follow the principles of either negative or positive feedback control. This is discussed in detail in Chapter 3. The majority of hormone secretion is reliant upon negative feedback mechanisms wherein hormones inhibit their own secretion or inhibit production to maintain a certain concentration (Figure 12.4).

Positive feedback (Figure 12.4.) is less common but occurs where the increasing concentration of one hormone results in another gland producing a hormone that further stimulates the production of the first. During female ovulation, luteinising hormone stimulates the production of estrogen by the follicle. The high levels of estrogen in turn stimulate secretion of luteinising hormone via the hypothalamus and the anterior pituitary gland. Mechanisms exist to prevent continuing positive feedback, otherwise these processes would continue unopposed. In this example, ovulation results in the termination of the estrogen-secreting follicle and therefore luteinising hormone. External factors such as stress may also affect certain hormonal feedback mechanisms (Figure 12.5).

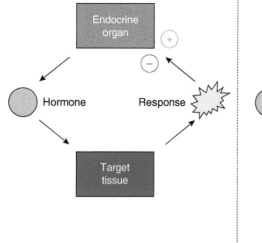

(a)

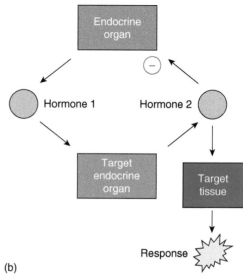

(b)

(a) The endocrine organ releases a hormone, which acts on the target tissue to stimulate a response. The response usually feeds back to inhibit (⊖) the endocrine organ to decrease further supply of the hormone. Occasionally, the feedback can act to enhance the hormone secretion (⊕, positive feedback). (b) The endocrine organ produces hormone 1, which acts on a second endocrine gland to release hormone 2. In turn, hormone 2 acts dually on the target tissue to induce a response and feeds back negatively onto the original endocrine organ to inhibit further release of hormone 1. This model is illustrative of the axes between the anterior pituitary and the peripheral end-organ targets.

FIGURE 12.4 Two models of feedback regulating hormone synthesis.

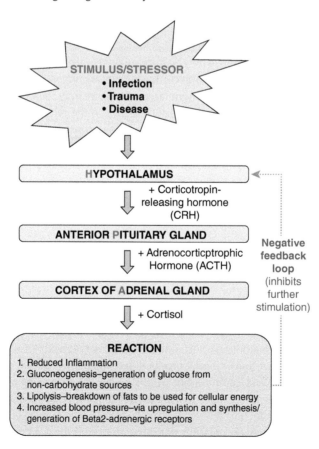

FIGURE 12.5 Effects of stress upon the hypothalamus, anterior pituitary, adrenal (HPA) axis. Source: Peate and Hill (2021)/John Wiley & Sons.

Introduction to Common Endocrine Pathologies

Endocrine pathology occurs due to abnormalities in plasma levels of hormones or in the responsiveness of the target cells. The concentration of circulating hormone is affected by:

- Hyposecretion or hypersecretion of the endocrine gland.
- Hyperfunction or hypofunction of the gland itself.
- Increased or decreased plasma protein binding.
- Increased or decreased excretion.

Hormone deficiency arises due to hypofunction or hyposecretion of the endocrine gland, while hormone excess conversely is due to hyperfunction or hypersecretion. Causes include congenital defects, immunological processes, lack of dietary intake, toxins or drugs, infection or inflammation, disruption of blood supply, tumours, iatrogenic (surgery) or idiopathic. The responsiveness of the target cell may be affected by the number of cell receptors, defects of the receptor, or the enzymes required for intracellular synthesis of specific hormones. The most common cause of endocrine disorders is hyposecretion.

Endocrine disorders may be classified as primary, secondary or tertiary. Primary problems arise due to a defect of the gland that produces the hormone. Secondary disorders occur due to abnormalities of the pituitary gland, with the target glands being essentially normal. Tertiary problems are caused by hypothalamus dysfunction, leading to under-stimulation of both the pituitary and target glands or tissues. It is beyond the scope of this chapter to discuss all endocrine pathology so only disorders that are relevant and pertinent to paramedic practice are included.

Clinical Features of Endocrine Disorders

Clinical features of endocrine pathology may be varied and non-specific due to the affect upon multiple anatomical sites and organ systems (Figure 12.6). Diagnosis may be incidental or secondary to investigations of other disease processes, and challenging due to potential coexistence with other endocrine pathology. Several conditions share common clinical symptoms including:

- Weight or appetite changes
- Sweating, flushing
- Lethargy
- Altered bowel habit
- Polyuria, polydipsia
- Hypertension
- Skin, hair and nail changes
- Neck swelling
- Erectile dysfunction, loss of libido
- Gynaecomastia, galactorrhoea
- Amenorrhoea
- Altered facial appearances or body habitus.

Pituitary Disorders

Hypopituitarism occurs due to the inability of the pituitary gland to produce hormones or as a result of a disorder of the hypothalamus, in which it is unable to release pituitary stimulating or inhibiting hormones. The causes of hypopituitarism include haemorrhage, infarction, surgery, radiation, congenital defects and, most commonly, tumours. The pituitary

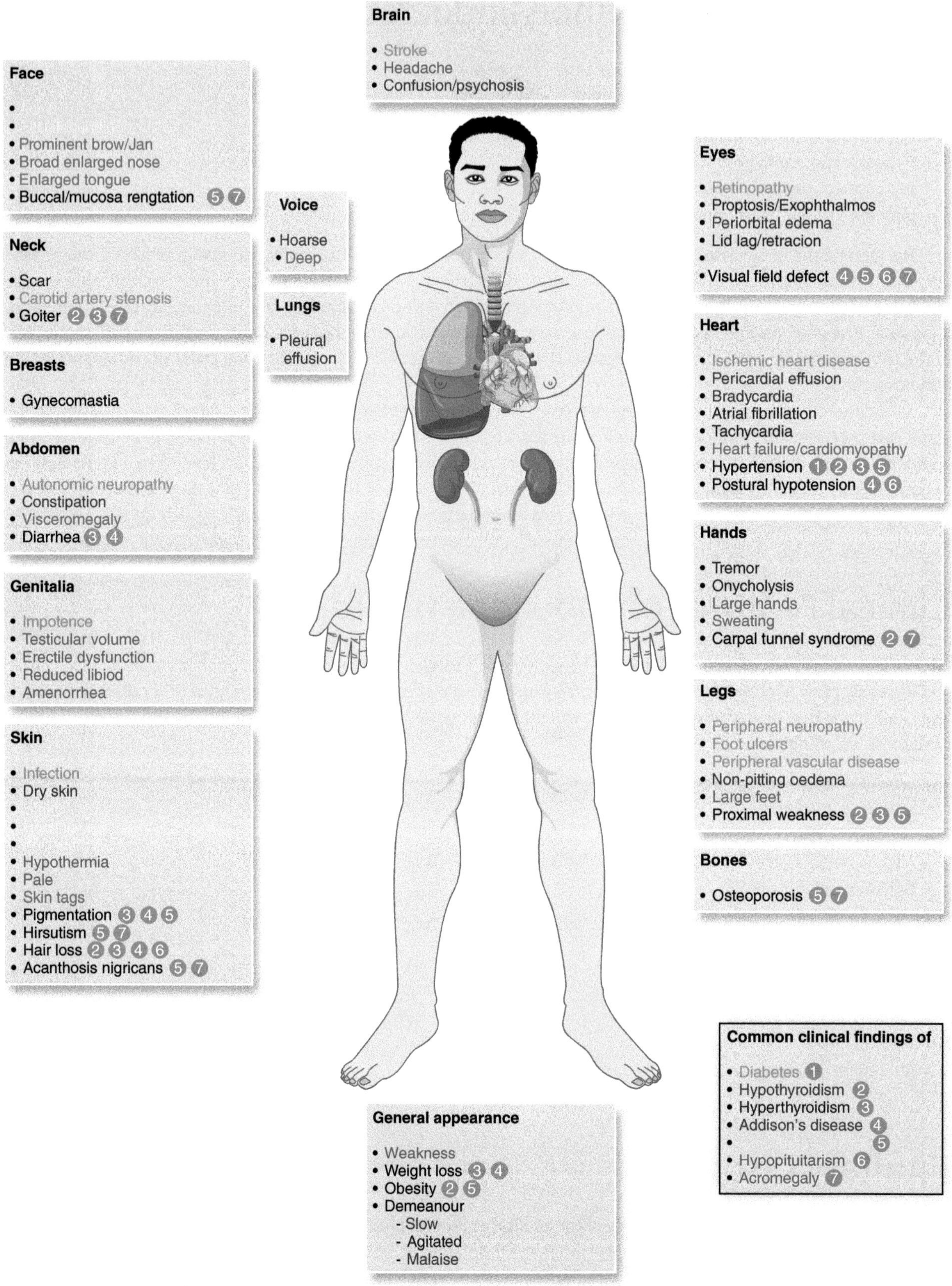

Brain

- Stroke
- Headache
- Confusion/psychosis

Face

-
-
- Prominent brow/Jan
- Broad enlarged nose
- Enlarged tongue
- Buccal/mucosa rengtation ⑤ ⑦

Voice

- Hoarse
- Deep

Neck

- Scar
- Carotid artery stenosis
- Goiter ② ③ ⑦

Lungs

- Pleural effusion

Breasts

- Gynecomastia

Abdomen

- Autonomic neuropathy
- Constipation
- Visceromegaly
- Diarrhea ③ ④

Genitalia

- Impotence
- Testicular volume
- Erectile dysfunction
- Reduced libiod
- Amenorrhea

Skin

- Infection
- Dry skin
-
-
-
- Hypothermia
- Pale
- Skin tags
- Pigmentation ③ ④ ⑤
- Hirsutism ⑤ ⑦
- Hair loss ② ③ ④ ⑥
- Acanthosis nigricans ⑤ ⑦

Eyes

- Retinopathy
- Proptosis/Exophthalmos
- Periorbital edema
- Lid lag/retracion
-
- Visual field defect ④ ⑤ ⑥ ⑦

Heart

- Ischemic heart disease
- Pericardial effusion
- Bradycardia
- Atrial fibrillation
- Tachycardia
- Heart failure/cardiomyopathy
- Hypertension ① ② ③ ⑤
- Postural hypotension ④ ⑥

Hands

- Tremor
- Onycholysis
- Large hands
- Sweating
- Carpal tunnel syndrome ② ⑦

Legs

- Peripheral neuropathy
- Foot ulcers
- Peripheral vascular disease
- Non-pitting oedema
- Large feet
- Proximal weakness ② ③ ⑤

Bones

- Osteoporosis ⑤ ⑦

Common clinical findings of

- Diabetes ①
- Hypothyroidism ②
- Hyperthyroidism ③
- Addison's disease ④
- ⑤
- Hypopituitarism ⑥
- Acromegaly ⑦

General appearance

- Weakness
- Weight loss ③ ④
- Obesity ② ⑤
- Demeanour
  - Slow
  - Agitated
  - Malaise

FIGURE 12.6   Clinical examination findings and features of common endocrine conditions. Source: Alexandra Gatehouse (co-author).

gland secretes several hormones, disorders of which may affect several endocrine glands, leading to adrenal and thyroid insufficiency, hypogonadism and diabetes insipidus. Adrenal and thyroid disorders are discussed later in the chapter, but diabetes insipidus may occur due to a lack of release of antidiuretic hormone from the posterior pituitary gland, resulting in dehydration secondary to polyuria, the most common cause of which is head injury. Management includes fluid replacement and careful fluid balance monitoring. Assessment of hypothalamic–pituitary function is required, with hormone replacement as necessary.

Thyroid Disorders

Thyroid disorders are the most common endocrine pathology diagnosed within primary care; approximately 2% of the UK population have hypothyroidism or hyperthyroidism (National Institute for Health and Care Excellence 2019). The two hormones, thyroxine (T_4) and tri-iodothyronine (T_3), released by the thyroid gland increase metabolic rate via thermogenesis. Hyperthyroidism or hypothyroidism occur either due to a primary thyroid gland problem or secondary due to changes in thyroid-stimulating hormone (TSH) from the pituitary gland or thyrotropin-releasing hormone from the hypothalamus.

Clinical Investigations: Measurement of Thyroid Hormone

Measurement of plasma TSH and thyroxine (T_4) aids in the diagnosis of hyperthyroidism or hypothyroidism:

- Hyperthyroidism – TSH low or undetectable, high T_3 or T_4.
- Hypothyroidism – TSH with low T_4.

Hyperthyroidism

Hyperthyroidism occurs due to thyroid gland overactivity, which results in high plasma levels of thyroid hormone. The most common cause is Grave's disease, an autoimmune condition where specific thyroid-stimulating antibodies imitate TSH, leading to an excessive release of thyroid hormone. Other causes of hyperthyroidism included cancer, drugs (amiodarone, thyroxine), infections, pregnancy, trauma or nutritional excesses or deficiencies (Malaty 2023). Treatment includes antithyroid drugs, surgery or radioiodine. Beta blockers are used to treat the enhanced β-adrenergic activity, which causes the most common symptoms of tachycardia and palpitations. If left undiagnosed, these symptoms may lead to cardiovascular disease and heart failure.

Thyroid crisis or storm is a life-threatening acute emergency that occurs as a result of partially, undertreated or, more rarely, undiagnosed hyperthyroidism. Precipitating factors include infection, radioactive iodine therapy, labour or eclampsia, surgery, drugs, diabetes, trauma, stress and overdose. It is associated with 8–25% mortality.

The clinical features of a hyperadrenergic state include tachycardia, hyperthermia, dehydration, agitation, confusion, nausea, vomiting and diarrhoea (Figure 12.7; Clare 2017, Leach 2014, Ross et al. 2016). Management includes an ABCDE approach, with specifically cooling measures, antithyroid drugs (propylthiouracil, carbimazole, thiamazole), steroids (hydrocortisone), betablockers (propranolol, esmolol, metoprolol) and iodine solution (Lugol's solution).

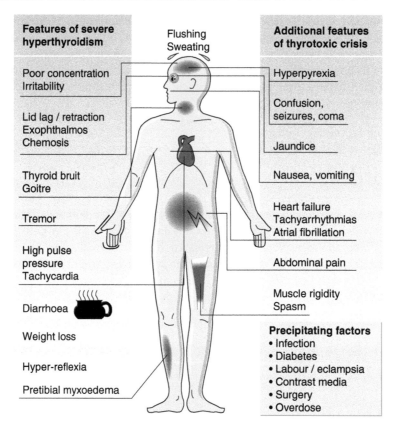

Features of severe hyperthyroidism	Flushing Sweating	Additional features of thyrotoxic crisis
Poor concentration Irritability		Hyperpyrexia
Lid lag / retraction Exophthalmos Chemosis		Confusion, seizures, coma
		Jaundice
Thyroid bruit Goitre		Nausea, vomiting
Tremor		Heart failure Tachyarrhythmias Atrial fibrillation
High pulse pressure Tachycardia		Abdominal pain
Diarrhoea		Muscle rigidity Spasm
Weight loss		Precipitating factors • Infection • Diabetes • Labour / eclampsia • Contrast media • Surgery • Overdose
Hyper-reflexia		
Pretibial myxoedema		

FIGURE 12.7   Clinical features of severe hyperthyroidism and thyrotoxic crisis.

Snapshot 12.1

Pre-arrival Information

You are dispatched to a 45-year-old patient who has been complaining of feeling generally unwell with palpitations, dizziness, diarrhoea and vomiting.

On Arrival with the Patient

On approaching the front door of the house, there are no signs of danger and it is safe to enter. You announce your arrival and the patient shouts to you that they are on the sofa in the living room. As you enter, you see the patient sitting on the sofa; they appear restless, tremulous and they are sweating.

Presenting complaint – palpitations, dizziness, diarrhoea and vomiting.

History of presenting complaint – the patient has felt generally unwell for a few days with worsening symptoms over the last four hours. They were due to see their general practitioner tomorrow as they had been feeling anxious over the previous two weeks, had been experiencing intermittent palpitations with unexplained weight loss of 3 stone over the past month.

Past medical history – nil of note, family history of Grave's disease.

Drug history – no regular medications, no known drug allergies.

Social history – full time teacher, non-smoker, occasional alcohol, lives with partner of 20 years.

Primary Survey

Danger – there is no danger and the scene is safe.

Response – the patient has called out therefore they are alert on the ACVPU scale.

Catstrophic haemorrhage – there are no signs of major haemorrhage.

Airway – the patient spoke to you, so the airway is patent; there are no added noises.

Breathing – the patient is breathing, respiratory rate 24 breaths/minute (NEWS2 = 2), oxygen saturations 96% on room air (NEWS2 = 0), auscultation; good air entry with no added sounds.

Circulation – the patient is sweating, appears well perfused and pink, heart rate is 107 beats/min (NEWS2 = 1), irregular, bounding; blood pressure 115/65 mmHg (NEWS2 = 0), capillary refill time < 2 seconds.

Paramedic actions – 12-lead ECG – atrial fibrillation; gain intravenous access, supplemental oxygen if saturations < 94%.

Disability – the patient is alert (NEWS2 = 0) and moving all four limbs; pupil size 3, equal and reactive to light, blood glucose 7.4 mmol/l

Exposure – there is no indication to expose the patient, temperature 39.3°C (NEWS2 = 2).

Total NEWS2 score prior to interventions = 5.

Assessment of patient's critical status = non-time critical.

Secondary Survey

Systems examination:
- Respiratory – palpable anterior neck mass over the thyroid gland
- Cardiac
- Neurological
- Gastrointestinal
- Musculoskeletal.

Last ins and outs – last ate 24 hours ago, drinking small amounts of water, bowels open today – diarrhoea, vomited prior to paramedic's arrival, passed urine this morning but very dark in colour.

Events leading up – as above.

Physical examination head to toe:
- No abnormal diagnosis – head, neck, upper limbs, chest, abdomen, pelvis, lower limbs.

Paramedic Actions

- Primary survey with interventions as required; time critical transfer not indicated.
- Secondary survey with monitoring of CABCD throughout the clinical assessment.
- Transfer to local hospital emergency department.
- Provide ATMIST handover to emergency department staff.

Diagnosis

- Patient presentation is that of a hyperadrenergic state, with signs and symptoms of thyroid storm including pyrexia, atrial fibrillation, mild agitation, tremors and gastrointestinal upset.
- The diagnosis is confirmed on biochemical tests with very low TSH and elevated free T_3 and T_4.

251

Hypothyroidism

Primary hypothyroidism occurs due to a deficiency of T_3 and T_4 caused by a thyroid gland disorder, most commonly autoimmune thyroiditis (Hashimoto), treatment for hyperthyroidism, tumours, radiotherapy, surgery, trauma, viral infection, pregnancy, autoimmune diseases or drugs (lithium, amiodarone). A lack of TSH produced by the pituitary gland leads to secondary hypothyroidism. Management of primary hypothyroidism is lifelong thyroid hormone replacement in the oral form of thyroxine with the aim of normalising TSH plasma levels.

Severe hypothyroidism or myxoedema coma is a rare endocrine emergency, usually precipitated by factors including illness, infection or drugs in pre-existing hypothyroidism. It is associated with multiorgan failure and a mortality rate of approximately 50% (Chaker et al. 2016, Leach 2014). Clinical features include hypothermia, hypotension, bradycardia,

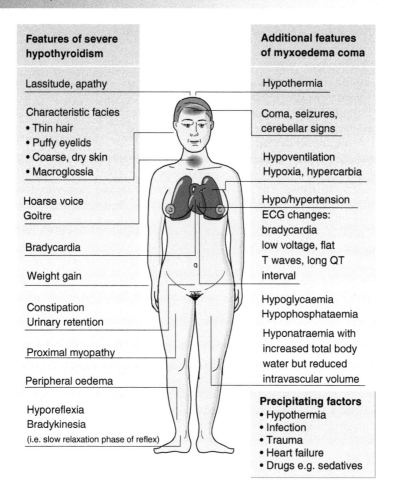

Features of severe hypothyroidism	Additional features of myxoedema coma
Lassitude, apathy	Hypothermia
Characteristic facies • Thin hair • Puffy eyelids • Coarse, dry skin • Macroglossia	Coma, seizures, cerebellar signs Hypoventilation Hypoxia, hypercarbia
Hoarse voice Goitre	Hypo/hypertension ECG changes: bradycardia low voltage, flat T waves, long QT interval
Bradycardia	
Weight gain	
Constipation Urinary retention	Hypoglycaemia Hypophosphataemia
Proximal myopathy	Hyponatraemia with increased total body water but reduced intravascular volume
Peripheral oedema	
Hyporeflexia Bradykinesia (i.e. slow relaxation phase of reflex)	**Precipitating factors** • Hypothermia • Infection • Trauma • Heart failure • Drugs e.g. sedatives

FIGURE 12.8   Severe hypothyroidism and myxoedema coma.

hypoventilation, hypoglycaemia, hyponatraemia and confusion leading to coma (Figure 12.8; Clare 2017, Holt and Hanley 2011). Management includes treatment of the cause, supportive care in the form of rewarming, correction of hypoglycaemia and invasive ventilation, in addition to immediate administration of intravenous levothyroxine and, if appropriate, liothyronine. Hydrocortisone should also be given until hypoadrenalism has been excluded, as this may precipitate an adrenal crisis.

Medications Management: Levothyroxine

Levothyroxine for long-standing hypothyroidism and ischaemic heart disease should be started with caution and a gradual increase in dose over several weeks is necessary because of the increased risk of exacerbation of angina in patients with coronary artery disease.

Orange Flag Alert: Thyroxine

Treatment of hypothyroidism requires lifelong medication, the most common of which is oral thyroxine. Evidence suggests that, despite this treatment, approximately 30–50% of patients are over- or undertreated, with subsequent adverse health implications (Eligar et al. 2016). Contributing factors include incorrect administration or dose, concordance with treatment, concomitant medications and comorbid conditions. Vigilance for monitoring clinical signs of overtreatment or undertreatment by both patients and healthcare practitioners is essential.

Parathyroid Disorders

The parathyroid glands contribute to plasma calcium homeostasis via the secretion of PTH The kidneys, gastrointestinal tract and bones contribute to this, in addition to vitamin D. Calcium is essential for many physiological processes including blood clotting, muscle contraction, nerve conduction, mineralisation of bone, intracellular signalling, enzyme activity and secretion of hormones (Leach 2014). Disorders of the parathyroid glands lead to either hypercalcaemia or hypocalcaemia.

Hyperparathyroidism

Over production of parathyroid hormone leads to primary hyperparathyroidism. There is a higher incidence in women and the most common cause cited is adenoma in 80% of cases (Holt and Hanley 2011). Secondary and tertiary hyperparathyroidism are usually caused by renal failure. Clinical features tend to be non-specific, including tiredness and fatigue, muscle weakness, abdominal symptoms and bony pain associated with high plasma calcium levels on blood testing. Definitive treatment is surgical removal of the parathyroid glands and conservative management with vitamin D replacement and bisphosphates pre-procedure. Acute hypercalcaemia is an emergency and requires intravenous fluids for hypovolaemia in the first instance.

Hypoparathyroidism

Hypothyroidism occurs due to a deficiency in the synthesis or secretion of plasma parathyroid hormone causing low calcium and raised phosphate levels in the blood. Although rare, one of the most common causes, in approximately 80% of cases, is thyroid surgery, due to the anatomical position of the parathyroid glands, and tumours (Shoback and Duh 2023). Genetic, autoimmune diseases or idiopathic pathologies are responsible for the remainder. Clinical features include tetany, paraesthesia, severe cramps, cardiac failure or arrhythmias, neuromuscular irritability and seizures. Calcium, vitamin D and magnesium replacement are the usual forms of treatment or in acute symptomatic management intravenous calcium replacement with electrocardiography monitoring.

253

Red Flag Alert: Calcium Gluconate

Intravenous calcium replacement with 10–20 ml of neat 10% calcium gluconate may be administered in an emergency but electrocardiography and plasma monitoring are recommended due to the risk of hypotension, bradycardia, arrhythmias or cardiac arrest (British National Formulary 2023a).

Adrenal Disorders

The adrenal glands secrete the hormones adrenaline and noradrenaline from the adrenal medulla, and mineralocorticoids, glucocorticoids and gonadocorticoids from the adrenal cortex. Adrenaline and noradrenaline are released as a result of sympathetic nervous stimulation.

The primary mineralocorticoid is aldosterone, which is responsible for the regulation of plasma sodium and subsequently water, potassium, chloride and bicarbonate, via excretion or absorption of sodium in the renal tubules. Its release is stimulated by plasma sodium or potassium levels, circulating blood volume and blood pressure via the renin–angiotensin–aldosterone system (Figure 12.9).

Cortisol is the primary glucocorticoid, which has effects upon metabolism and the immune system, facilitating gluconeogenesis and lipolysis in addition to tissue repair via protein catabolism. The adrenal glands are stimulated to release cortisol as a result of the pituitary gland producing adrenocorticotrophic hormone (ACTH). The secretion of cortisol occurs

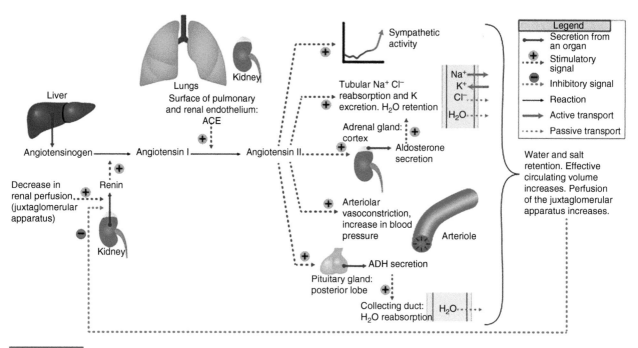

FIGURE 12.9   The renin angiotensin aldosterone system. Source: Soupvector/Wikimedia Commons/CC BY-SA 4.0.

in a physiological rhythm being highest in the hour after waking and lowest shortly before and following sleep. Stress can disrupt the usual mechanism of regulation of cortisol via CRH from the hypothalamus and ACTH from the pituitary gland (Figure 12.6).

Hyperadrenalism

Cushing's disease is caused by excess secretion of glucocorticoids, causes include pituitary adenoma producing ACTH, adrenal tumours or exogenous glucocorticoids. Treatment comprises surgical removal or titration of steroid therapy. Excess of mineralocorticoid is Conn syndrome, which is characterised by hyperkalaemic hypertension secondary to an adrenal adenoma.

Hypoadrenalism

Adrenal insufficiency is classified into primary and secondary but both occur as a result of reduced cortisol secretion by the adrenal gland. Primary adrenal insufficiency or Addison's disease is caused by intrinsic diseases of the adrenal glands such as autoimmune adrenalitis, or tuberculosis, infection or autoimmune diseases such as HIV or AIDS (Clare 2017, Leach 2014). Presenting complaints include fatigue, muscle weakness, hyperpigmentation and salt craving (Nematollahi and Arafah 2022). Lifelong oral replacement with glucocorticoids and mineralocorticoids is the main stay of management.

Secondary adrenal insufficiency occurs due to a lack of ACTH associated with hypothalamus or pituitary tumours or trauma, or more commonly, acute withdrawal of steroid therapy. Certain drugs may also inhibit steroid production (ketoconazole) or enhance hepatic metabolism (rifampicin, phenytoin) resulting in drug-induced adrenal insufficiency (Leach 2014).

An Addisonian or adrenal crisis is a life-threatening acute medical emergency with clinical features including shock, hypotension, hypovolaemia, hypoglycaemia, hyperkalaemia and hyponatraemia (Clare 2017, Leach 2014). Clinical features and precipitating factors are represented in Figure 12.10. Treatment includes fluid resuscitation and glucose, intravenous high-dose steroids (hydrocortisone) and inotropic support within critical care.

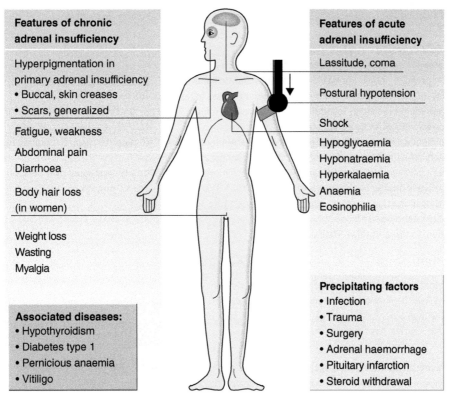

Features of chronic adrenal insufficiency

Hyperpigmentation in primary adrenal insufficiency
• Buccal, skin creases
• Scars, generalized

Fatigue, weakness

Abdominal pain
Diarrhoea

Body hair loss
(in women)

Weight loss
Wasting
Myalgia

Associated diseases:
• Hypothyroidism
• Diabetes type 1
• Pernicious anaemia
• Vitiligo

Features of acute adrenal insufficiency

Lassitude, coma

Postural hypotension

Shock
Hypoglycaemia
Hyponatraemia
Hyperkalaemia
Anaemia
Eosinophilia

Precipitating factors
• Infection
• Trauma
• Surgery
• Adrenal haemorrhage
• Pituitary infarction
• Steroid withdrawal

FIGURE 12.10 Acute adrenal (Addisonian) crisis.

255

Medications Management: Steroids

The anti-inflammatory effects of steroids may be used in anaphylaxis, airway oedema, exacerbation of asthma or chronic obstructive pulmonary disease, raised intracranial pressure due to cerebral tumour, Pneumocystis pneumonia or bacterial meningitis (*Streptococcus pneumoniae*). In acute critical illness or chronic disease states, cortisol may be depleted. Replacement with exogenous forms of corticosteroids may be required in adrenal crisis, myxoedema coma and peri- and postoperatively. Patients taking long-term steroids may wear a bracelet or have a card to make them identifiable, while those with Addison's disease who are at risk of an adrenal crisis may carry an emergency kit containing medical treatment.

Snapshot 12.2

Pre-arrival Information

You are dispatched to a 19-year-old patient who has been found by her flatmate incoherent and vomiting.

On Arrival with the Patient

On approaching the front door of the house there are no signs of danger and it is safe to enter. The flatmate shouts that they are in the bedroom. As you enter, you see the patient lying on the bed, her eyes open to your voice but she is making incoherent sounds. You notice a bracelet on the patient's wrist stating 'Addison's disease'. Her flatmate states that she has been generally unwell for a few days with nausea and vomiting;, she normally takes steroids.

Primary Survey

Danger – there is no danger and the scene is safe.

Response – the patient is V on the ACVPU scale as she opens her eyes to voice.

Catastrophic haemorrhage – there are no signs of major haemorrhage.

Airway – the airway is patent as the patient makes incoherent noises in response to voice.

Breathing – the patient is breathing, respiratory rate 12 breaths/minute (NEWS2 = 0), saturations 96% on room air (NEWS2 = 0), auscultation – good air entry with no added sounds.

Circulation – the patient is cool peripherally, heart rate 125 beats/minute (NEWS2 = 2), sinus tachycardia, blood pressure 89/56 mmHg (NEWS2 = 3), capillary refill time 3 seconds, 12-lead ECG: sinus tachycardia.

Paramedic actions – intravenous (IV) access access, 100 mg IV hydrocortisone, 500 ml IV crystalloid over 15 minutes.

Disability – the patient is drowsy but responds to voice (NEWS2 = 3); blood glucose is 4.7 mmol/l.

Exposure – there is no indication to expose the patient, temperature 36.5°C (NEWS2 = 0).

NEWS2 score prior to intervention = 8.

Assessment of patient's critical status = TIME CRITICAL.

Paramedic Actions

- Prepare patient for time critical transfer to local hospital emergency department.
- Reassessment of CABCD en route with interventions as required.
- Provide an ATMIST handover to the emergency department staff on arrival.

Diagnosis

- The patient is having an adrenal crisis due to gastroenteritis and is therefore not absorbing their usual enteral steroid.
- Treatment requires prompt treatment with hydrocortisone and fluid resuscitation.

Pancreatic Disorders

The pancreas produces both insulin and glucagon, which play an essential role in the control of blood glucose levels. They have directly opposite effects, with insulin reducing blood glucose levels via increased cell uptake of glucose for metabolism into energy or conversion into glycogen for storage, and glucagon increasing blood glucose levels via glycogen breakdown releasing glucose or synthesis of glucose within the liver. Disorders of the pancreas may lead to hyperglycaemia or hypoglycaemia. The latter is very rarely caused by hypersecretion of insulin and more is commonly due to overadministration of exogenous insulin as part of diabetes management or other disease processes such as sepsis, liver or renal failure, tumours, drugs or alcohol.

Hyperglycaemia

Hyperglycaemia is a common complication that may be encountered by the paramedic student. It is caused by pre-existing conditions such as diabetes mellitus, genetic disorders, infection, medications (steroids) or acute and critical-illness stress-induced hyperglycaemia. There are 4.9 million adults in the United Kingdom diagnosed with diabetes (Diabetes UK 2023), which is a metabolic condition resulting in hyperglycaemia due to insulin deficiency (type 1) or insulin resistance (type 2; Leach 2014). Secondary diabetes may occur due to other disease processes including endocrine conditions, steroids and pancreatitis.

Type 1 diabetes mellitus is associated with B cell destruction due to viral, autoimmune or genetic factors, presenting in younger individuals, resulting in insulin deficiency and ketoacidosis if left untreated. Insulin therapy is essential and regimens incorporate combinations of short-acting, biphasic and long-acting preparations. Insulin resistance occurs in type 2 diabetes mellitus occurring in older adults secondary to genetics and associated with poor diet and obesity. Treatment includes dietary control and oral hypoglycaemic medications including a combination of biguanides, sulphonylureas and sodium–glucose co-transporter-2 (abbreviated to SGLT2) inhibitors. The complications of diabetes are depicted in Figure 12.11.

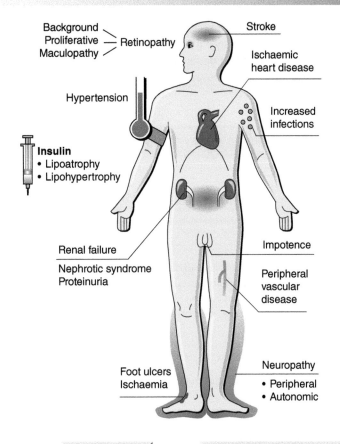

Background ⎫
Proliferative ⎬ Retinopathy
Maculopathy ⎭

Stroke

Ischaemic
heart disease

Hypertension

Increased
infections

Insulin
• Lipoatrophy
• Lipohypertrophy

Renal failure

Nephrotic syndrome
Proteinuria

Impotence

Peripheral
vascular
disease

Foot ulcers
Ischaemia

Neuropathy

• Peripheral
• Autonomic

Hypoglycaemia	Diabetic ketoacidosis/ hyperglycaemia
• Hunger • Jittery • Faint • Tachycardia • Sweaty • Headache • Neurological deficits • Coma	• Drowsy • Hypotension • Tachycardia • Dehydration • Kussmaul's respiration • Abdominal pain

FIGURE 12.11 Complications of diabetes.

Orange Flag Alert: Diabetes Emotional and Psychological Impact

The emotional and psychological impact of the diagnosis of diabetes should not be underestimated as individuals come to terms with lifestyle changes, potentially complex and invasive medications and monitoring. Education is paramount but with this comes knowledge of the condition and the long-term complications. Psychological support may be required at diagnosis and throughout the patient journey to care for the patient's mental health and in turn their quality of life.

There are two major hyperglycaemic diabetic emergencies – diabetic ketoacidosis (DKA) and hyperosmolar hyperglycaemic state (HHS). DKA occurs in type 1 diabetes mellitus, wherein insulin deficiency results in hyperglycaemia, metabolic acidosis, ketosis, electrolyte disturbance, dehydration and haemodynamic instability. Emergency treatment includes fluid resuscitation and intravenous insulin. Life-threatening hypokalaemia may occur following insulin therapy and should be replaced in early management.

HHS is uncommon, occurring in elderly patients with type 2 diabetes mellitus. It is characterised by hyperglycaemia, pseudo hypernatraemia and hyperosmolality, usually without ketosis and metabolic acidosis. Rapid fluid replacement and reduction of blood glucose may cause cerebral oedema and osmotic demyelination, so management should be conservative, with cautious fluid resuscitation and intravenous insulin.

Snapshot 12.3

Pre-arrival Information

You are dispatched to a 56-year-old patient who has been complaining of abdominal pain and nausea, as well as shortness of breath.

On Arrival with the Patient

On approaching the front door of the house there are no signs of danger and it is safe to enter. You announce your arrival and the patient shouts to you that they are in the kitchen. As you enter you see the patient sitting at the kitchen table, their work of breathing in increased, they look pale and generally unwell. The patient tells you that they have type I diabetes mellitus and their insulin pump stopped working last night; they have not taken any other form of insulin.

Primary Survey

Danger – there is no danger and the scene is safe.
Response – the patient is A on the ACVPU scale as they called out to you on arrival.
Catstrophic haemorrhage – there are no signs of major haemorrhage.
Airway – the airway is patent as the patient spoke to you; there are no added noises.
Breathing – the patient is breathing, respiratory rate 28 breaths/minute (NEWS2 = 3), saturations 92% on room air (NEWS2 = 2), auscultation – good air entry with no added sounds.
Paramedic actions – supplemental oxygen 2–6 l via nasal cannula.
Circulation – the patient is cool peripherally, heart rate 120 beats/minute (NEWS2 = 2), sinus tachycardia, blood pressure 78/42 mmHg (NEWS2 = 3), capillary refill time 4 seconds, 12-lead ECG: sinus tachycardia
Paramedic actions – IV access, 500 ml intravenous crystalloid over 15 minutes; do not delay transfer for fluid resuscitation.
Disability – the patient is alert (NEWS2 = 0), blood glucose is 34.1 mmol/l.
Exposure – there is no indication to expose the patient, temperature 36.5°C (NEWS2 = 0).
NEWS2 score prior to intervention = 10.
Assessment of patients critical status = TIME CRITICAL.

Paramedic Actions

- Prepare patient for time critical transfer to local hospital emergency department.
- Reassessment of CABCD en route with interventions as required.
- Conduct a secondary survey en route if the patient stabilises.
- Provide an ATMIST handover to the emergency department staff on arrival.

Diagnosis

Diabetic ketoacidosis due to lack of subcutaneous insulin.

Hypoglycaemia

The most common cause of hypoglycaemia is diabetic medications; other causes include renal and liver disease, sepsis and drug overdose. Clinical manifestations comprise neurological deterioration and management strategies incorporate oral glucose or carbohydrate, if the patient is conscious, or intravenous glucose.

Red Flag Alert: Recognition of Hypoglycaemia

Rapid recognition and correction of hypoglycaemia is vital to prevent seizures and coma, which can lead to permanent brain damage. There are several cardinal symptoms of hypoglycaemia that may proceed seizures and coma, including:

- Diaphoresis
- Tachycardia
- Confusion
- Visual changes
- Slurred speech
- Dizziness.

Clinical Investigations: Hypoglycaemia

- Urinalysis:
  - Glucose high in diabetes.
  - Presence of ketones in DKA.
- **Serum HbA1c** – an average of serum blood glucose levels over two to three months, ideally 48 mmol/l or less:
  - If raised, increased risk of developing type II diabetes.
- **Blood glucose** – using blood glucose monitor, normal measurement 4–10 mmol/l.
  - If raised could indicate DKA or HHS if associated with clinical deterioration.
  - If low could indicate over administration of insulin or acute illness.

259

Medications Management: Hypoglycaemia

Hypoglycaemia is defined as a blood glucose concentration of less than 4 mmol/l; it most commonly occurs as result of the treatment of diabetes mellitus. For patients who are conscious and able to swallow, management includes fast-acting carbohydrate such as glucose liquid, glucose tablets, glucose gel, pure fruit juice or sucrose dissolved in water (British National Formulary 2023b). Unresponsive hypoglycaemia, defined as a blood glucose of less than 4 mmol/l after 30–45 minutes or despite three treatment cycles, or an unconscious patient with hypoglycaemia, requires treatment with intramuscular glucagon or an intravenous infusion of 10% glucose.

Reflective Learning Activity

Reflect on what you understand about the emergency management of hyperglycaemia and hypoglycaemia as a paramedic.

Take Home Points

- The endocrine system plays a crucial role in homeostasis through regulation of hormones, via negative feedback mechanisms. A good understanding of the physiology and pathology is crucial in recognising common disorders.
- Diabetes mellitus and thyroid disease are the most common endocrine conditions.
- Clinical features of endocrine pathology may be varied and non-specific, in addition to affecting multiple anatomical sites and organ systems.
- Identification of life-threatening endocrine emergencies requires prompt identification and management.

Summary

As a student paramedic, you will undoubtedly be involved in the care of a number of patients with either a primary or secondary disorder of the endocrine system. Management strategies for this population can be very complex and have the potential to have detrimental effects. As such, it is crucial that the healthcare professionals involved in supporting this patient group have a sound understanding of the pathophysiological, pharmacological and evidence base that underpins the promotion of safe and effective care.

References

British National Formulary (2023a). Calcium gluconate. London: National Institute for Health and Care Excellence. https://bnf.nice.org.uk/drugs/calcium-gluconate/#indications-and-dose (accessed 8 October 2023).

British National Formulary (2023b). Medical emergencies in the community. London: National Institute for Health and Care Excellence. https://bnf.nice.org.uk/treatment-summaries/medical-emergencies-in-the-community (accessed 8 October 2023).

Chaker, L., Bianco, A., Jonklaas, J. et al. (2016). Hypothyroidism. *Lancet* 390: 1550–1562.

Clare, C. (2017). The endocrine system. In: *Fundamentals of Anatomy and Physiology for Nursing and Healthcare Students*, 2e (ed. I. Peate and M. Nair), 479–512. Chichester: Wiley.

Diabetes UK (2023). How many people in the UK have diabetes? www.diabetes.org.uk/professionals/position-statements-reports/statistics (accessed 8 October 2023).

Eligar, V., Taylor, P.N., Okosieme, O.E. et al. (2016). Thyroxine replacement: a clinical endocrinlologist's viewpoint. *Ann Clin Biochem* 53: 421–433.

Holt, R.I.G. and Hanley, N.A. (2011). *Essential Endocrinology and Diabetes*. Chichester: Wiley.

Leach, R. (2014). *Critical Care Medicine at a Glance*, 3e. Chichester: Wiley.

Malaty, W. (2023). Primary hypothyroidism. *BMJ Best Practice* 30 March. https://bestpractice.bmj.com/topics/en-gb/535 (accessed 8 October 2023).

National Institute for Health and Care Excellence (NICE) (2019). Thyroid Disease: Assessment and management. NICE Guideline NG 145. London: National Institute for Health and Care Excellence. www.nice.org.uk/guidance/ng145/chapter/Context (accessed 8 October 2023).

Nematollahi, L.R and Arafah, B. (2022). Primary adrenal insufficiency. *BMJ Best Practice* 3 May. https://bestpractice.bmj.com/topics/en-gb/56 (accessed 8 October 2023).

Peate, I. and Hill, B. (2021). Fundamentals of Critical Care: A Textbook for Nursing and Healthcare Students. Wiley-Blackwell.

Ross, D.S., Burch, H.B., Cooper, D.S. et al. (2016). 2016 American Thyroid Association Guidelines for diagnosis and management of hyperthyroidism and other causes of thyrotoxicosis. *Thyroid* 26 (10): 1343–1421.

Shoback, D. and Quan-Yang, D. (2023). Hypoprathyroidism. *BMJ Best Practice* 13 June. https://bestpractice.bmj.com/topics/en-gb/132#:~:text=The%20disorder%20is%20caused,the%20condition%20is%20permanent.&text=The%20disorder,is%20permanent.&text=is%20caused,the%20condition (accessed 16 October 2023).

Ward, J.P.T. and Linden, R.W.A. (2017). *Physiology at a Glance*. Chichester: Wiley.

Further Reading

BMJ Best Practice (2022). Overview of thyroid dysfunction. https://bestpractice.bmj.com/topics/en-gb/833 (accessed 8 October 2023).

Holmes, M. (2022). Thyroid storm. *RCEM Learning* 16 March. https://www.rcemlearning.co.uk/reference/thyroid-storm/#1646899559693-37304b99-1a81 (accessed 8 October 2023).

Vaidya, B. and Pearce, S.H.S. (2014). Diagnosis and management of thyrotoxicosis. *BMJ* 349: g5128.

Online Resources

Khan Academy. https://www.khanacademy.org/science/ap-biology/cell-communication-and-cell-cycle/cell-communication/v/intro-to-the-endocrine-system

Society for Endocrinology. https://www.endocrinology.org/

Glossary

Diaphoresis	Sweating, especially to an unusual degree as a symptom of disease or adverse effect of a drug.
Exogenous	Originates from outside or external to an organism.
Hormone	A regulatory substance produced in an organism and transported in tissue fluids such as blood or sap to stimulate specific cells or tissues into action.
Hypophysiotrophic	A stimulatory hormone that acts upon the pituitary gland.
Idiopathic	The cause is unknown.
Lipid soluble	The substance is able to pass through the cell membrane, which is comprised of phospholipids.
Metabolism	The chemical processes that occur within a living organism in order to maintain life.
Negative feedback loop	A biological process that occurs within our bodies that causes a decrease in the function of that pathway.
Phospholipid	A type of lipid molecule that is the main component of cell membranes.
Positive feedback loop	Occurs in nature when the product of a reaction leads to an increase in that reaction.

261

Multiple Choice Questions

1. Which of the following is NOT a function of the endocrine system?
    a. Regulation of electrolytes
    b. Growth and development
    c. Respiration
    d. Stress and adaptation

2. The hypothalamus exerts effects upon release of hormones from which gland?
    a. Thyroid gland
    b. Pituitary gland
    c. Adrenal glands
    d. Thymus gland

3. Hormones are classified according to their structure and include what?
    a. Steroids
    b. Peptides, polypeptides and proteins
    c. Amino acids
    d. All of the above

4. Hormones may have an autocrine effects where what happens?
   a. The hormone travels in the blood to the target cell
   b. The hormone produces an effect on the cells by which they are produced
   c. The hormone produces and effect upon nearby cells
   d. The hormone produces an effect upon the adjacent neuron

5. The majority of hormone secretion is regulated by what mechanism?
   a. Positive feedback mechanisms
   b. External factors
   c. Positive and negative feedback mechanisms
   d. Negative feedback mechanisms

6. What is the most common cause of diabetes insipidus resulting in a lack of release of ADH from the posterior pituitary gland?
   a. Head injury
   b. Diabetes mellitus
   c. Gestational diabetes insipidus
   d. Nephrogenic diabetes insipidus

7. Hyperthyroidism is confirmed by what biochemical investigations?
   a. Low TSH, low T3 and T4
   b. High TSH, high T3 and T4
   c. High TSH, low T3 and T4
   d. Low TSH, high T_3 and T_4

8. Which of the following is the most common cause of primary hyperparathyroidism?
   a. Renal failure
   b. Autoimmune thyroiditis
   c. Thyroid surgery
   d. Adenoma

9. Aldosterone is a mineralocorticoid which is responsible for the regulation of what?
   a. Sodium, potassium, chloride and bicarbonate
   b. Sodium, potassium, magnesium and bicarbonate
   c. Sodium, calcium, chloride and bicarbonate
   d. Sodium, calcium, magnesium and bicarbonate

10. The cardinal symptoms of hyperglycaemia include which of these combinations?
   a. Polyuria, weight loss, lethargy and polydipsia
   b. Diaphoresis, weight loss, lethargy and polydipsia
   c. Poluyuria, seizure, lethargy and polydipsia
   d. Diaphoresis, seizure, slurred speech and polydipsia

CHAPTER 13

The Reproductive Systems and Associated Disorders

Tim Millington and Aimee Yarrington

AIM

This chapter aims to provide an outline of the female and male reproductive systems as well as some commonly associated disorders.

LEARNING OUTCOMES

On completion of this chapter you will be able to:

- Identify the internal and external structures of the female and male reproductive systems.
- Describe the key functions of the female and male reproductive systems.
- Provide an explanation for the normal and abnormal pathological changes that can occur in the female and male reproductive systems.
- Outline the care and management of a number of conditions commonly seen in disorders of the female and male reproductive systems.

Test Your Prior Knowledge
1. Describe the multifaceted role of the paramedic when offering care to people with healthcare conditions associated with reproductive systems.
2. What is meant by the term miscarriage?
3. How can disorders of the reproductive system can impact the health and wellbeing of a person?

Fundamentals of Applied Pathophysiology for Paramedics, First Edition. Edited by Ian Peate and Simon Sawyer.
© 2024 John Wiley & Sons Ltd. Published 2024 by John Wiley & Sons Ltd.

The Female Reproductive System

The female reproductive system is divided into two distinct parts: internal and external structures/organs. The reproductive system comprises the organs required for fertilisation, gestation and reproduction. Often referred to as the genital organs, their specialised functions have the unique ability to adapt and accommodate a fetus during pregnancy, expel the fetus once labour starts, as well as commencing menses and menopause, all during the female life cycle.

Anatomy and Physiology

The external female genitalia comprise the area from the mons pubis to the anus. This area is termed the vulva; it is often mislabelled or mistermed the vagina, which is an internal structure (Figure 13.1).

The external genitalia is linked to the internal genitalia via the vagina. The vagina is a fibromuscular tube, capable of distention to allow the passage of a fetus, and is approximately 8.4–11.3 cm in length in the non-labouring woman. It is not visible from the external and sits within the pelvic cavity. The uterus sits at the top of the vagina, with the cervix, the lower pole of the uterus, protruding into the vault of the vagina. The cervix can only be seen with the use of a speculum examination, a procedure that should be performed by an appropriately trained practitioner. The uterus is divided into three areas: the fundus, body and cervix. As previously stated, the cervix sits into the vagina, but this is the section that, during labour, is drawn upward by the shortening of the muscle fibres, causing the effacement and dilation of the cervix. This action allows the passage of the fetus out of the uterus through the vagina or birth canal at birth.

Fertility and the Menstrual Cycle

The menstrual cycle will be individual for every woman. There are factors that can alter the length of the cycle, stress being one example. An average cycle is 28 days but normal ranges vary between 25 and 35 days (NHS England 2023). Periods can start from the age of 8 years, the average age of onset being 12 years, and end at the menopause from 50 to 55 years. During this time, a woman will have around 480 periods, but fewer if there are pregnancies or hormonal contraception that prevents periods.

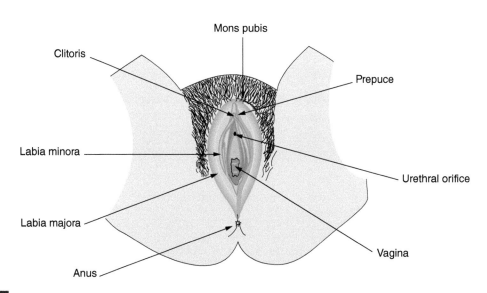

FIGURE 13.1   The external female genitalia.

Menstrual Cycle

The menstrual cycle is controlled by the sex hormones oestrogen and progesterone produced by the pituitary gland in the hypothalamus of the brain. The four main phases of the menstrual cycle are (NHS England 2023; Better Health 2018):

- Menstruation
- Follicular phase
- Ovulation
- Luteal phase.

Menstruation
Levels of oestrogen and progesterone fall and the endometrium (the lining of the uterus) is shed from the body as menstrual flow in a process commonly called a 'period'. The average length of a period is between three and seven days.

Follicular Phase
The follicular phase starts on the first day of menstruation and ends with ovulation. The pituitary gland releases follicle-stimulating hormone (FSH). This hormone stimulates the ovary to produce around 5–20 follicles on the surface of the ovary. Each follicle is an immature ovum, only one of which will mature to ovulation; the others will die. Progesterone is released, which helps the uterus to prepare for implantation of a fertilised ovum.

Ovulation
Rising levels of oestrogen cause the ovary to release an ovum at ovulation. The endometrium also starts to thicken. The hypothalamus recognises these rising levels and releases a chemical called gonadotrophin-releasing hormone. This hormone prompts the pituitary gland to produce raised levels of luteinising hormone (LH) and FSH. The ovum is collected by the fallopian tube and is moved towards the uterus by waves of small, hair-like projections called fimbra. The lifespan of the ovum is only around 24 hours. Unless it meets a sperm during this time, it will die. If fertilisation does not occur, the ovum is reabsorbed into the body.

Luteal Phase
During ovulation, the ovum bursts from its follicle but the ruptured follicle stays on the surface of the ovary. For the next two weeks or so, the follicle transforms into a structure known as the corpus luteum. This structure starts releasing progesterone, together with small amounts of oestrogen. This combination of hormones maintains the thickened lining of the uterus, waiting for a fertilised ovum to implant.

If a fertilised ovum implants in the endometrium, it produces the hormones that are necessary to maintain the corpus luteum. This includes human chorionic gonadotrophin, the hormone that is detected in a urine test for pregnancy. The corpus luteum keeps producing the raised levels of progesterone that are needed to maintain the thickened lining of the uterus.

If pregnancy does not occur, the corpus luteum withers and dies, usually around day 22 in a 28-day cycle. The drop in progesterone levels causes the lining of the uterus to fall away. This is known as menstruation. The cycle then repeats.

Fertile Window
Theoretically, there is a very small window where a woman can actually become pregnant. As it is difficult to pinpoint exactly when ovulation occurs, the woman's fertile window will be around 10–16 days before her next period, depending on when she has ovulated.

Physiological Changes of Pregnancy

Airway
- Hormonal changes lead to increased oedema to the neck, causing difficulties with airway management.
- Obesity in pregnancy compounds the issue further.
- Full dentition makes intubation difficult.

Breathing
There is an increase in tidal volume of 20% by 12 weeks and of 40% by 40 weeks of pregnancy. Capacity is unchanged; the increase is at the expense of the residual reserve capacity. This increased demand means that the woman has a reduced ability to compensate in injury or illness.

Pressure from the growing uterus causes splinting of the lower ribs, which in turn causes the diaphragm to be forced upward. This pressure also causes the rotation of the heart upwards and to the left. The pressure of fully engorged breasts causes further respiratory and ventilatory difficulty.

Circulation
By the end of pregnancy, the uterus and placenta receive approximately 20% of the maternal cardiac output. Maternal blood volume expands to approximately 7 l during pregnancy but red blood cell production does not increase, so there is a relative anaemia produced. Because of expanded blood volume, a pregnant woman can lose 1000–1500 ml of blood or experience 30–35% of total blood loss before exhibiting overt signs of shock.

The increased blood volume (hypervolaemia) meets the extra demands on the circulation, producing more heat. The extra blood flow to the skin helps with temperature regulation and safeguards a woman against haemorrhage at delivery. Decreased viscosity and increased cardiac force lead to decreased resistance to blood flow – increasing placental perfusion.

Gastrointestinal changes also occur. Progesterone decreases the tone and mobility of smooth muscle. This means that peristalsis of the intestine is slowed, the cardiac sphincter relaxes, reducing gastric emptying time (with a risk of aspiration).

Clinical Investigations: Reproductive Disorders

Most women are cared for in a primary care setting. Conditions mainly linked to pregnancy will require a knowledge of the reproductive system to manage the conditions.

Point of contact investigations:

- *Primary care*: appropriately trained clinicians in primary care settings may be able to perform internal examinations such as a speculum examination to assess the cervix.
- *Secondary care:* clinicians will have access to a full range of diagnostics including ultrasound, computed tomography and magnetic resonance imaging, as well as blood tests.

Vaginal Bleeding: Non-pregnant Causes

Endometriosis
Endometriosis is a condition where the endometrial cells from the lining of the uterus are found outside of the uterine cavity (Figure 13.2). Each month during the woman's menstrual cycle when the endometrial cells shed, bleeding occurs and because these cells are not in the correct location, the menstrual fluid has no way of escaping from the body. This process has a significant impact on the woman's life, with the resulting chronic pain, fatigue, depression, interruption to personal

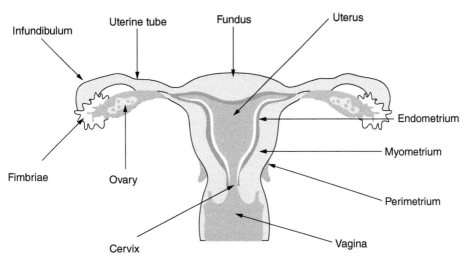

FIGURE 13.2 The uterus and associated structures.

relationships and fertility issues, as well as difficulty with work and social commitments (Endometriosis UK n.d.). There is no proven cause of endometriosis, although there are several theories about what contributes to its development:

- *Retrograde menstruation*: where the endometrium flows backwards during menstruation.
- *Genetic predisposition*: passed on from family members who are suffers.
- *Lymphatic or circulatory spread*: cells travelling around in the blood stream.
- *Immune dysfunction*: where there is a deficit within the immune system.
- *Environmental causes*: one theory suggests that exposure to dioxins can increase the risk of developing endometriosis.
- *Metaplasia*: where one cell morphs into a different type of cell; this type of cause would explain how endometrial cells have appeared in areas of the body such as the skin or lungs or in men who have taken hormone treatment.

There are several treatment options available that are appropriate to a woman's individual circumstances. This includes a holistic approach, taking several factors into account (Endometriosis UK 2010):

- Age
- The severity of symptoms
- The desire to have children, and when
- The severity of the disease
- Previous treatment
- Adverse effects of drugs
- Risks
- Intended duration of treatment.

Treatment options include:

- Surgery
- Hormone treatment
- Pain management
- Nutrition
- Complementary therapies
- Emotional support.

Reflective Learning Activity

Some myths still exist about treatment for endometriosis. Pregnancy and hysterectomy, for example, are not 'cures' for endometriosis. Awareness of this chronic and often misunderstood disease is very much needed. Endometriosis, a leading cause of infertility and its most common symptom is chronic, sometimes debilitating, pelvic pain. It can take, on average, eight years to get a diagnosis of endometriosis. The impact of delayed diagnosis on people's physical and mental health can not be overstated. If undiagnosed, treatment cannot be accessed and the condition may progress, negatively impacting careers, education, relationships and all aspects of the person's life.

Take some time to reflect on ways in which you can further develop your knowledge and understanding of endometriosis and how, in your role, you can offer support to people with this condition.

Sexually Transmitted Infections

Chlamydia trachomatis is the most common bacterial sexually transmitted infection (STI) in the UK (NHS England 2021a). It is transmitted via unprotected sex and is particularly prevalent in sexually active teenagers and young adults. Symptoms for women include:

- Dysuria
- Discharge and or bleeding from the vagina or rectum
- Abdominal pain
- Bleeding following sex or between periods.

If left untreated, STIs can lead to pelvic inflammatory disease and ectopic pregnancy, as well as infertility.

Treatment is with antibiotics, either doxycycline or azithromycin are most commonly used as a three-day course (NHS England 2021a). Prevention is the best way to avoid infection; condom use is recommended to avoid transmission during vaginal, anal and oral sex.

Other common STIs that paramedics may see in clinical practice (particularly within primary care) are described in Table 13.1.

268

TABLE 13.1   Showing signs, symptoms and treatment options for common STIs.

STI	Signs and symptoms	Treatment
Gonorrhoea	Vaginal discharge which may be thin or watery and green or yellow in colour; pain or a burning sensation when passing urine; bleeding between periods, heavy periods and bleeding after sex	Will depend on local antibiotic guidance, but will be: ceftriaxone or cefixime, azithromycin, ciprofloxacin or ofloxacin
Genital herpes	A first episode presents with multiple painful blisters, which quickly burst to leave erosions and ulcers, on the external genitalia. Lesions are usually bilateral and develop 4–7 days after exposure to herpes simplex virus infection. Around 50% of people with symptomatic lesions report headache, fever, malaise, dysuria, or tender inguinal lymphadenopathy. Other symptoms include vaginal discharge and local oedema. Tingling/neuropathic pain in the genital area, lower back, buttocks or legs. A primary episode can last up to 20 days and is often more severe than a recurrent episode	For initial episodes, treatment with oral aciclovir (200 mg five times a day) should be started within 5 days of the start of the episode or while new lesions are forming. This should be continued for 5–10 days, or longer if new lesions are still forming while on treatment
Genital warts	Caused by a virus called human papillomavirus (HPV). There are many types of HPV. The HPV virus can stay in your skin and warts can develop again. Warts may go away without treatment, but this may take many months. You can still pass the virus on, and the warts may come back	The type of treatment will depend on the type of wart, their appearance and where they are located. This includes creams, excision, freezing. There is no cure for genital warts

Source: adapted from NHS England (2021b) and National Institute for Health and Care Excellence (2022b).

Abnormal Uterine Bleeding

Regular vaginal bleeding is normal in females following puberty; however, around 14% of women can experience abnormal uterine bleeding (AUB). Various terminology exists to describe vaginal bleeding (Table 13.2).

Clinical Manifestations

When caring for a woman who is experiencing vaginal bleeding, two important details to establish rapidly are:

- Haemodynamic stability.
- Presence of pregnancy.

Haemodynamically unstable patients present with signs of hypovolaemic shock and require urgent resuscitation. Indicators of shock can be identified through history taking as well through as clinical examination and investigative tests. These tests will vary depending on the setting in which the paramedic is employed. Clinical examination and investigations performed by a paramedic in all settings will include manual pulse and capillary refill checks, abdominal examination, including palpation to ascertain areas of tenderness, blood pressure/pulse oximeter readings and ECG. Additional tests might include urinalysis for both infection and pregnancy, blood testing (more so in primary or secondary facilities) or point of care ultrasound. Clues to severe blood loss causing hypovolaemic shock include tachycardia, tachypnoea, pallor, hypotension, weak or absent pulses, syncope, diaphoresis, confusion due to end organ hypoperfusion and prolonged capillary refill (Taghavi and Askari 2021).

Considering pregnancy as a differential diagnosis is crucial, as this will guide subsequent management. This is because ectopic pregnancy is a life-threatening, time-critical emergency. As such, all post-pubescent females experiencing vaginal bleeding should be considered to be pregnant until proven otherwise.

Often, non-pregnant females will be stable but will require investigation as to the cause of their bleeding. The International Federation of Gynecology and Obstetrics uses the PALM-COEIN classification tool, an acronym describing causes of AUB in women of reproductive age, which divides causes into two groups: structural (measured via imaging or histopathology) or non-structural (cannot be measured; Munro et al. 2011; Table 13.3).

269

Treatment

Treatment of vaginal bleeding will depend on the presence of haemodynamic instability. Should instability be present, emergency resuscitation and rapid transport to an appropriate facility is required. Alternative treatments of patients with vaginal bleeding will depend on the cause and can include pharmacological therapies or surgical intervention.

TABLE 13.2 Definitions of vaginal bleeding.

Term	Description
Normal menstrual bleeding	Vaginal bleeding that occurs monthly (approximately), usually every 24–38 days, lasting 4–8 days, with an estimated volume of 5–80 ml or 1 soaked sanitary pad every 3 hours
AUB	Abnormal uterine bleed in non-pregnant females; 'abnormal' refers to frequency, volume or duration
Chronic	Frequent AUB for 6 months
Acute	Heavy bleeding requiring immediate treatment
Heavy menstrual bleeding	Menstrual bleed causing detriment to a person's quality of life. Estimated as being > 80 ml
Postmenopausal bleeding	Vaginal bleeding 1 year after the last menstrual period
Post-coital bleeding	Bleeding immediately after sexual intercourse that is not menstrual bleeding

AUB, abnormal uterine bleeding.
Source: adapted from Bhroin (2021).

TABLE 13.3   The International Federation of Gynecology and Obstetrics PALM-COEIN classification tool.

Classification	Definition
Structural:	
P	Polyp (AUB occurred in 68% of patients with endometrial polyps)
A	Adenomyosis (a process where the tissue lining of the uterus grows in the muscular wall causing AUB)
L	Leiomyoma; also known as fibroids, is a non-cancerous tumour
M	Malignancy
Bleeding can be an early symptom of uterine cancer or endometrial cancer. Studies have shown PMB present in 5–10% of endometrial cancer cases (Gredmark et al. 1995)	
Non-structural:	
C	Coagulopathy: 5–36% of adolescents presenting with AUB have bleeding conditions (Deligeroroglou and Karountzos 2018)
O	Ovulatory dysfunction: can be linked to polycystic ovary syndrome, extreme exercise, or thyroid imbalances
E	Endometrial: can have infective origins (e.g. due to endometritis)
I	Iatrogenic: Through medications or contraceptive devices
N	Not otherwise classified: describes AUB not related to pregnancy, structural pelvic alterations, hormonal imbalance, contraception or chronic disease

Source: adapted from Munro et al. (2011).

Female Genital Mutilation

The World Health Organization (WHO) defines female genital mutilation (FGM) as any non-medical procedure relating to partial or total removal of, or injury to, the external female genitalia. This includes removal of all or part of the clitoris, clitoral hood, inner and outer labia, or infibulation (describing closure of the vagina). 'FGM is recognized internationally as a violation of the human rights of girls and women. It reflects deep-rooted inequality between the sexes, and constitutes an extreme form of discrimination' (World Health Orgnization 2023).

An estimated 200 million females have been affected in 30 countries across Africa, South and Southeast Asia, as well as their communities worldwide (World Health Orgnization 2023). Reasons for FGM vary between regions and are formed from various sociocultural influences.

Clinical Manifestations

Clinical presentation will relate to when the FGM occurred. Similarly, treatments will vary depending on duration and nature of presentation. The WHO divides complications of FGM into immediate and long term complications (Table 13.4).

In Figure 13.3, types of FGM are detailed.

Paramedics have a statutory obligation under national safeguarding protocols to protect those at risk of FGM (Peate 2014). A consideration of any safeguarding measures is the assessment of the continued risk posed to a child born to a mother who has previously experienced FGM. FGM can occur at any time through childhood, so measures may remain in place for more than 15 years.

TABLE 13.4 The World Health Organization (2023) signs and symptoms associated with female genital mutilation.

Immediate	Long-term
Pain	Urinary issues (dysuria, infections)
Bleeding	Vaginal issues (pruritis, discharge, infections)
Swelling	Menstrual issues (abdominal or vaginal pain, difficulty passing blood)
Infections e.g. tetanus	Scar tissue
Urinary symptoms	Sexual issues (e.g. dyspareunia)
Genital tissue injury	Complications during childbirth
Complications of wound healing	Psychological issues (anxiety, post-traumatic stress disorder)
Shock (sepsis/blood loss), death	Need for corrective surgery

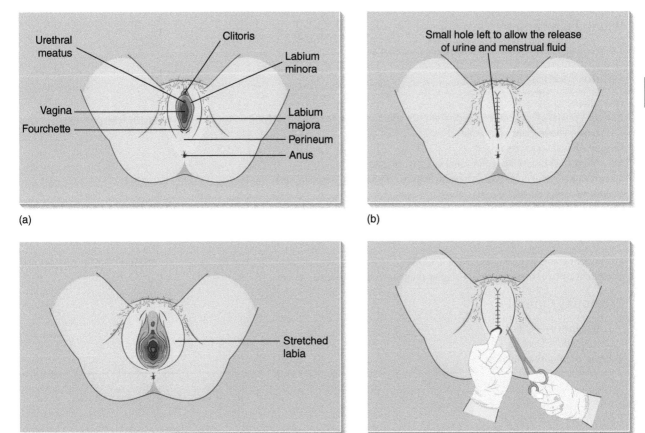

FIGURE 13.3 Types of female genital mutilation. (a) Type 2 FGM with key genitalia identified. (b) Type 3 FGM: infibulation. (c) Type 4 FGM: stretched labia. (d) Anterior episiotomy (deinfibulation) procedure.

Bleeding in the Pregnant Patient

Key facts about early pregnancy bleeding include:

- 50% of pregnant women will have some vaginal bleeding in the first 12 weeks of pregnancy.
- 75% of these women will carry on with their pregnancy.
- One in four pregnancies in the first trimester will miscarry.
- One in 80 pregnancies will result in an ectopic pregnancy.
- One in 600 is a molar pregnancy.
- One in 100 pregnancies in the second trimester miscarries.
- One in 100 women has recurrent miscarriage (Royal College of Nursing 2021).

Snapshot 13.1

Time of dispatch – 4.40 a.m.
On scene – 4.50 a.m.

Pre-arrival Information

Female patient, 22 years of age, with abdominal pain.

Windscreen Report

Terraced house in a residential street; appears well maintained.

Patient Assessment Triage

One patient.
Danger – no dangers observed or apparent to patient or crew; the patient is lying on the bed upstairs in the fetal position.
Response – she responds normally.
Airway – her airway is clear.
Breathing – her breathing is of normal rate rhythm and depth.
Circulation – radial pulse present; rapid, at approximately 100 beats/minute.
Disability – alert on ACVPU scale.
Exposure – consent will be required prior to exposure for examination.

Initial Questioning

The patient states that she has severe left lower quadrant abdominal pain; 10/10 on the pain score. She has been in constant and consistent pain for three hours. She denies pregnancy but is sexually active.

Promoting Curiosity

- Last menstrual period?
- Contraceptive use?
- Bowel or urinary symptoms

Ectopic Pregnancy

An ectopic pregnancy is where a fertilised ovum implants outside the uterine cavity. The most common place is within the fallopian tubes (95%), but there are other locations (Box 13.1; Figure 13.4).

The National Institute for Health and Care Excellence (2021) states that approximately 11 000 pregnancies each year in the UK are ectopic, giving a risk factor of 11 : 1000 pregnancies.

BOX 13.1 Ectopic Pregnancy: Locations Outside the Uterine Cavity.

3% are interstitial (inside the part of the fallopian tube that crosses into the uterus).
<1% are within a caesarean section scar on the uterus.
<1% are cervical (on the cervix).
<1% are cornual (within an abnormally shaped uterus).
<1% are ovarian (in or on the ovary).
<1% are intramural (in the muscle of the uterus).
<1% are abdominal (in the abdomen).
<1% are heterotopic pregnancies.

Source: Ectopic Pregnancy Trust (2022).

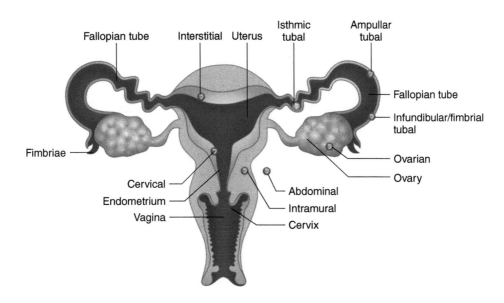

FIGURE 13.4 Ectopic pregnancy. Source: Ectopic Pregnancy Trust (2022).

Symptoms may be atypical, and ectopic pregnancy should always be excluded in any female with reproductive ability with abdominal pain. Even if the woman states that she is using or has a contraceptive device (intrauterine device or implant) no type of contraception is 100% effective. Atypical symptoms may be mistaken for urinary tract infection or gastrointestinal disturbance. Common symptoms include abdominal or pelvic pain, amenorrhoea or missed period and vaginal bleeding, which can be minimal or just spotting.

Immediate hospital admission via the emergency department or an early pregnancy assessment unit should be sought without delay, especially if signs of haemodynamic instability are present.

Medicines Management: Contraceptive Implants

A contraceptive implant is a small plastic rod that is inserted under the skin by a general practitioner or sexual health clinic. It works by the steady release of progesterone, which prevents ovulation as well as thickening cervical mucus (NHS England 2021b). The implant is claimed to be 99% effective but can lead to adverse effects including headaches, nausea, breast tenderness and mood swings. For the implant to remain effective, it must be replaced every three years or there is a risk of pregnancy (Brook 2022).

Pregnancy Loss

Attending cases of baby and infant death is a challenging area of paramedic practice. Paramedics experience a range of issues from resuscitation to dealing with bereaved parents and relatives.

Orange Flag Alert: Dealing with Pregnancy Loss

Dealing with pregnancy loss is a traumatic event for the patient and the attending clinician. Remember to observe your own feelings and that mental wellbeing services are available for clinicians either through your trust or the College of Paramedics.

Pregnancy loss can occur for a number of reasons, such as:

- *Miscarriage* is the spontaneous loss of a pregnancy before 24 weeks of gestation. Unfortunately, miscarriage is a common complication of pregnancy, with about 10–24% of clinically recognised pregnancies ending in miscarriage, but it is thought many more end prior to their recognition (National Institute for Health and Care Excellence 2022a). The majority occur within the first trimester; however, the Royal College of Obstetricians and Gynaecologists estimates that approximately 1% occur before the second trimester (Regan et al. 2023).
- *Molar pregnancy* (also called a *hydatidiform mole*) is a pregnancy where an abnormal fertilised egg implants in the uterus. The cells that should become the placenta grow far too quickly and take over the space where the embryo would normally develop. The consequences of a molar pregnancy include persistent trophoblastic disease, a type of cancer, and the possible need for chemotherapy (Miscarriage Association 2023).
- *Pregnancy of unknown location* occurs when a woman has a positive pregnancy test, but there is no evidence of an intrauterine or extrauterine pregnancy or retained products of conception on transvaginal ultrasound examination. Management options that will be offered to the woman include:
  - Expectant management (wait and observe for deterioration), as 44–69% of such pregnancies settle without intervention.
  - Medical management: methotrexate may be used to absorb the pregnancy cells, but this involves several weeks of monitoring.
  - Surgical management: a laparotomy may be indicated for the unstable patient with signs of rupture (Royal College of Nursing 2021).

Clinical Investigations: Examination Scenario

A woman attends for her 12-week pregnancy dating scan but no fetus is located within the uterus. A transvaginal scan is performed by a trained sonographer and no evidence of a fetus is located. The woman is appropriately counselled and offered expectant or surgical management. She is discharged home with advice to contact the gynaecology unit if her condition deteriorates or to call 999 in the case of collapse.

Antepartum Haemorrhage

An antepartum haemorrhage (APH) is any frank blood loss from the genital tract, after 24 completed weeks of pregnancy, until the onset of labour. APH occurs and complicates 2–5% of pregnancies. It is often unpredictable and, because of the nature of compensation in a pregnant woman, deterioration is often rapid and unexpected.

The Royal College of Obstetricins and Gynaecologists (2011) cites the following as common causes of APH:

- Minor APH (<50 ml that has settled) include cervical erosion, marginal placental bed bleeding or a bloodstained show.
- Major APH (50–1000 ml) are mainly due to placental abruption and placenta praevia. Uterine rupture can also lead to major haemorrhage by either the forces of labour or blunt trauma, road traffic collision or assault.

Snapshot 13.2

Time of dispatch – 3.09 p.m.
On scene – 3.18 p.m.

Pre-arrival Information

Female patient, 40 years of age, with abdominal pain; she is 32 weeks' pregnant and has vaginal bleeding.

Windscreen Report

Detached house in a residential street.

Patient Assessment Triage

One patient.
Danger – no dangers observed or apparent to patient or crew, patient is on the toilet.
Response – she responds normally.
Airway – her airway is clear.
Breathing – her breathing is of normal rate, rhythm and depth.
Circulation –radial pulse present rapid at approximately 120 beats/minute.
Danger – alert on ACVPU scale.
Exposure – consent will be required prior to exposure for examination.

Initial Questioning

The patient states that she has had an increasing pain in the right side of the abdomen. She has bled around 200 ml of dark blood but thinks this has stopped now.

Promoting Curiosity

- Any recent trauma?
- Any hypertensive disorders?
- Any pregnancy complications or placental issues?

The blood loss from an APH can be either revealed or concealed. The revealed blood loss is more commonly caused by placental praevia as the location of the placenta allows an easy exit for blood loss to occur. A concealed haemorrhage is normally caused by trauma, assault or any blunt force to the uterus causing the placenta to shear off the uterine wall.

Medicines Management: Tranexamic Acid

Tranexamic acid (TXA) is often given in cases of major bleeding in relation to trauma. The current Joint Royal Colleges Ambulance Liaison Committee (JRCALC 2022) guideline on the administration of TXA states that it should only be administered to pregnant women in cases of life-threatening haemorrhage in relation to a trauma or postpartum haemorrhage situation. For bleeding not involving trauma TXA cannot be administered.

Risk factors for APH according to the Advance Life Support Group (2019) include:

- Maternal age over 40 years
- Presence of complex medical problems
- Multigravida
- Previous caesarean section
- Known as placenta previa

TABLE 13.5   Placental abruption and placenta praevia.

Clinical sign	Placenta abruption	Placenta praevia
Pain	Yes, can be severe	No, usually painless
Blood loss colour	Dark red/brown	Frank fresh red
Warning haemorrhage	No not commonly	Yes
Consistency of uterus	Tense, hard or wooden	Soft/non-tender
Onset	Usually a cause/trauma	At rest/post-coital

- Use of crack cocaine
- Coagulopathies
- Previous history of APH
- Hypertension
- Polyhydramnios.

Table 13.5 may assist with differential diagnosis to establish the cause of the bleeding.

Red Flag Alert: Bleeding in a Pregnant Woman

- Continuous abdominal pain at any gestation of pregnancy.
- Bleeding at any gestation.
- Non-pregnant bleeding which has led to haemodynamic instability

The Male Reproductive System

The male reproductive system serves to enable sperm, full name; spermatozoa (singular; spermatozoon), and semen to be produced, stored, and exit the body via ejaculation. With regards to reproduction, the intention of ejaculation is to deposit semen within the female reproductive tract to enable fertilisation of the female egg.

Anatomy and Physiology

Male reproductive anatomy consists of internal and external structures. Internally, there are the testes (singular testis/testicle), epididymis, vas deferens (or ductus deferens) and prostate gland, and externally, the penis and scrotum. The head of the penis is called the glans penis (Figure 13.5).

The scrotal sac is a pouch-like collection of skin, inferior to the penis, which contains two reproductive glands called the testes. Technically external to the body, testes begin life within the abdominal cavity, descending through the inguinal canal during fetal development, towards the end of the third trimester, where they are suspended externally, within the scrotum. Failure to descend is termed cryptorchidism.

The scrotum houses two muscular layers – the dartos and cremaster muscles. The dartos muscle divides the scrotum in two, forming the scrotal septum. The cremaster muscles form a thin, net-like layer of striated muscle around each testis. They originate laterally in the inguinal canal from the internal oblique muscle and inguinal ligament, and medially from the pubic tubercle. When the dartos and cremaster muscles contract, they elevate the testes, pulling the

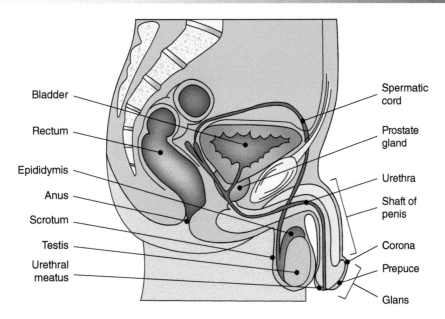

Bladder

Rectum

Epididymis

Anus

Scrotum

Testis

Urethral
meatus

Spermatic
cord

Prostate
gland

Urethra

Shaft of
penis

Corona

Prepuce

Glans

FIGURE 13.5 The male reproductive system.

scrotum closer to the body. This is an important function in thermoregulation. The optimum temperature for sperm production is around 34°C. In cold conditions, these muscles receive signals to contract and pull the testes closer to the body to retain heat.

The cremasteric reflex can be elicited when stroking the inner thigh of males. Stimulating these sensory neurons innervates the genitofemoral nerve causing the contraction and elevation of the ipsilateral testis. This should be included in clinical examination of patients presenting with scrotal pain, as testicular torsion can result in loss of cremasteric reflex. It is important to note that this reflex can remain present in some cases of torsion or might be absent as a normal variant, so its lack is not diagnostic (Mellick et al. 2021).

The testes produce sperm and hormones called androgens, testosterone being an important example. Testes are egg shaped, 4–5 cm long and housed within two layers of protective, connective tissue (outer: tunica vaginalis, inner: tunica albuginea). The dense layers of the tunica albuginea surround and penetrate the testes, dividing them into smaller structures called lobules. These lobules contain coiled, seminiferous tubules, within which are located specialised spermatogenic (or germ) cells, responsible for sperm production. Leydig cells present in the connective tissue produce testosterone and LH (Figure 13.6).

Once produced, the immotile sperm cells pass into the epididymis, where they begin their journey of maturation through its coils. The epididymis is a long, coiled tube that, if extended fully, would be around 6 m long. Sperm take an average of 12 days to navigate its length, gaining motility as they are pushed along by smooth muscle contraction of the epididymal lining. The fully mature sperm are then stored in the tail of the epididymis ready for ejaculation.

At ejaculation, contraction of the smooth muscle of the epididymis moves the sperm into the vas deferens, a muscular tube approximately 40 cm long. From the tail of the epididymis, the vas deferens becomes straighter as it ascends, joining the other structures of the spermatic cord at the deep inguinal ring. It dilates as it terminates at the ampulla. The ampulla then narrows at the prostate before converging with seminal vesicle ducts to form the ejaculatory duct.

The vas deferens is a favoured target during male sterilisation surgery due to its accessibility within the scrotum. The procedure (vasectomy) involves removal of a length of the vas deferens to disrupt transport of sperm during ejaculation.

The prostate gland sits in front of the rectum, just behind the bladder, and contains a portion of the urethra, which passes directly through it. The prostate's milky secretions make up a proportion of the seminal fluid volume. These enzyme-rich secretions contain prostate-specific antigen (PSA), which acts to make the semen thinner and plays an import role in male fertility.

277

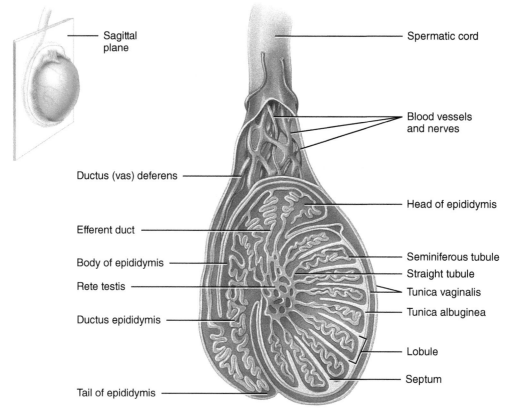

Sagittal plane

Spermatic cord

Blood vessels and nerves

Ductus (vas) deferens

Head of epididymis

Efferent duct

Seminiferous tubule

Straight tubule

Body of epididymis

Rete testis

Tunica vaginalis

Tunica albuginea

Ductus epididymis

Lobule

Septum

Tail of epididymis

FIGURE 13.6   The testicle.

Pathophysiology

Abnormalities of the scrotum usually present with pain and/or swelling. Patients might not seek medical advice until symptoms have progressed significantly or may not divulge an issue due to embarrassment. A thorough systems enquiry and open mind will enable paramedics to identify the issue behind the patient seeking assistance, be that in an ambulance, primary or secondary care setting.

Testicular Torsion

Testicular torsion is an important differential diagnosis in any patient with testicular pain, owing to its time-critical nature. Torsion occurs when the spermatic cord twists, resulting in the blood supply being cut off. This leads to ischaemia which, left unchecked, can cause tissue necrosis and eventual loss of the testis. Delays in treatment must be avoided, so immediate surgical review and exploration override diagnostic testing such as ultrasound.

Typically, testicular torsion affects younger males aged 12–18 years, although it can affect men of any age. Estimates suggest an incidence of 1 in 4000 under 25-year-olds, increasing slightly in those below 18 years of age (Thakkar et al. 2021).

Clinical Manifestations

Patients often describe severe, unilateral pain of sudden onset, with nausea, vomiting and abdominal pain. These associated symptoms might cause the less vigilant clinician to focus on gastrointestinal pathology. This referred abdominal pain originates from the extensive nerves supplying the testis and scrotum. Examination should therefore include both the abdomen and the genitals.

Tenderness is usually severe, seen on palpation of the affected testis. It may appear higher (termed 'high riding') with an absent cremasteric reflex. If presentation is delayed, scrotal discoloration and swelling may be present. Elevation of the testis will not reduce the pain – a negative Prehn's sign.

Intermittent pain could be indicative of periods of spontaneous untwisting then retorsion. Other symptoms such as dysuria, discharge from the penis or pyrexia are not usually associated with torsion and might give clues to an alternative infective pathology.

Risk Factors

A bell-clapper deformity, involving an abnormally high testicular attachment of the tunica vaginalis, is an anatomical variant associated with increased incidence of torsion. It occurs during fetal development as the testes descend, resulting in two superior attachments and horizontal lie of the testes, meaning that there is more room for them to be mobile, swinging like a bell clapper. Trauma is a less frequent cause (4–10% incidence) and the exact aetiology can remain a mystery.

Testes gain weight during puberty, which in turn leads to them becoming more pendulous, an affect exacerbated by contraction of the cremasteric muscle. A bell-clapper deformity increases a person's vulnerability to torsion when the cremaster muscle contracts. Studies have shown increased incidence of torsion during the cold winter months, explained by the increased frequency in the body's natural response to the changing temperatures (Gomes et al. 2015; Molokwu et al. 2020).

Treatment

Testicular torsion is a condition that must be diagnosed clinically; a thorough history and clinical examination are critical. Patients presenting within six hours of symptom onset have the greatest chance of salvaging a viable testis. Once 48 hours has been breached, chances of avoiding testicular loss are almost nil; hence diagnostic imaging being forfeited for exploratory surgery. Surgical management varies with age and aims to detorsion and anchor a salvageable testis.

Reflective Learning Activity

If you see someone in pain – think analgesia. Make an assessment and respond appropriately.

Epididymitis

Epididymitis involves inflammation of the epididymis. Usually infective in origin, epididymitis is characterised by a swollen and painful scrotum. Pain is usually unilateral and gradual, typically taking three to five days to reach peak intensity. Acute epididymitis describes symptoms present for less than six weeks and the term acute epididymo-orchitis is used when both the epididymis and testis are affected.

Epididymitis is a common cause of scrotal pain in sexually active men. Causative agents can be organisms associated with STIs such as *Chlamydia trachomatis* and *Neisseria gonorrhoeae*, or enteric pathogens attributed to anal sex, such as *Escherichia coli*.

Medicines Management: Gonorrhoea

Pharmacological treatment for gonorrhoea includes the use of cephalosporins (e.g. ceftriaxone, cefixme), quinolones (e.g. ciprofoxacin, ofloxacin) or azithromycin. Prescribing considerations for review prior to commencing treatment include:

- Local guidelines and formularies
- The patient's allergy status
- Cautions or contraindications
- Antimicrobial susceptibility/resistance following cultures.

In later life, conditions such as benign prostatic hyperplasia or bladder neck obstruction can lead to bladder outflow inefficiencies. Partial bladder emptying and increases to voiding pressures can lead to reflux or regurgitation of urine, which enables pathogens to enter the ductal system and epididymis.

Clinical Manifestations

History taking must include a detailed sexual history, ensuring that enquiries about recent viral infective symptoms, penile discharge, fever, and any urinary symptoms are included. On examination, the epididymis is located posterior to the testis and is a palpable tubular structure. Tenderness at this site can be indicative of epididymitis. The condition demonstrates a positive Prehn's sign, observed when pain is eased by elevation of the testes. It is important to consider findings such as these alongside a detailed history and other clinical findings. If the testis feels swollen and tender, epididymo-orchitis should be considered.

Treatment

Management of epididymitis begins with treatment of the presenting symptoms. Treatment options will depend on the setting in which a paramedic sees the patient and also their prescribing status. Analgesia will be a priority and should follow a stepwise approach to pain management as recommended by JRCALC. Then, should circumstances allow, progress to identification of the causative agent and its elimination via the prescribing of an appropriate antibiotic.

Balanitis, Posthitis and Balanoposthitis

In non-circumcised males, the prepuce (foreskin) covers the glans penis like a sheath, either partially or fully. *Balanitis* involves inflammation of the glans penis and can affect approximately 4% of uncircumcised boys aged two to five2 – 5 years. *Posthitis* refers to inflammation of the prepuce. Owing to the proximity of the prepuce to the glans penis, one is rarely affected without the other. When both are affected, it is termed *balanoposthitis.* As it is a condition affecting penile skin, other causes in adults include dermatitis (possibly secondary to candidal or bacterial infection), trauma, STIs or premalignant skin changes.

Clinical Manifestations

Patients might complain of a sore, itchy, penis that appears red and swollen, possibly with exudate. The foreskin might be tight and meatal stenosis (narrowing of urethral entrance) may also be present.

Treatment

A tailored assessment and treatment plan, depending on the cause, must be adopted. Paramedics who identify balanitis, posthitis or balanoposthitis when attending a patient at their own address should consult the patient's primary care provider.

Primary-care based paramedics should initiate discussion and advice regarding hygiene practices to explore and eliminate possible allergens and irritants. Swabs, screening for STIs and the use of topical steroid creams may also be considered to aid diagnosis and improve symptoms. If the diagnosis is uncertain, transport or referral to an appropriate specialist should be considered to rule out a premalignant condition.

Phimosis

Phimosis is an inability to retract the foreskin; it affects 1% of boys. Causes can be divided as primary (without scarring) or secondary (with scarring). Primary causes are rare and caused by congenital abnormalities. Secondary causes include recurrent balanitis, previous trauma or balanitis xerotica obliterans (BXO). BXO is chronic inflammatory condition and is a common cause of secondary phimosis. It is thought to be brought on by friction or burns, so it is theorised that the area under the foreskin that is frequently exposed to urine can create conditions contributing to BXO. Persistant BXO can lead to squamous cell carcinoma of the penile skin (Pietrzak et al. 2006).

Treatment

Treatment of phimosis can be either conservative or surgical. Conservative treatment uses a 'wait and see' approach plus topical steroids to help loosen scar tissue. Surgical correction via circumcision removes the foreskin, eliminating the urine-rich environment previously contributing to BXO, so reoccurrences rates are low. Paramedics should assess severity and consider signposting less severe cases to primary care facilities, where they can be referred for specialist outpatient review, should it be required. If diagnosis is uncertain or complications are noted (e.g. infection, urinary retention), transport or referral for same-day review should be considered.

Penile Trauma

Examples of penile trauma include penile fracture and frenulum tears, injuries typically occurring as a result of sexual misadventure. Fractures are caused by rapid, bending forces to the erect penis.

Clinical Manifestations

- *Penile fracture*: patients report severe pain, loss of erection and a 'popping' sensation. Patients note severe bruising and swelling to the penile shaft due to subcutaneous bleeding, referred to as an 'eggplant' deformity. Investigations include urinalysis, where blood (either microscopic or macroscopic) could signify a urethral tear, a more severe symptom.
- *Frenulum tear:* the frenulum refers to the skin at the underside of the penis that attaches the foreskin to the tip of the penis. It can become tight and so be vulnerable to tearing during vigorous repetitive activities, usually of a sexual nature, but can also be caused by sports such as cycling or rugby, work-related accidents, or by being caught when grooming. Tearing can be painful but can go unnoticed initially, not identified until the bleeding is seen, which can be significant, and worrisome to the patient.

Treatment

- *Penile fracture*: paramedics should attempt to reduce the patient's pain with an appropriate analgesic. It is important always to gain consent prior to any examination, to be chaperoned by a colleague and to maintain patient dignity throughout. It is good practice to document these elements in detail, remembering to include the full name and role of the chaperone. Patients will require transport to hospital for an urgent urological review and possible surgical repair. A surgical approach aims to improve penile curvature and mitigate erectile dysfunction, which might result from untreated injury. Surgery incorporates drainage and defect repair, with patients often discharged that day, so reassurance will be important.
- *Frenulum tear*: initially, patients need to be examined, remembering to gain consent, to maintain dignity and to use a chaperone. The patient could be incredibly worried or embarrassed, so a paramedic should maintain the highest levels of professionalism – a minimal expectation in all patient interactions. Adopting an open mind and empathetic approach will build rapport with the patient. If pain is present, analgesia should be administered. Wound management should include application of a sterile dressing to minimise risk of infection. Patients should then be transported to the emergency department to undergo a full review. However, often these wounds will require minimal medical intervention and will heal of their own accord. As such, reassurance is key. In certain cases, notably if bleeding persists, a urological specialist review might be required and a frenuplasty could be indicated. This a relatively straightforward surgical procedure to repair the frenulum.

Benign Prostatic Hyperplasia

The prostate naturally grows with age, starting during puberty, then from 25 years and throughout a man's life. This should not cause a problem, but when the rate of growth results in urinary symptoms, it is referred to as benign prostatic hyperplasia (BPH). Benign, as it is a non-cancerous enlarging of the prostate. It is very common, affecting 50% of men aged 51–60 years and 90% of men over 80 years (Prostate Cancer UK 2022). The prostate is usually 4 cm wide, 3 cm high and 2 cm thick, often compared to a walnut. It can grow much larger than this, impacting the structures around it, particularly the urethra, squeezing it and inhibiting urine flow. This causes the bladder wall to become thicker and weaken over time, eventually losing its ability to fully empty.

Clinical Manifestations

Symptoms can be divided into either urethral obstruction or secondary bladder changes. Obstructive symptoms include a weak urinary stream, difficulty starting to urinate even with straining, or dribbling when trying to stop. Changes to bladder functioning might present as changes to frequency, urgency, nocturia (urinating more at night) or a feeling of incomplete emptying of the bladder.

Treatment

Treatment options will depend upon the setting in which a paramedic will see these patients. Severe cases of urinary retention will require symptom management, namely analgesia and catheterisation. Specialist paramedics might be able to perform catheterisation in the community, but transport to hospital may be required.

Specific guidelines exist for the treatment of BPH with lower urinary tract symptoms. Conservative management in the form of fluid intake advice (i.e. avoiding certain drinks such as alcohol and caffeine or reducing evening fluid intake by aiming to drink 1.5–2 l daily) might be used in non-urgent cases; for example, if a paramedic sees patients in clinics within a general practice. In addition, pharmacological management is available and takes various forms, each with their own array of adverse effects for which patients should be counselled (Madersbacher et al. 2019).

Prostate Cancer

Malignant growth of the prostate with metastatic spread can be life threatening. Globally, prostate cancer is the fifth leading cause of cancer deaths in men (Prostate Cancer UK 2022). The prostate has three zones, named the central, peripheral and transition zones. Most cancers start in the peripheral zone located near the rectum – hence why the digital rectal examination is commonly used in screening (Figure 13.7).

Clinical Manifestations

Symptoms of prostate cancer can mimic that of BPH but can also be painful. Pain might be present on urination (dysuria), ejaculation, in the lower back, pelvis, thighs or bones, and can be associated with haematuria or weight loss, although these are late symptoms.

Risk Factors

Risk factors for prostate cancer include age (men over 50 years old), ethnicity or previous family history.

Health Education for Prostate Cancer

282

Importantly, patients are usually asymptomatic, with diagnosis achieved by identification of risk factors and entering into testing programmes. Black men over 45 years are encouraged to enter testing programmes (data regarding ethnicity included statistics measured from men who recorded their ethnicity as either 'black Caribbean', 'black other' or 'black African'). Research suggests including early PSA testing in this patient population (40–44 years) can be prognostic (Prostate Cancer UK 2023).

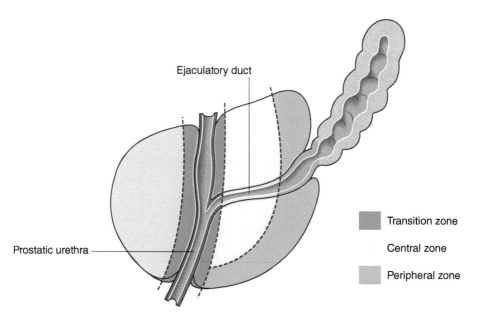

Ejaculatory duct

Transition zone

Central zone

Peripheral zone

Prostatic urethra

FIGURE 13.7   The prostate gland.

Treatment

Treatment of prostate cancer depends on its severity described by its staging. Early-stage asymptomatic prostate cancer is conservatively managed with observation through regular PSA testing, biopsies or imaging. Late-stage prostate cancers can be surgically removed or undergo radiotherapy with hormone treatments. When metastatic spread is present, chemotherapy may also be used.

An understanding of the stage of a patient's cancer and the risks associated with its treatment will enable paramedics to identify possible differential diagnoses and treat these patients appropriately. A patient with active prostate cancer receiving hormone replacement therapy might present with shortness of breath and tachycardia. An important differential to consider is pulmonary embolism. Once this is confirmed, treatment will include anticoagulation or thrombolysis. Useful tools exist for risk stratifying patients suspected of pulmonary embolism, two examples being the Wells and PERC (pulmonary embolism rule-out criteria; Table 13.6).

TABLE 13.6 Wells and PERC criteria for pulmonary embolism.

Criteria	Present	Points score[a]
Wells criteria		
Clinical signs/symptoms of DVT	Yes	+3
PE most likely diagnosis	Yes	+3
Heartrate above 100 beats/min	Yes	+1.5
Immobilised for 3 days/surgery in past 4 weeks	Yes	+1.5
Previous diagnosed PE or DVT	Yes	+1.5
Haemoptysis	Yes	+1
Malignancy with treatment in past 6 months	Yes	+1
Score greater then 4 = PE likely		
PERC criteria		
Age 50 years or over	Yes	+1
Heart rate 100 beats/min or more	Yes	+1
Oxygen saturations on air less then 95%	Yes	+1
Unilateral leg swelling	Yes	+1
Haemoptysis	Yes	+1
Recent surgery or trauma	Yes	+1
Previous PE or DVT	Yes	+1
Hormone use	Yes	+1

DVT, deep vein thrombosis; PE, pulmonary embolism.
[a] Score of 1 or more: pulmonary embolism cannot be ruled out.
Source: adapted from Kline (2023).

Alternatively, a patient with metastatic spread from primary prostate cancer receiving chemotherapy might present as pyrexic and generally unwell. In this instance, the paramedic should consider neutropenic sepsis and the immediate need for further investigation and intravenous antibiotics.

Medicines Management: Brachytherapy

Brachytherapy is a targeted form of radiotherapy used in the treatment of certain cancers such as prostate, in which a radioactive source (usually in the form of seeds or capsules) is placed within the body, next to or inside the cancer, to shrink it. As it is localised, it enables higher doses of radiation to be used. Radiation is given off for some time after insertion and, in certain cases, very high doses of radiation might be used. In these instances, certain safety measures need to be considered, particularly by paramedics when attending these patients. These safety measures include:

- Isolating the patient wherever possible.
- Minimising patient contact – by treating them quickly then maintaining a significant distance away to hold conversations.
- Use of protective clothing where available.
- Not attending if the paramedic is pregnant.

Red Flag Alert: Neutropenic Sepsis

Neutropenic sepsis potentially fatal condition in people with low neutrophil counts (neutropenia), seen in immunosuppressed patients undergoing chemotherapy. The mortality rate is 20%. A diagnosis of neutropenic sepsis should be suspected in anyone with risk factors for neutropenia and symptoms or signs indicating possible infection (note that these signs/symptoms can be minimal, atypical or absent). Signs include:

- Feeling generally unwell.
- Temperature greater than 38°C (but may be afebrile or low temperature).
- Clinical features of possible sepsis (might be minimal or absent).
- Relative or carer concern regarding change in a patient's appearance or behaviour.

In unwell patients who have received chemotherapy in the past six weeks, assume neutropenic sepsis until proven otherwise. This is time critical. Intravenous antibiotics are required within one hour of identification (National Institute for Health and Care Excellenc 2020).

Hydrocele

Hydrocele is painless swelling of the scrotum caused by the collection of clear fluid between the layers of the tunica vaginalis. Communicating hydroceles are where an opening (or a communication) remains between the scrotum and the abdomen (specifically the peritoneum) following descent of the testis during fetal development, allowing abdominal fluid to flow into the scrotum. This opening is called the processus vaginalis. If the opening is large enough, abdominal contents can enter the scrotum, as is seen in inguinal hernias.

A non-communicating hydrocele occurs due to inflammation. The processus vaginalis is closed, more fluid is produced, then absorbed and so causes swelling (Huzaifa and Moreno 2023).

Treatment

Urological surgeons treat symptomatic hydroceles by draining the fluid. The important consideration from a paramedic perspective is identifying the origin of the underlying cause and treating any symptoms (e.g. pain with analgesia). The underlying cause might be due to cancer, torsion, trauma or epididymo-orchitis; however, hydroceles can be idiopathic.

The suspected pathology will dictate the speed of response and emergency hospital admission might be indicated if testicular torsion is suspected. If torsion is not suspected but the testes cannot be palpated, or the patient is aged 18–40 years of age, an urgent ultrasound must be arranged.

Varicocele

Dilation of blood vessels within the spermatic cord, called the pampiniform plexus, is termed varicocele. It presents as a soft, worm-like lump and is common, affecting 15% of men over 18 years, and is most prevalent in males aged 15–25 years. The exact cause remains unclear but is thought to be due to venous valvular incompetence, although varicoceles have been reported in men with patent valves. Ninety per cent are left sided because the left testicular vein is around 10 cm longer than the right (Sandlow and Kansal 2021). It inserts at a right angle to the left renal vein whereas the right testicular vein inserts directly into the inferior vena cava. This differing anatomy leads to higher back pressures on the left side, hence the assumed cause of varicocele being valvular failure. Hyperthermia due to increased volumes of warm abdominal blood in these dilated vessels can result in infertility, with varicocele thought to contribute to 35% of male infertility cases.

Treatment

Treatment of varicocele is usually conservative and involves regular growth checks in adolescents. Should growth arrest be identified, surgery is indicated. From a paramedic perspective, patients experiencing varicoceles that are of sudden onset and painful, or do not drain when the patient is laid flat, should be referred for specialist review by a urologist. Similarly, if there are concerns regarding the appearance of the testes, referral should be considered.

Red Flag Alert: Testicular Pain

Sign or symptom	Differential diagnosis
Sudden onset	Torsion
Severe	Torsion
Nausea/vomiting	Torsion
	Epididymo-orchitis
	Epididymitis
Fever	Torsion
	Epididymo-orchitis
	Epididymitis
Haematuria	Torsion
	Epididymo-orchitis
	Epididymitis
	Testicular cancer

Snapshot 13.3

Time of dispatch – 11.45 p.m.
On scene – 12.08 p.m.

Pre-arrival Information

Passed from NHS 111 – male patient, 13 years of age, abdominal pain and vomiting. No previous medical history.

Windscreen Report

Terrace house in residential area.

Patient Assessment Triage

One patient.

Primary Survey

Danger – No dangers identified; patient is laid on a sofa, mother is with patient, good interaction between mother and son noted.
Response – responds appropriately.
Airway – airway is patent and self maintained.
Breathing – respiration rate 20 breaths/minute. Chest auscultation: clear breath sounds heard throughout.
Circulation – radial pulse present at 102 beats/minute. Blood pressure 128/67 mmHg.
Disability – orientated, alert on ACVPU; appears in pain.
Exposure – temperature 36.7°C, blood glucose 4.7 mmol/l. Consent gained, chaperoned examination. Tender left lower quadrant abdomen, no guarding.

Initial Questioning

Mother called 111 concerned her son, who was unable to sleep due to stomach pain, having vomited once, following 750 mg of paracetamol at 11.30 p.m. He was fine earlier, having gone swimming that evening, and went to bed well. He was woken by severe left quadrant abdominal and left testicular pain. Normal stool passed that afternoon. No urinary symptoms.

Review of the patient

Consented and chaperoned testicular examination performed using personal protective equipment. High-riding left testis noted, no erythema or swelling, severe tenderness on palpation and loss of cremasteric reflex. Negative Prehn's sign.

Reflective Learning Activity

How might you approach examination of the patient in Snapshot 13.1?
Would taking a sexual history be appropriate?
What would be your analgesia strategy?

Conditions of the male reproductive system typically present with either testicular pain or swelling, or both. Clues to the underlying pathology will be found by taking a thorough history of the presentation. Testicular torsion is an important, time-critical condition that presents with sudden onset of severe pain, often with gastrointestinal symptoms including abdominal pain and vomiting. When performing clinical examinations consent, dignity and a chaperone should always be considered.

Take Home Points

- Vaginal bleeding can be a normal occurrence in women who are pregnant and those who are not.
- Paramedics must establish two important details in patients presenting with vaginal bleeding: haemodynamic stability and the presence of pregnancy.
- The PALM-COEIN tool can be used to classify causes of non-pregnant, vaginal bleeding. This includes polyps, adenomyosis, leiomyoma, malignancy, coagulopathy, ovarian dysfunction, iatrogenic and other causes such as STIs or endometriosis.
- FGM is a non-medical procedure performed to the external female genitalia and requires safeguarding if suspected.
- Ectopic pregnancy is a life-threatening emergency and can present with atypical symptoms. It should always be considered and excluded in females with reproductive ability who present with vaginal bleeding and abdominal pain, regardless of contraception use.
- Antepartum haemorrhage is unpredictable and can be associated with rapid deterioration in pregnant patients due to compensatory mechanisms masking symptoms. It is defined as any frank blood loss from the genital tract.
- Testicular torsion is a time-critical presentation in males, where the spermatic cord twists, resulting in ischaemia and necrosis. Delays in treatment must be avoided; immediate surgical review overrides diagnostic testing.
- Patient dignity and consent are essential considerations in all presentations of the reproductive system.
- Owing to the sensitive nature of the reproductive system, patients may present with alternative complaints. Building rapport with patients through being empathetic, caring and keeping an open mind will best equip paramedics to identify potentially hidden complaints.

Summary

Having read this chapter, you will have developed your understanding of the female and male reproductive systems. Traditionally, paramedics work on emergency ambulances and attend patients in a prehospital setting. The role has evolved significantly due to the versatility of paramedics and the many transferable skills they possess. As such, paramedics now feature in a variety of primary and secondary care clinical teams. This chapter has described some of the common conditions of the male and female reproductive systems that a paramedic might come across when working in any of these settings. It is important to remember the sensitive nature of these presentations. Patients may delay seeking help or may not feel comfortable in disclosing their symptoms at the first time of asking. Adopting a sensitive approach, being empathetic, professional and keeping an open mind will better equip paramedics in gaining the vital clues required to identify the patient's presenting complaint.

287

References

Better Health Channel. (2018). Menstrual cycle. https://www.betterhealth.vic.gov.au/health/conditionsandtreatments/menstrual-cycle (accessed 9 October 2023).

Bhroin, S. U., (2021). Vaginal Bleeding in the Non-Pregnant Patient. *RCEM Learning*. www.rcemlearning.co.uk/reference/vaginal-bleeding-in-the-non-pregnant-patient/#1635517374271-f0d27a8f-80f9 (accessed 9 October 2023).

Brook Young People. (2022). Contraceptive implant. www.brook.org.uk/your-life/contraceptive-implant (accessed 9 October 2023).

Deligeoroglou, E. and Karountzos, V. (2018). Abnormal uterine bleeding including coagulopathies and other menstrual disorders. *Best Practice and Reseach: Clinical Obstetrics and Gynaecology* 48: 51–61.

Ectopic Pregnancy Trust (2022). What is an ectopic pregnancy? https://ectopic.org.uk/what-is-an-ectopic-pregnancy (accessed 9 October 2023).

Endometriosis UK (2010). *Treatment options*. London: Endometriosis UK. https://www.endometriosis-uk.org/files/files/Treatment%20Options%20August%202018%20edit.pdf (accessed on 1/3/22)

Endometriosis UK (n.d.). Causes. https://www.endometriosis-uk.org/causes-endometriosis (accessed 9 October 2023).

Gomes, D., Vidal, R.R., Foeppel, B.F. et al. (2015). Cold weather is a predisposing factor for testicular torsion in a tropical country. A retrospective study. *Sao Paulo Medical Journal* 133 (3): 187–190. https://doi.org/10.1590/1516-3180.2013.7600007.

Gredmark, T., Kvint, S., Havel, G., and Mattsson, L.A. (1995). Histopathological findings in women with postmenopausal bleeding. *British Journal of Obstetrics and Gynaecology* 102 (2): 133–136.

Huzaifa, M. and Moreno, M.A. (2023). *Hydrocele*. Treasure Island, FL: StatPearls Publishing https://www.ncbi.nlm.nih.gov/books/NBK559125/#_NBK559125_pubdet_ (accessed 9 October 2023).

Joint Royal Colleges Ambulance Liaison Committee (2022). *JRCALC Guidelines*. London: Class Publishing.

Kline, J. (2023). PERC rule for pulmonary embolism. *MD+CALC* https://www.mdcalc.com/perc-rule-pulmonary-embolism (accessed 9 October 2023).

Madersbacher, S., Sampson, N., and Culig, Z. (2019). Pathophysiology of benign prostatic hyperplasia and benign prostatic enlargement: a mini-review. *Gerontology* 65: 458–464. https://doi.org/10.1159/000496289.

Mellick, L.B., Mowery, M.L., and Al-Dhahir, M.A. (2021). *Cremasteric Reflex*. Treasure Island, FL: StatPearls Publishing https://www.ncbi.nlm.nih.gov/books/NBK513348 (accessed 9 October 2023).

Miscarriage Association (2023). *Molar Pregnancy (Hydatidiform Mole)*. London: Miscarriage Association.

Molokwu, C.N., Ndoumbe, J.K., and Goodman, C.M. (2020). Cold weather increases the risk of scrotal torsion events: results of an ecological study of acute scrotal pain in Scotland over 25 years. *Scientific Reports* 10: 17958. https://doi.org/10.1038/s41598-020-74878-0.

Munro, M.G., Critchley, H.O.D., Broder, M.S., and Fraser, I.S. (2011). FIGO classification system (PALM-COEIN) for causes of abnormal uterine bleeding innongravid women of reproductive age. *International Journal of Gynecology and Obstetrics* 113: 3–13. http://dx.doi.org/10.1016/j.ijgo.2010.11.011.

National Institute for Health and Care Excellence (2021) Ectopic pregnancy. Clinical Knowledge Summary. https://cks.nice.org.uk/topics/ectopic-pregnancy (accessed 9 October 2023).

National Institute for Health and Care Excellence (2022a) Miscarriage: how common is it? Clinical Knowledge Summary. https://cks.nice.org.uk/topics/miscarriage/background-information/prevalence (accessed 21 October 2023).

National Institute for Health and Care Excellence (2022b). *Reducing Sexually Transmitted Infections*. NICE Guideline NG221. London: National Institute for Health and Care Excellence. https://www.nice.org.uk/guidance/ng221 (accessed 21 October 2023).

National Institute for Health and Care Excellence. (2020) Neutropenic sepsis. Clinical Knowledge Summary. https://cks.nice.org.uk/topics/neutropenic-sepsis/#:~:text=Neutropenic%20sepsis%20is%20a%20potentially,109%2FL%20or%20lower. (accessed 9 October 2023).

NHS England (2021a). Chlamydia. https://www.nhs.uk/conditions/chlamydia (accessed 9 October 2023).

NHS England (2021b). Contraceptive implant: your contraceptive guide. https://www.nhs.uk/conditions/contraception/contraceptive-implant (accessed 9 October 2023).

NHS England (2023). Periods and fertility in the menstrual cycle. https://www.nhs.uk/conditions/periods/fertility-in-the-menstrual-cycle (accessed 9 October 2023).

Peate, I. (2014). FGM: the role of front-line staff. *Journal of Paramedic Practice* 6 (5): https://doi.org/10.12968/jpar.2014.6.5.221.

Pietrzak, O., Hadway, P., Corbishley, C.M., and Watkin, N.A. (2006). Is the association between balanitis xerotica obliterans and penile carcinoma underestimated? *BJU International* 9((1): 74–76.

Prostate Cancer UK. (2022). About prostate cancer. https://prostatecanceruk.org/prostate-information/about-prostate-cancer. [accessed on 15/4/22]

Prostate Cancer UK. (2023). Black men and prostate cancer. https://prostatecanceruk.org/prostate-information/are-you-at-risk/black-men-and-prostate-cancer (accessed 9 October 2023).

Regan, L., Rai, R., Saravelos, S., and Li, T.-C. (2023). Recurrent miscarriage. Greentop Guideline No. 17. *BJOG* 130: e9–e39.

Royal College of Nursing (2021). *Clinical Nurse Specialist in Early Pregnancy Care*. London: Royal College of Nursing.

Royal College of Obstetricians and Gynaecologists. (2011) *Antepartum Hemorrhage*. Green-top Guideline No. 63 London: Royal College of Obstetricians and Gynaecologists.

Sandlow, J.I., Kansal, J.K. (2021). Varicocele. *BMJ Best Practice* https://bestpractice.bmj.com/topics/en-gb/1103 (accessed 9 October 2023).

Taghavi, S. and Askari, R. (2021). *Hypovolemic Shock*. StatPearls. Treasure Island, FL: StatPearls Publishing. https://www.ncbi.nlm.nih.gov/books/NBK513297

Thakkar, H., Lee, R., Kang, C. et al. (2021). Testicular torsion. https://bestpractice.bmj.com/topics/en-gb/506 (accessed 9 October 2023).

World Health Organization. (2023). Female genital mutilation. Fact sheet. https://www.who.int/news-room/fact-sheets/detail/female-genital-mutilation (accessed 9 October 2023).

Further Reading

Hudson, R. (2023). *Hydrocele in Adults*. Leeds: Egton Medical Information Systems https://patient.info/mens-health/scrotal-lumps-pain-and-swelling/hydrocele-in-adults (accessed 9 Otober 2023).

Online Resources

NHS England. Female Genital Mutilation (course on e-learning for healthcare): https://portal.e-lfh.org.uk/Component/Details/390922
World Health Organization. Female genital mutilation: https://www.who.int/news-room/fact-sheets/detail/female-genital-mutilation

Glossary

Antepartum haemorrhage	A condition involving frank blood loss from the genital tract, after 24 completed weeks of pregnancy, until the onset of labour.
Benign prostatic hyperplasia	Non-cancerous enlarging of the prostate gland associated with urinary symptoms (e.g. retention).
Brachytherapy	A targeted form of radiotherapy used in patients with late-stage prostate cancer, where a radioactive source is placed within the body, next to or inside the cancer.
Ectopic pregnancy	A life-threatening condition where the fertilised ovum implants outside the uterine cavity.
Endometriosis	A condition where the endometrial cells from the lining of the uterus are found outside of the uterine cavity.
Female genital mutilation (FGM)	Any non-medical procedure relating to partial or total removal, or injury, to the external female genitalia. FGM is illegal in the UK.
Miscarriage	The spontaneous loss of a pregnancy before 24 weeks of gestation.
Molar pregnancy	A rare complication of pregnancy that involves rapid, abnormal growth of cells of the placenta known as trophoblasts.
Tranexamic acid (TXA)	An antifibrinolytic medication used to control bleeding in certain presentations.
Testicular torsion	A time-critical presentation whereby the spermatic cord twists, resulting in reduced blood supply and ischaemia to the testis.

289

Multiple Choice Questions

1. What is the correct order of the four phases of the menstrual cycle?
   a. Luteal phase – menstruation – ovulation – follicular phase
   b. Menstruation – follicular phase – ovulation – luteal phase
   c. Ovulation – menstruation – follicular phase – luteal phase
   d. Follicular phase – luteal phase – menstruation – ovulation

2. Which of these statements is the correct description of post-coital bleeding?
   a. A heavy menstrual bleed
   b. Bleeding that occurs after pregnancy
   c. Bleeding that occurs after sexual intercourse
   d. An absence of menstrual bleeding

3. Which of the following statements is FALSE regarding endometriosis?
   a. Diagnosis can be difficult and can take as long as eight years
   b. Pregnancy and hysterectomy are cures for endometriosis
   c. Symptoms can impact a patient's physical and mental health
   d. Causes are not clearly understood

4. Which of the following is NOT a sign or symptom of haemodynamic instability associated with heavy vaginal bleeding?
   a. Syncope
   b. Tachycardia
   c. Prolonged, central capillary refill times
   d. Jaundice

5. Which of these early pregnancy bleeding facts is FALSE?
   a. 50% of pregnant women will experience vaginal bleeding in the first 12 weeks of pregnancy
   b. 1 in 80 pregnancies will result in ectopic pregnancies
   c. 1 in 600 pregnancies are molar pregnancies
   d. Bleeding in early pregnancy always leads to miscarriage

6. Which is not a sign or symptom of ectopic pregnancy?
   a. Pain on neck flexion
   b. Light or heavy vaginal bleeding
   c. Diarrhoea or rectal pressure
   d. Abdominal pain

290

7. Which of these statements about molar pregnancies is true?
   a. Molar pregnancies are common
   b. Molar pregnancies are viable
   c. Molar pregnancies may need chemotherapy
   d. Molar pregnancies are identifiable in the third trimester

8. JRCALC states what about tranexamic acid?
   a. Can be given to shocked patients when ectopic pregnancy is suspected
   b. Should only be used in traumatic causes of bleeding
   c. Can be used routinely in all hypovolaemic patients secondary to bleeding
   d. Should only be administered to pregnant women in cases of life threatening haemorrhage in relation to a trauma or postpartum haemorrhage

9. Which of these statements about regarding testicular torsion is true?
   a. The absence of the cremasteric reflex is diagnostic
   b. Presentation may involve abdominal pain and vomiting
   c. CT urogram with contrast is the gold standard investigative tool to aid diagnosis
   d. Only males under 18 years of age are affected

10. Prostate cancer risk includes which of these factors?
    a. Age over 50 years
    b. Ethnicity
    c. A positive family history
    d. All of the above

CHAPTER 14

Pain

Rory Prevett

AIM

The aim of this chapter is to provide the reader with an understanding of the physiology and pathophysiology of pain.

LEARNING OUTCOMES

Upon completion of this chapter, you will to be able to:

- Describe the physiology and pathophysiology of pain.
- Explain the difference between acute and chronic pain.
- Discuss pain assessment models.
- Explain the influence of biopsychosocial factors.
- Identify appropriate pain management strategies.

Test Your Prior Knowledge

1. Describe pain pathways.
2. How do you assess a patient's pain level?
3. How would you recognise pain symptoms in a patient?
4. What are the non-pharmacological methods for pain relief?
5. What is your understanding of the difference between acute and chronic pain?

Introduction

Defined as an 'unpleasant sensory and emotional experience associated with actual or potential tissue damage, or described in terms of such damage' (International Association for the Study of Pain 2021), it should be noted that the concept and interpretation of pain may not be solely physical, as a result of injury or disease, but also from an emotional

Fundamentals of Applied Pathophysiology for Paramedics, First Edition. Edited by Ian Peate and Simon Sawyer.

source. The paramedic practitioner should note that 'Pain is whatever the experiencing person says it is, existing when they say it exists' (McCaffrey 1979).

This definition which was recommended by the Subcommittee on Taxonomy and adopted initially in 1979 by the International Association for the Study of Pain is widely accepted by the healthcare community and is the definition used by numerous governmental and non-governmental organisations such as the World Health Organization (WHO).

As a paramedic practitioner, you need to be acutely aware of the consequences of unmanaged pain. Failure to resolve the pain to at least a tolerable level can increase the adverse effects on a patient's respiratory, cardiovascular and gastro-intestinal body systems. It can also increase anxiety (MacIntyre and Schug 2015).

The Physiology and Pathophysiology of Pain

Pain is sensed within four processes (McCaffrey and Pasero 1999; Figure 14.1):

1. A sensation, such as one caused by injury, is stimulated in the peripheral nervous system. This occurs at receptors called nociceptors.
2. This sensation is then transmitted as an action potential from the peripheral nervous system to the central nervous system.
3. A third process known as modulation occurs. This is where the transmitted message is either enhanced or inhibited by other central nervous system activity.
4. Finally, there is perception. Once received in the brain, the stimulus would be perceived as painful.

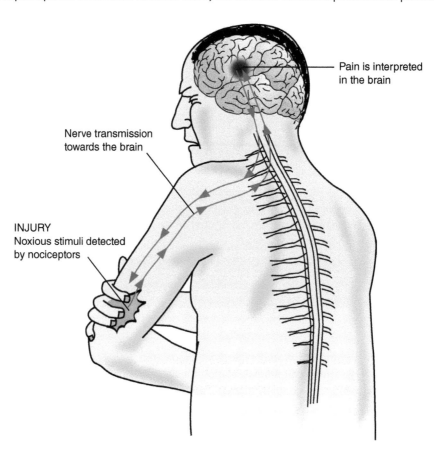

Pain is interpreted in the brain

Nerve transmission towards the brain

INJURY
Noxious stimuli detected by nociceptors

FIGURE 14.1   The pain pathway. Source: Peate (2021) pg. 505/John Wiley & Sons.

Nociceptor Transduction

With the exception of the brain, nociceptor transduction free nerve endings are located in all tissues in the body. When tissue damage or inflammation occurs, the nociceptors are activated by a noxious stimulus occurring within A-delta fibres and C fibres in the primary afferent neurons. Broadly speaking, this stimulus can be classified into three groupings (Table 14.1). At the cell membranes, exchange of potassium and sodium ions results in the generation of an action potential, thus allowing transmission.

Transmission

Known as 'the ascending pain pathway', the transmission phase can be subdivided into three stages:

- Transduction site to spinal cord dorsal horn (Figure 14.2).
- Spinal cord to brain stem.
- Brain stem to thalamus and somatosensory cortex.

Located at the spinal cord dorsal horn, the A-delta fibres and C fibres terminate here at the presynaptic terminal. Synaptic transmission is then required to facilitate transmission across the synaptic cleft, between the fibres and the nociceptive dorsal neurons.

Neurotransmitters such as adenosine triphosphate, glutamate, serotonin and substance P maintain this synaptic transmission (MacLellan 2006).

The speeds at which synaptic transmission occurs here is dependent on the makeup of the nerve fibres. These nerve fibres can be either myelinated or non-myelinated. Myelinated fibres which are surrounded by a sheath of myelin and conduct the action potential faster due to the presence of the 'nodes of Ranvier' (Figure 14.3). The A-delta fibres are myelinated whereas C fibres are not, so sensations transmitted via the A-delta fibre would be sensed first.

Modulation

Within the spinal cord, pain impulses are either inhibited or excited. There are numerous pathways in this stage of the process, which will result in either an increase in the transmission of pain as a result of excitatory impulses or a decrease in pain transmission as a result of inhibitory action. Certain analgesia provided by the paramedic practitioner can affect modulation by inhibiting nociceptor terminal sensitisation.

People naturally produce inhibitory transmitters. These endogenous opioids can prevent the release of excitatory transmitters, so they inhibit transmission of pain impulses. This may explain why different people sense

TABLE 14.1 Types of noxious stimulus.

Stimulus	Causation
Mechanical	Tissue damage
Thermal	Heat/cold sensation
Chemical	Presence of chemicals (e.g. prostaglandins)

Source: adapted from Loeser and Treede (2008).

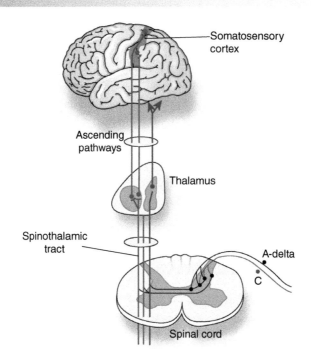

FIGURE 14.2 Spinal cord dorsal horn (spinothalamic tract). Source: Peate (2021) pg. 505/John Wiley & Sons.

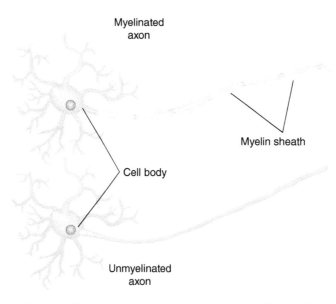

FIGURE 14.3 Myelinated and non-myelinated axon. Source: Peate (2021) pg. 504/John Wiley & Sons.

different levels of pain. These endogenous opioids are located within descending pain pathways and are divided into three groups:

1. Encephalins
2. Endorphins
3. Dynorphins.

There are four categories of opiate receptors:

1. **Mu**
2. **Kappa**
3. **Sigma**
4. **Delta.**

Whereas the ascending pathways bring the sensation to the higher centres in the brain, the descending pathways set out to inhibit pain perception.

Perception

Elicited responses occur in multiple cortical areas of the brain when a painful stimulus is received (Figure 14.4). One of the initial structures to receive pain stimuli is the reticular formation. Neurotransmission here can influence those vital signs that are associated with a pain response. These signs can include cardiovascular changes such as heart rate increase, blood pressure increase, increased myocardial oxygen consumption and respiratory system changes, including decreased alveolar ventilation leading to hypoxaemia, hypercapnia, and increased oxygen consumption. This centre also controls the initial response to that noxious stimulus, (e.g. to remove your hand from a source of heat) or, conversely, if adequate distraction is present, this area of the brainstem will allow the painful stimulus to go unnoticed.

From the reticular formation, pain impulses are transmitted to various other brain structures via the thalamus. One such area is the somatosensory cortex. This structure assesses the pain for its intensity, the location of the sensation and the type of pain. It is also known to be involved in memory and past experiences of painful episodes (Godfrey 2005).

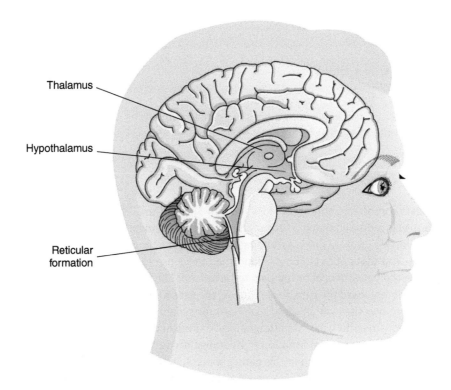

Thalamus

Hypothalamus

Reticular formation

FIGURE 14.4 Location of the thalamus, hypothalamus and reticular formation. Source: Peate (2021) pg. 508/John Wiley & Sons.

The limbic system of the cortex area has also been shown to be involved in the emotional aspects of pain perception. This system is also responsible for the behavioural responses exhibited by a person to pain. However, research has shown that a situation will influence a person's emotional response and the risk of causing pain to themselves (e.g. rescuing a family member from a house fire, knowing that exposure to heat and flame will have an extremely high probability of causing themselves pain; Johnson 2005).

Pain Theories

Several theories of pain have been proposed, which aim to explain pain physiology:

- Specificity
- Intensity
- Pattern
- Gate Control.

Specificity Pain Theory

The specificity theory of pain hypothesises that there are specific dedicated pathways for modality. Each modality has a specific receptor that is sensitive to a specific stimulus (Dubner et al. 1978).

Intensity Pain Theory

Intensity theory postulated that pain was not uniquely sensory, but rather an emotion which occurred when a stimulus was applied that was more intense than usual. Many of the studies related to this theory were carried out in the 1850s by the pathologist Naunyn.

The Pattern Control Theory

The pattern control theory was based on research conducted by Nafe, an American psychologist, who dismissed the theories of specificity and intensity. This theory supported the belief that the firing of neurons occurred within distinct patterns once a significant stimulus was received.

Gate Control Theory

In 1965, the theory of gate control was proposed. This theory by Melzack and Wall completely changed the perception of the physiology of pain. It was proposed that the sensation of pain, ergo, perception, would be determined based on which fibre, the A-delta or C fibre, was involved in the ascending pathway, and a third fibre, the A-beta fibre, which is involved in the descending pathway, was thought to inhibit or diminished the sensation. To liken this theory to the 'gate' concept, A-delta and C fibres push the gate open, allowing pain to be sensed. The wider the opening the greater the intensity of pain, whereas the A-beta fibres closed the gate, thus reducing the sensation. This theory was specific in that Melzack and Wall stated that there were two sites within the dorsal horn for synaptic transmission, the substantia gelatinosa and transmission cells. The theory hypothesised that modulation occurred in the substantia gelatinosa within the dorsal horn at the spinal cord, allowing this sensory information to be transmitted to the transmission cells within the spinal cord. Large and small afferent fibres were involved in this gating process, in that the large fibres closed the gate whereas the small fibres opened the gate (Figure 14.5). Melzack and Wall believed that nociception had to reach a specific threshold to allow the gate to open. Once open, pathway activation would occur which would result in pain perception. What is significant about this theory is that it allowed for the grounding of a neural basis in pain perception. This theory currently and most accurately accounts for the physical and psychological aspects of pain perception.

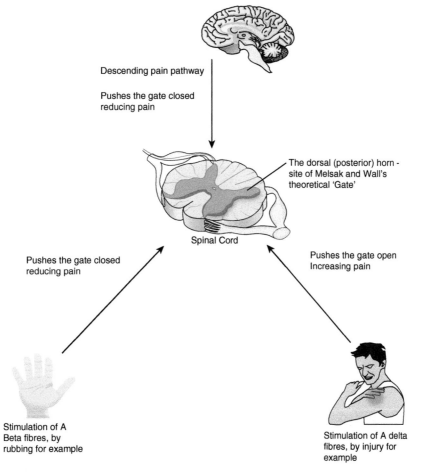

Descending pain pathway

Pushes the gate closed
reducing pain

The dorsal (posterior) horn -
site of Melsak and Wall's
theoretical 'Gate'

Spinal Cord

Pushes the gate closed
reducing pain

Pushes the gate open
Increasing pain

Stimulation of A
Beta fibres, by
rubbing for example

Stimulation of A delta
fibres, by injury for
example

FIGURE 14.5 Gate control theory of pain transmission. Source: Peate (2021) pg. 510/John Wiley & Sons.

Pathophysiology

Many of the patients to whom a paramedic practitioner responds will present with one of three classifications of pain. Their pain may be either transient, acute or chronic. The classification is based on the duration of pain. Transient pain is generally of very short duration (e.g. standing on a child's small building brick). Here, the pain, although possibly initially intense, will be short lived and will not require medical attention by the paramedic.

Acute Pain

Acute pain, like transient pain, will be of sudden onset, but the difference here is that duration is longer and generally to the point that intervention by the paramedic is made or healing occurs. Acute pain is usually caused by a noxious stimulation. Common examples that a paramedic will encounter as causes of acute pain would include:

- Myocardial infarction
- Orthopaedic trauma
- Acute medical illnesses, such as appendicitis.

It is with acute episodes of pain that the systemic changes seen in vital signs can be observed.

Chronic Pain

Chronic pain has a complex pathophysiology that is believed to result from alterations in nociception injury or disease. This alteration may be due to current or past injury to the peripheral nervous system, the central nervous system or, indeed, may have no organic cause (Calvino and Grilo 2006). As such, it is often considered as a syndrome in its own right (Melzack and Wall 1988). It is thought that the pathophysiology involves long-term changes to the modulation and transmission phases of pain pathways (Ko and Zhou 2004).

Red Flag Alert: Pain Is What the Patient Says

Chronic pain may not present with the same vital signs that are present in acute pain episodes. There may be no:

- Hypertension
- Grimace
- Guarding
- Tachycardia.

Remember: pain is what the patient says, so intensity ascertained during assessment may be of a significance that warrants appropriate high levels of analgesia.

Referred Pain

Occurring because of a 'shared space' of the nerves in the spinal cord where the actual damage is and where the pain is sensed, referred pain is where damage in one part of the body results in pain being sensed elsewhere. One of the classic examples of referred pain that the paramedic may encounter will be when dealing with patients who are experiencing myocardial infarction. In addition to the typical chest pain, patients can report painful sensations in the left arm, jaw and shoulder blades (Figure 14.6).

Cancer Pain

There is an extremely high incidence of pain experienced by those patients who have cancer. Studies have shown that cancer pain can occur in up to 96% of this patient cohort (Solano et al. 2006). Cancer pain can divide into two classifications: nociceptive or neuropathic. The WHO states that the aim of palliative care is to reduce pain to a level that the patient can tolerate at the most minimal level. By doing this, associated symptoms may also be alleviated. Within cancer treatment, pain can be classified under five headings, described in Table 14.2.

Neuropathic Pain

Neuropathic pain is often described as a burning or tingling sensation and is a result of damage occurring at the neurons and nociceptors. Patients may complain of this pain being constant or spasmodic. Sensitivity of the nociceptors is believed to change, which results in the patient experiencing what is thought to be a noxious stimulus when, in actual fact, a non-noxious stimulus has been applied. Because the neurons are damaged, the level of pain experienced is often greater than the level of stimulus being applied. An example of this type of pain, the paramedic may commonly encounter, is seen in those patients with sciatic pain.

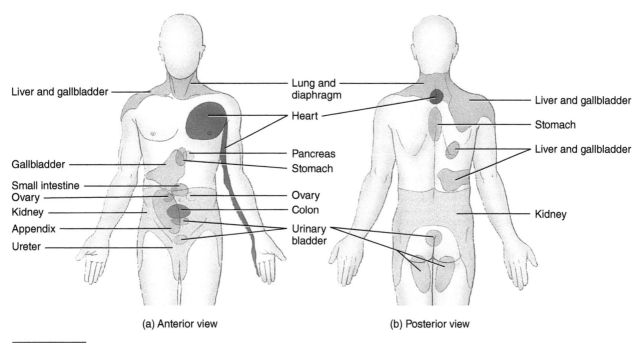

FIGURE 14.6 Examples of referred pain and the origin of tissue damage. Source: Peate (2021) pg. 513/John Wiley & Sons.

TABLE 14.2 Cancer pain descriptions.

Pain	Description
Nerve	Caused by pressure on the nerves or spinal, described as 'burning, shooting or tingling'
Bone	Also called 'somatic', described as 'aching, dull or throbbing' it's as a result of cancer spreading into bone
Soft tissue pain	As a result of damage to organs or muscles, often described as 'cramping, sharp or aching'
Phantom	Pain experienced in a part of the body where that body part has been removed, for example, pain in the breast area after a mastectomy
Referred	Pain felt in an alternative location in the body.

Source: adapted from Cancer Research UK (2020).

Clinical Investigations: Magnetic Resonance Imagining

Magnetic resonance imaging (MRI) is a scan that produces detailed internal images of the body using radio waves and strong magnetic fields. During the scan, the patient will be required to lie flat and still on a bed, which is then moved through the scanner. Depending on which body system is being scanned, the patient may enter the tube either head or feet first. Operated by a radiographer, the patient can communicate through an intercom. An MRI scan generally takes about 15–90 minutes, depending on the area being scanned and how many images are taken. It works by aligning and distributing protons within hydrogen atoms in the body. The radio waves disrupt the proton alignment, whereas the magnets in the scanner realigns them.

Pain Assessment

Analgesia provision within the prehospital setting is recognised as a key area of patient care and its significance can be seen in that many ambulance services use pain management as a key performance indicator. Paramedics need to be able to apply recognised robust measurement systems to ascertain the level of pain that the patient is experiencing as correctly or as accurately as possible. This will allow them to determine the most appropriate analgesic pathways.

Assessment of pain is very much dependent on the age of the patient and, within that, the cognitive ability of the patient. Standardised questioning of the patient should be employed. The paramedic practitioner should be familiar with whatever method their service employs. One of the most common questioning patterns used is the pneumonic OPQRST (Table 14.3). Other questions that the paramedic can include here concern any self-management strategies that the patient may have employed:

- Have you taken any medication to help with the pain?
- Do you use any devices to help with pain levels?
- Are you attending any pain management clinics/specialists?

Orange Flag Alert: Pain Is What the Patient Says

Avoid TRAPS:

- Do not assume that one method of assessment has more validity or is more reliable than others.
- The most valid measure is one that fits the purpose.
- Account for both physical measures of pain AND self-reported instruments.
- The patient's psychological state can influence a physical assessment.
- The paramedic MUST interpret accurately to allow adequate pain diagnosis and treatment.

Adult Assessment

Remembering that 'pain is what the patients says', the easiest and most common way to ascertain the severity of the pain is to employ the 0 to 10 point verbal numerical scale, as recommended by Joint Royal Colleges Ambulances Liaison Committee (JRCALC). Within this scale, 0 would refer to no pain whereas a reported score of 10 would indicated the worst imaginable pain experienced. Broadly speaking, scores of:

TABLE 14.3   The OPQRST mnemonic for pain assessment.

Mnemonic	Questions
Onset	What was the patient doing when the pain started? Was this onset sudden or gradual? Is this an exacerbation of a chronic condition?
Provocation	Does anything make this pain worse or is there anything that the patient does that helps relieve the pain?
Quality	Describe the characteristic of the pain. For example, is the pain a sharp sensation or a dull ache? Is it a constant pain or is it intermittent?
Region/**R**adiation	Where is the pain located? Does this pain move anywhere or can it be felt in another location?
Severity	How bad/ severe is the pain that the patient is experiencing.
Time	When did this start? How long has this painful episode been experienced?

TABLE 14.4 TEACH mnemonic for patients with communication difficulties.

Mnemonic	Definition
Time	Spend more time on the assessment of the patient. Assess the person in front of you using a structured approach irrespective of ethnicity, religion or age.
Environment	What is the environmental impact on your assessment? It is too noisy, is it unfamiliar to the patient? Is your patient too distracted?
Attitude	Adjust your attitude towards this assessment. Make no presumptions about the patient or their quality of life.
Communication	What is best method to communicate with your patient? Is it more appropriate to use signs or symbols. What is the normal method of communication for the person?
Help	Is there anyone present that can assist you with your assessment? Is there family present or a carer? In a school setting is the child's special needs teaching assistant present?

- 1–4 may indicate a mild level of pain.
- 5–7 indicate a moderate level of pain.
- 8–10 suggest severe pain.

As pain perception is an individual experience specific to the patient, it is important to focus the patient on comparing previous experiences of pain, to allow a comparison to be made. In addition to this, the trending of pain scores is an important factor for the paramedic, to ensure that management strategies are appropriate, thus ensuring effective pain reduction for the patient.

In adult patients where there may be dementia or cognitive impairment, an altered level of consciousness or those with communication difficulties, the scoring of pain severity can prove to be somewhat difficult. A change in behaviour may be the only manifestation to signal that your patient is in pain (Cipher et al. 2006). Intensity and frequency of facial activity has been shown to increase by three times in those patients with Alzheimer's disease when in pain compared with healthy controls (Mustafa et al. 2017).

It is important to remember the TEACH mnemonic, as recommended by the JRCALC, which may aide the paramedic in this cohort of patients (Table 14.4).

For this cohort of patients, it may be prudent to use the Abbey pain scale (Abbey et al. 2004). This scale is based on scoring from six different sets of questions asked while observing the patient. Each question is allocated a pain score, which is then totalled and attributed to a pain classification (Figure 14.7).

301

Snapshot 14.1

Pre-arrival Information

Control has requested you respond to an urgent call. Incident details passed to you state that an elderly lady has been found lying on the ground in her house by a family member. The lady is unable to get up from her position.
Dispatched: 9.50 a.m.
Arrival: 10:05 a.m.

On Arrival with the Patient

Airway: clear.
Breathing: bilateral chest rise, lung sounds clear, no extra effort required.
Cardiac: pulses present, weak, fast.
Disability: alert as per baseline with confusion due to dementia.

Exposure: no immediate life threats found.
Background: age: 84 years, female.
Weight/height: approximately 50 kg and 157 cm.
Medical history: hypertension, coronary artery bypass graft, atrial fibrillation, dementia, duodenal ulcerations.
Medications: warfarin, lansoprazole, bisoprolol, bendroflumethiazide, donepezil.

Examination

On specific examination of this patient, you see that she is inclined slightly to the right hand side, propped from the left. She indicates that this is the most comfortable position. You notice her right leg is bent at the knee and she refuses to move the leg for you. On palpation of the leg, you notice swelling and deformity in the upper third of the thigh. You form a working diagnosis of a suspected fracture to the upper third of the right femur.

Vital Signs

Vital signs taken are:

Vital sign	Observation	Normal range
Pulse (beats/min)	110	80–100 regular
Respiration (breaths/min)	18	12–20
O_2 saturation (%)	96 (on room air)	94–98
Blood pressure (mmHg)	108/60	120/80
Temperature (°C)	36.1	37
Eyes	4	4 – spontaneously
Verbal	5	5 – orientated
Motor	6	6 – obeys commands
Total GCS score	15	14
Pupils	4 and PEARRL	Equal, round, reactive
ECG	Sinus tachycardia	
Pain score	9/10	

Reflective Learning Activity

Take some time to reflect on Snapshot 14.1. Then consider the following:

1. How would you assess this patient's pain?
2. What would be your initial approach to pain management here?
3. What considerations must you be acutely aware of with this patient in relation to analgesia? Is it best to give standard adult or specific weight-based doses here?
4. What would be appropriate analgesia options during transport to hospital?

Abbey Pain Scale

For measurement of pain in people with dementia who cannot verbalise.

How to use scale: While observing the resident, score questions 1 to 6

Name of resident: ....

Name and designation of person completing the scale: ....

Date:...**Time:** ....

Latest pain relief given was..**at**..............**hrs.**

Q1.	**Vocalisation** eg. whimpering, groaning, crying *Absent 0 Mild 1 Moderate 2 Severe 3*	**Q1** ☐
Q2.	**Facial expression** eg: looking tense, frowning grimacing, looking frightened *Absent 0 Mild 1 Moderate 2 Severe 3*	**Q2** ☐
Q3.	**Change in body language** eg: fidgeting, rocking, guarding part of body, withdrawn *Absent 0 Mild 1 Moderate 2 Severe 3*	**Q3** ☐
Q4.	**Behavioural Change** eg: increased confusion, refusing to eat, alteration in usual patterns *Absent 0 Mild 1 Moderate 2 Severe 3*	**Q4** ☐
Q5.	**Physiological change** eg: temperature, pulse or blood pressure outside normal limits, perspiring, flushing or pallor *Absent 0 Mild 1 Moderate 2 Severe 3*	**Q5** ☐
Q6.	**Physical changes** eg: skin tears, pressure areas, arthritis, contractures, previous injuries. *Absent 0 Mild 1 Moderate 2 Severe 3*	**Q6** ☐

Add scores for 1 – 6 and record here ⟹ **Total Pain Score** ☐

Now tick the box that matches the Total Pain Score ⟹

0 – 2 No pain	3 – 7 Mild	8 – 13 Moderate	14+ Severe

Finally, tick the box which matches the type of pain ⟹

Chronic	Acute	Acute on Chronic

FIGURE 14.7 Abbey pain scale. Source: Abbey et al. (2004)/MA Healthcare.

303

Paediatric Assessment

There is no validated prehospital method for pain assessment in children. It is therefore deemed acceptable to use emergency department tools. Two such methods that are used are Wong–Baker FACES© (Figure 14.8) and the FLACC scales (Figure 14.9).

Wong–Baker is a method that maybe useful for younger children, as it involves the child attributing their experience to a similar face shown as an image. A correlating pain score is then taken from this face shape.

Wong-Baker FACES® Pain Rating Scale

0	2	4	6	8	10
No Hurt	Hurts Little Bit	Hurts Little More	Hurts Even More	Hurts Whole Lot	Hurts Worst

FIGURE 14.8   The Wong Baker Faces Scale for paediatric pain assessment. Source: adapted from Wong and Baker (1988).

FLACC Score			
CATEGORY	**0 POINTS**	**1 POINT**	**2 POINTS**
Face	Disinterested	Occasional grimace, withdrawn	Frequent frown, clenched jaw
Legs	No position or relaxed	Uneasy, restless, tense	Kicking or legs drawn up
Activity	Normal position	Squirming, tense	Arched, rigid, or jerking
Cry	No crying	Moans or whimpers	Constant crying, screams or sobs
Consolability	Content, relaxed	Distractible	Inconsolable
SCORES ADD UP IN RANGE FROM 0–10			

FIGURE 14.9   The FLACC pain assessment tool. Source: adapted from Merkel et al. (1997).

JRCALC states that the Wong–Baker FACES scale can be used with children aged three years and older. To use this scale correctly, the patient must be able to comprehend the instructions given. The paramedic will point to each face using the words to describe the level of pain. The child is then asked to choose the face that best describes their pain (Hockenberry et al. 2005).

The FLACC scale is used for pain assessment in children under the age of seven years, the preverbal child or older children if required (JRCALC 2022). This scale is scored on a range from 0 to 10 based on five criteria for assessment (Figure 14.9; Malviya et al. 2006). The paramedic will observe the patient's:

- Face
- Legs
- Activity
- Cry
- Consolability.

Medications Management: Nitrous Oxide

Commonly known as 'laughing gas', nitrous oxide is a colourless gas with a sweet odour and taste. It is a self-administered preparation that has a rapid onset with minimal adverse effects. Long-term use can lead to vitamin B_{12} deficiency.

Snapshot 14.2

Pre-arrival Information

You are tasked as a solo responder to a football match. Ambulance control informs you that you are responding to a single male patient with a leg injury. They inform you that an ambulance has been dispatched but their journey time is approximately 50 minutes, while your journey time will be approximately 20 minutes.
Dispatched: 1.30 p.m.
Arrival: 1.47 p.m., estimated time of arrival for ambulance: 2.20 p.m.

On Arrival with the Patient

Airway: clear.
Breathing: bilateral chest rise, lung sounds clear, no extra effort required.
Cardiac: pulses present, fast.
Disability: alert.
Exposure: no immediate life threats found.
Background: age 12 years, male; weight/height approximately 43 kg and 160 cm.
Medical history: none.
Medications: none; however, the patient's parent states that when he was younger, 'a grey-blue inhaler' was used when exercising.

Examination

On specific examination of the patient, you observe deformity and tenderness to the patient's lower left leg. The patient has a decreased circulation and motor function on the left foot with capillary refill approximately three to four seconds. The position of the foot/ankle is angulated with a noticeable difference from that of the right foot. You also notice an open wound on the tibial aspect of the leg where an obvious fracture can be seen. You form a working diagnosis of a tibial fracture and possible fibula fracture.

Vital Signs

Vital signs taken are:

Vital sign	Observation	Normal values
Pulse (beats/min)	127	80–100 regular
Respiration (breaths/min)	23	12–20
O_2 saturation (%)	98 (on room air)	94–98
Blood pressure (mmHg)	131/86	120/80
Temperature (°C)	35.8	37
Eyes	4	4 – spontaneously
Verbal	5	5 – orientated
Motor	6	6 – obeys commands
Total GCS score	15	15
Pupils	4 and PEARRL	Equal, round, reactive
ECG	Sinus tachycardia	
Pain score	10/10	

The journey to hospital time is around 45 minutes. Upon arrival of the ambulance, you are informed that the crew model is both technician level.

Reflective Learning Activity

Take some time to reflect on Snapshot 14.2, then consider the following:

1. Which method of pain assessment would you use and why?
2. What is the best approach to use here to provide adequate analgesia as a solo responder?
3. What level of analgesia can the technician crew provide during the long journey by road?
4. What would be your long-term pain management plan?
5. Is the helicopter emergency medical service an appropriate option? If considered so, why? If ruled out, why?

The Biopsychosocial Approach

In the supplementary revision of *Pain Management in Adults* (Association of Ambulance Chief Executives 2017), the JRCALC recommends a multimodal approach whereby the practitioner should pay consideration to biopsychosocial factors. This approach may be best defined where pain is viewed as a dynamic interaction within the biological, social and psychological factors that are unique to each individual patient (Gatchel and Howard 2021). This model therefore uses these factors in addition to cognitive, affective and behavioural influences and interactions to determine the patient's pain condition. We have already seen that the same or similar noxious stimulus can illicit a different response in individuals, so use of this approach in both assessment and management may allow for a tailored individualistic regimen.

Pain Management

Orange Flag Alert: Pain Relief

- Pain relief will not affect subsequent diagnosis.
- Appropriate management of pain will have clinical benefits.
- Do not withhold analgesia.
- Reassessments must be frequent to measure effectiveness.
- Where possible, treat the cause.
- Where appropriate, use weight-based calculations.

In both adult and paediatric patients, the biopsychosocial factors that were employed during assessment should be applied for management strategies. Where this model is of particular benefit is when managing exacerbations of chronic pain. Remember that it is important to tailor the treatment to the patient. As a paramedic, it is prudent to remember that two patients with the same diagnosis may have different social setups, psychological influences and physical differences, so providing both these patients with an identical treatment regimen in comparison with an individualistic analgesic plan may not be an appropriate response for the patients (Gatchel 2005).

As a paramedic, it is important to adhere to the guidance laid down by JRCALC and to possess intimate knowledge of the local NHS trust guidelines.

Pain management can occur in two ways: non-pharmacological and pharmacological:

- Non-pharmacological methods will encompass both psychological and physical applications, such as distracting a small child with their favourite teddy, or applying a vacuum splint to an fractured limb or a burns dressing to the affected area.
- Pharmacological methods, on the other hand, involve the administration of drugs to the patient.

A balanced pain management plan should be employed by the paramedic for all patients, where it has been shown that a combination of both pharmacological and non-pharmacological methods proves to be most effective for the patient (Hader and Guy 2004).

When using pharmacological methods, a multimodal approach may be beneficial as it will allow different analgesics with different mechanisms of action to have an oversynergistic effect. An example of this may be combining both morphine and paracetamol. Studies have shown that combination of these two analgesics results in analgesia improvement with significant opioid-sparing effect (Zeidan and Saifan 2014).

An opioid-sparing effect may be defined as interaction which enables a reduced opioid dose without loss of efficacy (Neuropsychopharmacology 2017).

Within the prehospital setting, strict following of the WHO guidance is not as common as would be seen in other clinical settings. In the prehospital environment, especially with acute pain management, rapid analgesia is often required, which may be either from strong opioids or short-acting fast-onset preparations such as Entonox® (50% nitrous oxide, 50% oxygen; BOC Healthcare, Manchester). Once initial control of pain has been gained, the paramedic then can decide to introduce a simpler analgesic such as paracetamol instead of maintaining an opioid regimen. Analgesic options include those noted in Table 14.5.

Within paediatrics, based on your pain assessment and depending on the nature of the injury, it may be prudent to begin analgesia with a stronger, more potent preparation such as oral morphine as opposed to oral paracetamol. This may enable the child to become more at ease, thus allowing physical treatment to occur. An example of this would be a child with a fractured tibia. The distress caused by the pain may make it difficult to allow adequate splinting of the leg without causing further psychological stress. Appropriate strong pain relief and the addition of other non-pharmacological adjuncts (allowing the parents to comfort the child, distraction techniques) may facilitate splint application. Conversely, the child with a small superficial burn that is not time sensitive may find adequate relief from an oral preparation of paracetamol or an non-steroidal anti-inflammatory drug. Giving that patient oral opioids could be inappropriate. In paediatrics, providing pain relief should always be undertaken alongside careful explanation to those children who can comprehend in addition to parents/guardian or caregivers.

TABLE 14.5 Options for analgesia.

Pain severity	Analgesia options
Mild	Oral preparations[a]
Moderate	Oral preparations[a] Methoxyflurane Intravenous paracetamol Nitrous oxide
Severe	Intravenous morphine Intravenous paracetamol Methoxyflurane Nitrous oxide

[a] Paracetamol and non-steroidal anti-inflammatory drugs.

Red Flag Alert: Opioid Administration

Providing patients with opioids can be accompanied with adverse effects. These include:

- Respiratory depression
- Significant nausea and/or vomiting
- Hypotension
- Bradycardia
- Drowsiness.

Slow administration of analgesia can mitigate these effects.

In the United Kingdom, in addition to helicopter emergency medical services (HEMS), there are appropriately trained paramedic practitioners within trusts who can administer additional analgesia to both adult and paediatric patients above the normal scope of practice. These regimens include:

- Ketamine
- Intranasal opioids (e.g. fentanyl)
- Local anaesthetic techniques.

As a paramedic practitioner, you should be aware of the additional services you can use for the benefit of the patient while adhering to the local policy and procedure. These can include HEMS teams, British Association for Immediate Care providers, critical care paramedics, urgent care paramedics, community nursing teams (palliative care).

Medicines Management: Opioids

Opioids are drugs that are indicated for severe pain. Available to paramedics in both oral and intravenous preparations, they work by binding to opiate receptors in the central nervous system, thus mimicking endogenous opiates. However, because they are not broken down quickly by the body, the opioids that the paramedic administers can have long effects. Careful consideration of this length of action must taken into account by the paramedic when treating patients who require this class of medication.

Snapshot 14.3

Pre-arrival Information

You are dispatched to a call of a 47 year old male patient with cancer. Ambulance control informs you that the nature of the call is breathing difficulty. You are also informed that a community palliative care team is not available for this call.
Dispatched: 10.10 p.m.
Arrival: 10.36 p.m.

On Arrival with the Patient

Airway: clear.
Breathing: bilateral chest rise, lung sounds have crackles, marked increased respiratory effort with some intercostal muscle movement.
Cardiac: pulses present, slow.
Disability: voice responsive.
Background: age: 47 years, male; weight/height approximately 80 kg and 173 cm.
Medical history: stage 4 terminal lung cancer, currently home palliative care, diverticulitis, urinary catheter in place.
Medications: morphine sulphate tablets, morphine solution, haloperidol, cyclizine, home oxygen at 4 l/minute via nasal cannula.

Background

The patient's wife, who is present, informs you and presents a 'Do not attempt resuscitation' form. You confirm that the form is recent and is from a reliable clinical source. The wife informs you that her husband has been in a lot of discomfort for the past hour and it is getting worse. The patient nods his head in agreement when you ascertain a pain score confirming a high level of pain.

Vital Signs

Vital signs taken are:

Vital sign	Observation	Normal range
Pulse (beats/min)	52	80–100 regular
Respiration (breaths/min)	19	12–20

Vital sign	Observation	Normal range
O_2 saturation (%)	92 (on 4 l/min)	94–98
Blood pressure (mmHg)	118/64	120/80
Temperature (°C)	37.1	37
Eyes	3	4 – spontaneously
Verbal	4	5 – orientated
Motor	6	6 – obeys commands
Total GCS score	13	15
Pupils	4 and PEARRL	Equal, round, reactive
ECG	Sinus bradycardia	
Pain score	9/10	

Background

The patient's wife informs you that they currently do not have a supply of medication at home. Both the patient and his wife express that they will not be travelling to an emergency department.

Reflective Learning Activity

Take some time to reflect on Snapshot 14.3 then consider the following:

1. What options do you have for analgesia?
2. What is your role here with regards the service you offer?
3. How is this patient best managed at home?
4. What options have you in terms of extra help?

Take Home Points

- Treat each patient individually.
- Carry out a detailed measured assessment.
- Try to minimise the patient's pain level to that which is tolerable.
- Select appropriate analgesic options that best fit the patient.
- Prehospital care is one aspect of the overall holistic patient-centred approach in patients with chronic pain.
- Use additional supportive resources when required.
- Be acutely aware of pharmacological interactions.

Summary

As a paramedic, the analgesic suite of medication available for pain management is significant. However, to maximise the effectiveness of this suite, pathways that are employed must be tailored to individual patient needs. It is important to remember that pain is what the patient says it is. Unmanaged pain in patients that are encountered within the prehospital setting will result in physiological changes and, left uncorrected, may result in the transformation from acute to chronic pain. The paramedic is ideally placed to deal with episodes of acute pain and exacerbations of chronic pain. Dealing with these presentations will require both an accurate patient-centred assessment and a balanced approach in treatment combining both non-pharmacological techniques and pharmacological pathways.

References

Abbey, J., Piller, N., De Bellis, A. et al. (2004). The Abbey pain scale: a 1-minute numerical indicator for people with end stage dementia. *International Journal of Palliative Nursing* 10 (1): 6–13.

Association of Ambulance Chief Executives (2017). *Pain Management in Adults Supplementary Revision 2017*. Bridgwater: Class Professional Publishing.

Calvino, B. and Grilo, R.M. (2006). Central pain control. *Joint, Bone, Spine* 73 (1): 10–16.

Cancer Research UK (2020). Causes and types of cancer pain. http://www.cancerresearchuk.org/about-cancer/coping/physically/cancer-and-pain-control/causes-and-types (accessed 10 October 2023).

Cipher, D.J., Clifford, P.A., and Roper, K.D. (2006). Behavioural manifestations of pain in the demented elderly. *Journal of the American Medical Directors Association* 7: 355–365.

Dubner, R., Sessle, B.J., and Storey, A.T. (1978). *The Neural Basis of Oral and Facial Function*. New York, NY: Plenum.

Gatchel, R.J. (2005). *Clinical Essentials of Pain Management*. Washington DC: American Psychological Association.

Gatchel, R.J. and Howard, K.J. (2021). The biopsychosocial approach. *Practical Pain Management* 8 (4): 28–39.

Godfrey, H. (2005). Understanding pain part 1; physiology of pain. *British Journal of Nursing* 14 (6): 846–852.

Hader, C.F. and Guy, J. (2004). Your hand in pain management. *Nursing Management* 35 (11): 21–28.

Hockenberry, M.J., Wilson, D., and Winkenlstein, M.L. (2005). *Wongs Essentials of Paediatric Nursing*, 7e, 1259. St. Louis: Mobsy.

International Association for the Study of Pain (2021). Terminology. http://www.iasp-pain.org/resources/terminology/#pain (accessed 10 October 2023).

Johnson, M. (2005). Physiology of chronic pain. In: *Chronic Pain Management* (ed. C. Banks and K. Mackrodt), 75–91. London: Whurr.

Joint Royal Colleges Ambulance Liaison Committee, Association of Ambulance Chief Executives (2022). JRCALC Clinical Guidelines.

Ko, S.M. and Zhou, M. (2004). Central plasticity and persistent pain; drug discovery today: disease models. *Pain and Anaesthesia* 1 (2): 101–106.

Loeser, J.D. and Treede, R.D. (2008). The Kyoto protocol of IASP basic pain terminology. *Pain* 137 (3): 473–477. https://doi.org/10.1016/j.pain.2008.04.025.

MacIntyre, P.E. and Schug, S.A. (2015). *Acute Pain Management: A Practical Guide*, 4e. Boca Raton, FL: CRC Press.

MacLellan, K. (2006). *Expanding Nursing and Health Care Practice: Management of Pain*. Cheltenham: Nelson Thrones.

Malviya, S., Voepel-Lewis, T., Burke, C. et al. (2006). The revised FLACC observational pain tool: improved reliability and validity for pain assessment in children with cognitive impairment. *Paediatric Anaesthesia* 16 (3): 258–265.

McCaffrey, M. (1979). *Nursing Management of the Patient with Pain*, 2e. New York, NY: Lippincott.

McCaffrey, M. and Pasero, C. (1999). *Pain: A Clinical Manual*. St. Louis, MO: Mosby.

Melzack, R. and Wall, P. (1988). *The Challenge of Pain*, 2e. London: Penguin.

Merkel, S., Voepel-Lewis, T., Shayevitz, J.R. et al. (1997). The FLACC: a behavioural scale for scoring postoperative pain in young children. *Pediatric Nursing* 23: 293–797.

Mustafa, A., Kreshnik, H., Parsons, P., and Hughes, J. (2017). Pain assessment in dementia: evaluation of a point of care technological solution. *Journal of Alzheimer's Disease 2017* 60 (1): 137–150.

Neilsen, S., Sabioni, P., Trigo, J.M. et al. (2017). *Neuropsychopharmacology* 42 (9): 1752–1765.

Peate, I. (ed.) (2021). *Fundamentals of Applied Pathophysiology: An essential guide for nursing and healthcare students*, 4e. Oxford: Wiley Blackwell.

Solano, J.P., Games, B., and Higginson, I.J. (2006). A comparison of symptom prevalence in far advanced cancer, AIDS, heart disease, chronic obstructive pulmonary disease (COPD) and renal disease. *Journal of Pain and Symptom Management* 31 (1): 58–69.

Wong, D. and Baker, C. (1988). Pain in children: comparison of assessment scales. *Pediatric Nursing* 14 (1): 9–17.

Zeidan, A. and Saifan, A. (2014). Median effective dose (ED50) of paracetamol and morphine for postoperative pain: a study of interaction. *British Journal of Anaesthesia* 112 (1): 118–123.

Further Reading

Faculty of Pain Medicine (2021) (2nd Ed). Core Standards for Pain Management Services in the UK. Royal College of Anaesthetists. London.
Mears, J. and Mears, L. (2023). The Pathophysiology, Assessment, and Management of Acute Pain. *British Journal of Nursing* 32 (2): 58–65.
Scottish Intercollegiate Guidelines Network (2019) Guidelines: Management of chronic pain. https://www.sign.ac.uk/our-guidelines/management-of-chronic-pain/

Online Resources

British Pain Society: www.britishpainsociety.org
Includes information for patients.
International Association for the Study of Pain: http://www.iasp-pain.org
Leading global organisation supporting the study of pain and pain relief.
NHS Choices: http://www.nhs.uk/condition/back-pain
Guidance on care of patients who are experiencing pain.
Live well with pain: www.liewellwithpain.co.uk
Developed by clinicians for clinicians providing information to support patients who live with chronic pain.
Practical Pain Management: www.practicalpainmanagement.com
Eevidence-based strategies for the treatment of chronic pain.

Glossary

Central nervous system	The brain and spinal cord.
Dorsal horn	Grey matter found on either side of the spinal cord.
Dynorphin	Neuropeptide found in the central nervous system.
Endorphin	Neuropeptide that inhibits substance P.
Hypertension	Elevated blood pressure.
Limbic system	Controls feelings of emotion and behaviour; part of the forebrain.
Myelinated	Covered by a protective sheath of myelin.
Neuron	A nerve cell.
Nociceptor	Special cell that detects pain due to damage and irritation.
Neurotransmitter	Molecule that transmits neural messages across the synapse.
Reticular formation	Neural network found in the central part of brainstem.
Substance P	Neurotransmitter found in sensory nerves.
Substantia gelatinosa	Part of the spinal cord grey matter containing large amounts of nerve cells.
Synapse	The junction where two neurons meet or neurons meet tissue.

Multiple Choice Questions

1. Wong–Baker FACES is applicable for paediatric patients from what age?
   a. 2 years
   b. 3 years

   c. 4 years

   d. 5 years

2. What is the third process in pain sensation?

   a. Modulation

   b. Transformation

   c. Transmission

   d. Stimulation

3. Noxious stimulation occurs in which fibres?

   a. A delta

   b. B delta

   c. D delta

   d. E delta

4. Pain can fall under how many classifications?

   a. 2

   b. 4

   c. 3

   d. 5

5. T in the TEACH pneumonic equates to what?

   a. Temperature

   b. Thalamus

   c. Touch

   d. Time

6. Which of these lists explains the meaning of FLACC?

   a. Face, legs, arms, cry, consolability

   b. Face, look, activity, cry, consolability

   c. Face, legs, activity, cry, consolability

   d. Face, look, arms, cry, consolability

7. Long term nitrous oxide use can result in deficiency of which vitamin?

   a. A

   b. B_{12}

   c. C

   d. D

8. The biopsychosocial approach allows for what?

   a. Rapid pain score assessment

   b. Individual tailored approach

   c. Differentiate between acute or chronic pain

   d. Correct analgesic dose

9. Opioid administration can result in which condition?

   a. Hypotension

   b. Hypertension

   c. Tachypnoea

   d. Tachycardia

10. Neuropathic pain occurs as a result of what?

   a. Increased synaptic transmission

   b. Decreased synaptic transmission

   c. Excitation of the reticular formation

   d. Damage to the nociceptors

CHAPTER 15

The Musculoskeletal System and Associated Disorders

George Bell-Starr and Ashley Ingram

AIM

The aim of this chapter is to introduce the reader to the pathophysiology associated with musculoskeletal system and associated disorders.

LEARNING OUTCOMES

On completion of this chapter, you will be able to:

- Confidently discuss the formation and development of bones.
- Describe the functions of the musculoskeletal system.
- Outline common musculoskeletal presentations and have an understanding of assessment strategies.
- Understand some of the treatment options available to paramedics for these common pathophysiological changes.

Test Your Prior Knowledge

1. How many bones make up the musculoskeletal system, and does this change with age?
2. What is the purpose of the musculoskeletal system?
3. Discuss the types of musculoskeletal disorders that paramedics might encounter.
4. What long-term musculoskeletal conditions might reduce someone's ability to mobilise?
5. How many types of joints are there, and can you name them?

Introduction

The musculoskeletal (MSK) system is a system that provides the body with support, protection and structure and allows movement. It is a crucial system; without it, we would be unable to sustain life. Our hearts would not beat, and we would be unable to breathe, run or smile without the MSK system.

Fundamentals of Applied Pathophysiology for Paramedics, First Edition. Edited by Ian Peate and Simon Sawyer.

The World Health Organization (WHO) estimates that at least 1.7 billion people worldwide suffer from disorders of the musculoskeletal system (World Health Organization 2022). These disorders are the primary cause of disability, with lower back pain being the leading cause in 160 countries worldwide (World Health Organization 2022). The prevalence of these MSK-caused disabilities has risen by almost 30% in the first 15 years of this century (Sebbag et al. 2019). MSK injury is among the most common clinical presentations to the ambulance service, equating to almost 10% of attendances (Rosser 2020).

For paramedics to provide safe and effective care, it is imperative that they have a fundamental understanding of the issues relating to the MSK system. This chapter provides an overview of the MSK system, commonly associated disorders and the care or treatment they require.

The Musculoskeletal System

The MSK system is widely referred to as the locomotor system. It is then divided into two: the axial skeleton and the appendicular skeleton (Figure 15.1). The axial skeleton comprises the bones along the body's long axis, such as the skull and vertebral column. The appendicular skeleton is the portion that supports appendages such as the pelvic girdle and limb bones. A baby is born with 300 bones; as we age, some of these bones fuse, leaving adults with 206. Most of a baby's bones are made out of cartilage; as the baby ages, they turn into bone through ossification.

As well as having 206 bones, the human skeleton consists of a wide range of joints (such as the knee and shoulder); without these joints, movement would be impossible. These joints are supported by cartilage and ligaments. Cartilage is a tough yet flexible type of tissue that provides protection for joints against the forces exerted during movement. Ligaments are attached bone to bone and provide strength and structural support during moving actions. These elements work in conjunction to provide a range of fundamental functions that are essential to life, including:

- **Protection** – the bones within the skeleton afford protection against injury from impact and safeguard the internal organs.
- **Support** – the skeleton gives the body shape and keeps us upright.
- **Blood** – certain bones contain marrow; red and white blood cells and platelets are produced within this bone marrow – haemopoiesis.
- **Storage** – bones act as a reservoir for minerals that are vital to bodily function; these include calcium, phosphorus and potassium.
- **Movement** – the skeleton allows movement as a whole as well as individual elements.

Bone Development and Structure

Bone is a living tissue, made primarily of collagen and calcium phosphate. Collagen is a protein that provides a soft, flexible framework. Calcium phosphate is a mineral that adds a strength element to bones. This combination allows bones to be strong and flexible enough to survive day-to-day activities. More than 99% of all the body's calcium is stored within bones and teeth, and the other 1% is found in the blood.

Bone formation or ossification is essentially a replacement process. In the early phases of embryonic development, the embryo's skeleton consists primarily of hyaline cartilage and fibrous membranes. By the seventh week of development, the bone formation process begins in two processes – intramembranous and endochondral ossification. Continuing ossification is then controlled by osteoblast and osteoclast activity. Osteoblasts control bone formation and osteoclasts are responsible for bone breakdown. Various factors influence bone structure, including exercise type and amount, diet and gait.

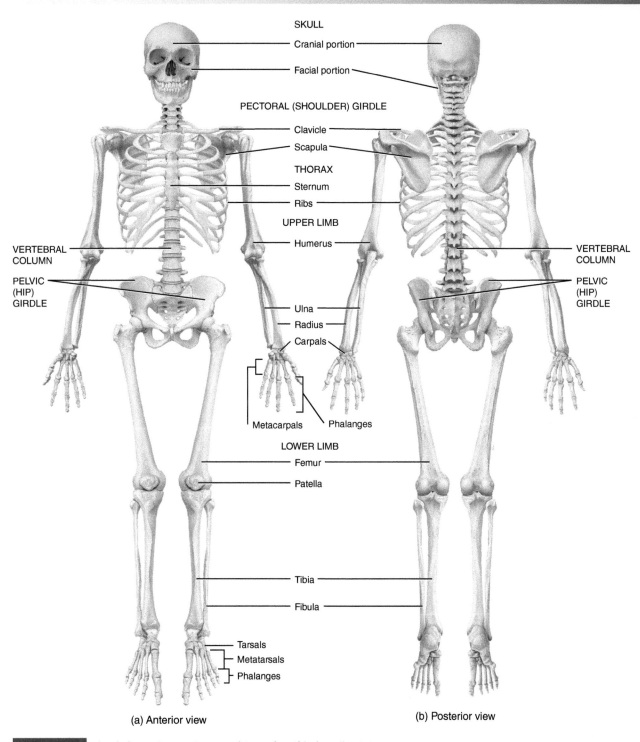

SKULL
— Cranial portion —
— Facial portion —

PECTORAL (SHOULDER) GIRDLE
— Clavicle —
— Scapula —

THORAX
— Sternum —
— Ribs —

UPPER LIMB
— Humerus —

VERTEBRAL
COLUMN

PELVIC
(HIP)
GIRDLE

— Ulna —
— Radius —
— Carpals —

Metacarpals   Phalanges

LOWER LIMB
— Femur —
— Patella —

VERTEBRAL
COLUMN

PELVIC
(HIP)
GIRDLE

— Tibia —
— Fibula —

— Tarsals
— Metatarsals
— Phalanges

(a) Anterior view

(b) Posterior view

FIGURE 15.1   The skeleton. Source: Peate and Evans (2020)/John Wiley & Sons.

315

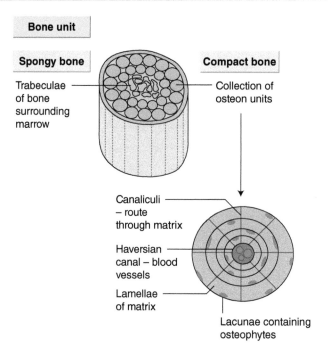

FIGURE 15.2   Bone structure. Source: Peate (2021)/John Wiley & Sons.

Bone is made up of two different types of tissue: cancellous bone and cortical bone. The cortical bone is often referred to as the compact bone. It is the hard, dense outer layer of the bone, which provides protection and support for the inner, cancellous structure. The cortical bone comprises three components: the periosteum, intracortical areas and the endosteum (Figure 15.2). There are five types of bone within the skeleton:

1. Long bones: femur, tibia.
2. Short bones: hand bones.
3. Flat bones: Skull, ribs.
4. Irregular bones: pelvis.
5. Sesamoid bones: patella.

Joints

A joint is described as a point in the skeleton where two bones meet, permitting them to move. There are three types of joints found within the human body. They are categorised by the type of movement that they allow:

- *Immovable* (synarthroses) are fixed or fibrous joints; two (or more) bones in contact that have little or no movement, such as the bones of the skull.
- *Slightly moveable* (amphiarthrosis) joints are sometimes known as cartilaginous joints. These joints are where bones are held so tightly together that movement is limited, such as spinal vertebrae.
- *Freely moveable* (diarthrosis) joints are usually known as synovial joints, because of the synovial fluid within the joint that aids smooth movement. These are the most common joints within the body, such as the knee and shoulder.

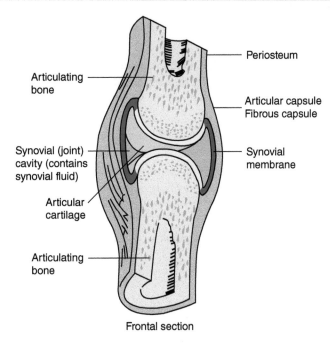

FIGURE 15.3 A synovial joint. Source: Peate (2021)/John Wiley & Sons.

Synovial Joints

There are six types of synovial joint within the human body, which allow the body to move in a variety of ways. A key characteristic of the synovial joint is the joint cavity (Figure 15.3). This cavity is fluid filled, with the fluid being found in the spaces between the articulating bones. This synovial fluid allows the joints to articulate in a smooth manner.

1. *Plane joints* are essentially flat and offer only a short range of movement in a non-axial, gliding fashion. Examples include the intertarsal joints.
2. *Hinge joints* (uniaxial) allow a bending motion to occur through a single axis. The convex end of one bone joins with the concave end of an adjoining bone. A good example of this would be the elbow joint. Others include the knee and interphalangeal joints.
3. *Pivot joints* (unilateral) only allow movement in a unilateral plane around their own longitudinal axes. An example of this type of joint is the joint between the atlas (C1) and the dens of an axis (C2), which allows rotational movement of the skull left and right.
4. *Saddle joints* (biaxial) allow a fuller range of motion, such as the movement of a thumb. The articulating surfaces for both adjoining bones have a saddle shape in a concave and convex manner.
5. *Ball and socket joints* (multiaxial) allow free movement in all directions, including rotation. A spherical head of one bone articulates within a cuplike socket of another bone. The only examples are the shoulders and hips.
6. *Condyloid joints* (biaxial) are similar to saddle joints. They allow movement in two directions; however, they also allow axial rotation. Examples of condyloid joints include the radiocarpal joint within the wrist.

317

Muscle

There are thought to be over 650 muscles found within the human body. Each of these muscles is made up of thousands of smaller muscle fibres; these fibres are then made up of many smaller strands called fibrils. There are three types of muscle skeletal, smooth and cardiac. Each of these types has the ability to contract and relax at various speeds.

Skeletal Muscle

Skeletal muscles give the body shape by sitting atop the skeleton; they are also responsible for movement and limb control (Figure 15.4). They comprise approximately 35% of the total body mass. All skeletal muscles work in pairs as they only pull in one direction, such as the biceps and triceps. One muscle in the pair contracts and flexes (the flexor) and the opposing muscle relaxes and extends (the extensor).

Muscles such as the neck, back and trunk work together to provide stability and support posture. Without these muscles, sitting and standing would be impossible.

Cardiac Muscle

Commonly known as the myocardium, the only function of cardiac muscle is to keep the heart pumping. The cardiac muscle is the only muscle that moves involuntarily. This involuntary movement is controlled by specialised cells called pacemaker cells. The autonomic nervous system alters heart rate automatically, with both the parasympathetic and sympathetic branches having an impact.

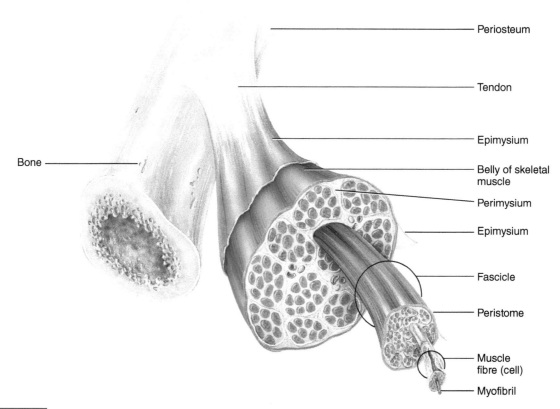

FIGURE 15.4   Gross anatomy skeletal muscle. Source: Peate (2021)/John Wiley & Sons.

Smooth Muscle

Smooth muscle contracts without any voluntary action. It is formed of thin layers of unstriated cells. These muscles perform several vital functions and are found throughout the body; they are controlled by the nervous system. Functions include regulating blood pressure and aiding in digestion within the gastrointestinal tract.

With blood pressure regulation and oxygen demand, the nervous system will independently control the smooth muscle by regulating hormones and neurotransmitters among other receptors.

The Nervous System

Almost all aspects of the body are controlled or impacted by the nervous system (see Chapter 6). It is essential for regulating autonomic processes such as breathing and heart rate, as well as movement, coordination and balance. The primary motor cortex connects to and controls the movement of various parts of the body. The primary motor cortex is broken down into smaller areas, controlling different parts of the body. The various areas are 'mapped' in a cortical homunculus; the larger the area mapped the higher level of fine motor control that body part has. A large portion of the motor cortex is devoted to thumbs and fingers.

Coordination, movement or balance can be disrupted by any number of disorders that impact the primary motor cortex. If the neurons within the primary cortex are damaged, as they would be in a cerebrovascular event, they will never regrow or repair. If this damage was to occur in a specific area of the homunculus, it will affect the associated area of the body.

Common Musculoskeletal Presentations

Fractures

Commonly called breaks by patients, fractures are a common presentation to ambulance paramedics. It is estimated that there are over 76 000 hip fractures every year (Healthcare Quality Improvement Partnership 2021). It is safe to assume that a large proportion of these fractures are seen by the ambulance service.

Fractures are defined as a break into the continuity of the bone. Common causes include direct or indirect trauma, repetitive stress or disease. Treatment for these fractures is generally limited to pain management, including splinting.

There are several different classifications of fractures. Common types include:

- Stress – small cracks in the bone, usually not full thickness.
- Compound – more commonly known as an open fracture.
- Transverse – a break at a right angle to the long aspect of the bone.
- Displaced – a transverse fracture where the broken bones have come out of alignment.
- Spiral (torsion) – a break along two planes, causing a spiral fracture along the bone.
- Greenstick – most common in children, where the bone is malleable and therefore bends, then breaks.
- Compression – caused by excessive axial load, common in vertebrae.
- Pathological – when the bone is weakened by malignancy, infection or lack of nutrition.

Cervical Spine

Blunt force trauma can lead to a fracture of the cervical vertebrae in 2–4% of incidences (Armstrong et al. 2007). This means that the vast majority of patients who are seen with MSK neck presentations are unlikely to have any serious pathology; however, the risk of missing any neck injury is serious. It is important for paramedics to remember that cervical spine immobilisation is not a risk-free procedure and comes with a significant increase in morbidity.

319

Dislocations

A dislocation is a condition that happens when a joint is knocked out of its usual position. Joints can be either partially dislocated or fully dislocated. Usually, they are caused by trauma or external forces but can be caused by chronic diseases or the weakening of muscles and tendons.

Dislocations are very common, Nabian et al. (2017) suggests that shoulder dislocations are the most common. Other common dislocation sites include fingers, patellae and ankles.

Signs and Symptoms

Signs and symptoms will be similar for both fractures and dislocations, they include:

- Pain
- Swelling
- Bruising
- Obvious deformity
- Joint instability
- Reduced range of movement.

Snapshot 15.1

Pre-arrival Information

You are working solo on a rapid response vehicle and are called to the local rugby football club.

On Arrival with the Patient

Ultan, a 49-year-old man, has been playing rugby. Immediately following a tackle, he felt a pop in his right shoulder, which was accompanied by severe pain. Since this incident, he has not been able to move from the field of play and cannot move his right arm. It becomes clear from the history of events that Ultan was conscious throughout and has had this happen before. He has no cervical spine tenderness and has been freely moving his head and neck without pain before your arrival.

Examination

On examination, you note that his right shoulder is deformed anteriorly.

Diagnosis

Your working diagnosis is of anterior dislocation to the right shoulder.

Reflective Learning Activity

Take some time to reflect on the presentation in Snapshot 15.1, then consider:

- How might you support this dislocation?
- What management options do you have, and what might be effective in this scenario?

Sprains/Strains

Often confused, sprains and strains are disorders that affect soft tissue. They are found within the musculoskeletal system and usually arise following trauma.

Sprains

A sprain is the stretching or tearing of the ligaments connecting two bones together. The most common type of sprain is the ankle. Patients can easily roll their ankles, stretching or tearing the lateral collateral ligaments. Sprains can be categorised into three grades, with one being stretching with small tears to three being completely torn.

Strains

A strain is an injury to a muscle or the fibrous connective tissues – the tendons. More commonly known as pulled muscles, these injuries can range in severity. Minor strains might simply overstretch a muscle or tendon, while severe strains could involve complete tears in these soft tissues. Similarly to sprains, strains are graded. A grade 1 strain involves less than 5% of the fibres and causes minimal functional loss, while grade 3 is a complete rupture or tear of the muscle or tendon.

Lower Back Pain

Lower back pain is the world's leading cause of disability. Most of these cases are classed as non-specific lower back pain (more than 90%). This means that clinicians cannot attribute one single pathological or anatomical cause of the pain. Less than 1% of low back presentations are due to serious pathology such as cauda equine syndrome. Although this condition is rare, if missed it can have devastating consequences for the patient. Symptoms include:

- Urinary retention.
- Urinary and/or faecal incontinence.
- Weakness or paralysis in lower extremities.
- Pain in the low back and/or legs similar to sciatica pain.
- Saddle anaesthesia – sensory change involving the genitals, anus or buttocks.

Arthritis

Arthritis is not a single condition; it is an umbrella term that encompasses a range of conditions. It generally describes pain, swelling and stiffness in singular or multiple joints. It can affect many people, including children and teenagers, although some types of arthritis are more prevalent in older generations. It is estimated that more than 350 million people suffer from arthritis globally; in the United Kingdom, over 10 million people (one in six adults) have arthritis (Versus Arthritis 2023).

Osteoarthritis

Osteoarthritis is the most common joint disease in the world, affecting 18% of women over the age of 60 years worldwide (Glyn-Jones et al. 2015). It is a chronic condition that causes pain, stiffness and reduced joint function when the cartilage between bones begins to wear down. It is most common in the hands, feet, knees and spine, but can occur in any joint in the body. Osteoarthritis can be divided into four stages (Table 15.1).

Rheumatoid Arthritis

Unlike osteoarthritis, which is degenerative, rheumatoid arthritis is an autoimmune disorder which attacks the lining (synovium) of the joints. The start of the autoimmune process may occur in other parts of the body, but the symptoms will

TABLE 15.1   The four stages of osteoarthritis.

Stage	Severity	Description
1	Minor	Minor wear and tear, little, to no pain or dysfunction
2	Mild	Increased stiffness following sedentary periods; more prominent bone spurs (osteophytes)
3	Moderate	Joint cartilage starts to erode; inflammation and discomfort impacts on day-to-day activities
4	Severe	Significant pain; cartilage has almost completely gone; overgrowth of osteophytes occurs increasing pain

usually be most noticeable in the joints. The autoimmune process causes inflammation and thickening of the synovium and, over time, this inflammation becomes chronic. As rheumatoid arthritis progresses, the thickened synovium causes long-term damage to the cartilage and bones within joints. This then impacts the surrounding tissues destabilising the joints and causing further issues.

The exact cause of rheumatoid arthritis is unclear, but it is believed that a combination of environmental factors and genes starts the developmental process of rheumatoid arthritis.

Gout

Gout is a common form of arthritis that is exceptionally painful. Gout occurs as a response to the monosodium urate (MSU) crystals found in the bones and soft tissues. Hyperuricaemia (an elevated uric acid level in the blood) is the key risk factor for gout and is considered a prerequisite for MSU crystal formation. These crystal depositions trigger an immune response, releasing several inflammatory cytokines. Over time, the joint is irreversibly damaged leading to disability, deformed joints and chronic pain.

Gout is usually categorised by the rapid development of monoarticular pain, associated with swelling and redness. It often starts with the metatarsophalangeal joint of the great toe.

Risk factors include age, sex and diet. Over the age of 80 years, prevalence peaks at 12% (Zhu et al. 2011). Female sex hormones increase the urinary excretion of uric acid. Women who are premenopausal therefore have a significantly lower prevalence of gout compared with men (Reginato et al. 2012). Alcoholic drinks, especially beer, increase the risk by over 200% compared with drinking no beer (Roddy and Doherty 2010).

Pseudogout

Formally known as calcium pyrophosphate disease, pseudogout is very similar to gout; however, rather than MSU crystals, it is calcium crystals that form and cause damage to joints and soft tissues. Unlike gout, the causation of these calcium crystals is relatively unknown. There may be a genetic cause, but some risk factors might include kidney failure and thyroid or calcium metabolism disorders.

Osteoporosis

Osteoporosis is a metabolic bone disease that develops due to a decrease in bone mass and mineral density. This can lead to an increased risk of fractures with the decrease in bone strength. On a cellular level, osteoporosis results from osteoclastic bone resorption not being compensated for by osteoblastic bone formation; essentially, the formation of new bone is unable to keep up with the breakdown of old bone.

There are numerous risk factors, some of which are unchangeable and some of which can be altered on a personal level. Unchangeable risk factors include age, sex, ethnicity and familial history. As age increases, so does the risk of osteoporosis. Women, those of white or Asian descent and those with a familial history of osteoporosis all have a higher risk of developing the disease.

Snapshot 15.2

Pre-arrival Information

While working on a duel-crewed ambulance, you are called to Rebecca, a 75-year-old woman who has fallen and is now reporting hip pain.

On Arrival with the Patient

Rebecca's husband gives you her medications; you note that among other medications, she is taking alendonric acid.

Reflective Learning Activity

Taking the information in Snapshot 15.2 into consideration:

- What condition is Rebecca likely to have if she is taking alendronic acid?
- Would this change your management of Rebecca's condition?

Assessing Musculoskeletal Presentations

Paramedics need to be able to perform a thorough and comprehensive assessment. Performing such an assessment competently requires excellent communication skills. A competent paramedic will be able to identify any presenting conditions that require immediate interventions or onward referral, clinicians can be aided by using the clinical flag system (Table 15.2).

Clinical Investigations: Examination

When examining a patient presenting with an MSK disorder, a thorough physical assessment is imperative. Following a logical approach, it is essential to keep an open mind and generally assess before focusing on the obvious disorder, comparing the affected and unaffected side of the body to understand what is normal for that patient.

With some conditions, such as gout, history is just as important as a physical assessment. When assessing pain, using a mnemonic such as SOCRATES (Table 15.3) is an effective way for paramedics to avoid missing any key factors relating to that patient's pain (see also Chapter 14). Using simple assessments such as this can yield enough information for effective treatment to be started (Swift 2015).

In 1992, a team of doctors at a Canadian hospital created a list of rules to reduce the number of plain film x-rays being undertaken for possible ankle fractures. Dubbed the 'Ottawa ankle rules' (Box 15.1) and expanded to include the knee (the Ottawa knee rules), these rules comprise some simple questions and examinations that indicate a requirement for an x-ray (and likely fracture) or no requirement for an x-ray (and a reduced likelihood of a simple fracture).

TABLE 15.2   **Clinical flag system.**

Flag	Nature	Examples
Red	Signs of serious pathology	CES, sudden weight loss, night sweats, previous cancers
Orange	Psychiatric symptoms	Depression, personality disorders
Yellow	Psychosocial issues	Unhelpful beliefs about pain, anxiety, lack of job satisfaction
Blue	Perceptions about health between work and the patient	Belief that work may further worsen the injury; belief that work colleagues and management are unsupportive
Black	Systemic obstacles	Legislation that restricts options for returning to work

TABLE 15.3   **SOCRATES pain assessment mnemonic.**

Mnemonic	Definition
S	Site
O	Onset
C	Characteristics – sharp/stabbing/dull/pulling
R	Radiation of pain
A	Associations – symptoms linked to the pain
T	Time course – does the pain follow any pattern
E	Exacerbating/relieving factors
S	Severity – Pain out of 10

Source: Adapted from National Institute for Health and Care excellence (2020).

BOX 15.1   **Ottawa ankle rules.**

An ankle x-ray is only required when there is:

- Pain in the malleolar zone

and

- Any of the following:
  - Bone tenderness along the distal 6 cm of the posterior edge of the tibia or tip of the medial malleolus, OR
  - Bone tenderness along the distal 6 cm of the posterior edge of the fibula or tip of the lateral malleolus, OR
  - An inability to bear weight both immediately and in the emergency department for four steps.

Source: National Institute for Health and Care Excellence (2020).

Knee x-ray indications after acute knee injury, based on the Ottawa knee rules, are:

- Age 55 years or over.
- Tenderness at the head of the fibula.
- Isolated tenderness of the patella.
- Inability to flex knee to 90 degrees.
- Inability to bear weight (defined as an inability to take four steps; i.e. two steps on each leg, regardless of limping) immediately and at presentation.

Treating Musculoskeletal Presentations

Fractures

Treating fractures is a common skill for paramedics working on an ambulance. Limb trauma, while at times dramatic, is seldom life threatening. It is essential to not over-triage limb trauma and thus miss more life-threatening presentations in the immediate patient or other patients who may be on scene and involved in the same incident. Fractures are common and may lead to reduced mobility and increasing mortality, with falls associated with deaths as high as 14 000/year in the UK (Office for Health Improvement and Disparities 2022).

Snapshot 15.3

Pre-arrival Information

While working solo on a rapid response vehicle, you are tasked to Abdul, a 49-year-old man who has fallen from his push bike.

On Arrival with the Patient

The accident was witnessed by Abdul's friends, who reported that he was flung over the handlebars and landed head first. He was wearing a helmet.

Patient Assessment

On your initial assessment of the patient, he is alert and talking, repeatedly stating that he cannot feel his legs.

Reflective Learning Activity

Taking the information in Snapshot 15.3 into consideration:

- What would your initial actions be in this scenario?
- When your backup has arrived, how might you manage this patient's condition?

Treating fracture in the initial phases is very similar to other conditions. Consider whether there is an immediate <C>ABCDE issue that needs to be addressed. Examples of these would include a catastrophic haemorrhage that may be suspected in a pelvic fracture. An airway and breathing issue could be attributed to a rib fracture or a circulatory fracture attributed to a complex ankle fracture.

Closely followed by this is early pain management. Relieving pain and suffering is one of the most important tasks paramedics perform (Lord and Nicholls 2014). Patient management and patient outcome measures found that the measurement and relief of pain was one of the most highly rated patient outcome measures (Turner et al. 2019).

The National Institute for Health and Care Excellence (2016) suggests oral paracetamol or non-steroidal anti-inflammatory drugs (NSAIDs) for mild pain. For moderate pain, add codeine; for severe pain, intravenous paracetamol and morphine are titrated to effect.

Red Flag Alert: Non-steroidal Anti-inflammatory Drugs

The risk of bleeding associated with aspirin, ibuprofen and other NSAIDs increases in the elderly and is more likely to lead to a serious or fatal outcome. It should be noted that NSAIDs are particularly hazardous to those with cardiac disease or renal impairment. It is recommended that clinicians use other options, such as physiotherapy, exercise and paracetamol, to treat MSK presentations such as osteoarthritis and low back pain before using NSAIDs.

Once pain relief has been established, splinting is often also an effective analgesic. A splint is a device that is used to support an injury that has caused a body part (normally an extremity) and the associated joints not to function in a normal manner; it achieves this by restraining, immobilising and/or supporting the injured body part (McKelvin 2018).

Complex Fractures

Complex fractures are complicated breaks in bones, which usually need care by a specialist team. They include open fractures, pelvic fractures and severe ankle fractures that may have vascular compromise (National Institute for Health and Care Excellence 2022).

Clinical Investigations: Six Ps of Suspected Vascular Compromise

Pain – will occur at rest, although a patient with a viable limb may present with acute-onset short-distance claudication. Rest pain is usually worse in the most distal part of the limb (toes) since this has the worst perfusion and may be relieved on dependency (hanging legs over bed). Pain that is worse on passive movement of the muscles indicates potential compartment syndrome (see below) and is a poor prognostic sign.

Pallor – useful in comparison to the opposite limb; it is also useful to check venous filling. Acutely ischaemic limbs are classically white rather than blue. Chronic critically ischaemic limbs may appear pink due to compensatory vasodilation, the so-called sunset foot. In this situation, Buerger's test may also be useful (pallor on the elevation of the limb, with erythema on dependency).

Paraesthesia – present in over 50% of cases. Sensory nerves are smaller than motor nerves and more sensitive to ischaemia so tend to be affected first.

Paralysis – a poor prognostic sign; it indicates an element of irreversible ischaemia.

Perishingly – cold is a helpful sign when comparing with the uninjured limb. Check the temperature using the back of your hand.

Pulselessness – checking pulses is notoriously unreliable. In patients who are obese or incredibly muscular, palpating distal pulses such as the dorsalis pedis can be very challenging. Checking for capillary bed refill can provide reassurance for adequate blood flow (Darwood 2022).

Clinicians should consider hospital services for the specific type of injury and convey or refer to the hospital with the correct services.

Open fractures have a high risk of infection. Intravenous prophylactic antibiotics should be administered as soon as possible, ideally within one hour of injury. Gross contamination may be removed from the wound. Irrigation should not be performed in the prehospital setting as this may drive contaminants further into the wound and risk further infection.

Cervical Spine

Immobilisation is a routine procedure in the prehospital environment. Its potentially serious adverse sequelae and the litigious nature of modern medicine have seen the development of an extraordinarily conservative approach to immobilisation, where it is applied in many cases in which neither the mechanism of injury nor the clinical findings would support its use. Rigid cervical spine immobilisation collars have been commonplace in prehospital care for decades now, although the evidence base is shifting, seeing many ambulance services removing them from service completely. Manual in-line stabilisation and vacuum mattresses are slowly being adopted as the norm across ambulance services in the United Kingdom.

Sprains and Strains

Sprains and strains are treated in much the same way as a suspect fracture, as it may be challenging to ascertain whether the injury is a fracture or a strain/sprain.

Dislocation

Treatment of dislocation is often the same as fracture treatment in the prehospital setting, and mainly revolves around appropriate pain management and stabilisation of the injury. Actively reducing dislocations is not frequently undertaken by frontline ambulance staff; however, Fennelly (2020) suggests that, with adequate training, anterior shoulder dislocations can be carried out in the prehospital arena with a success rate of over 90% with no reported complications during follow-up examinations.

Cauda Equina Syndrome

Although there is no specific prehospital treatment for caude equina syndrome, staff must quickly identify the condition and transport the patient to an appropriate receiving facility to allow prompt investigation. In hospital, investigations are likely to include magnetic resonance imaging or computed tomography, followed by spinal decompression surgery.

Orange Flag Alert: Lower Back Pain

A significant amount of adults who suffer with lower back pain will also go on to suffer from depression or depressive episodes (Wong et al. 2019). Paramedics assessing patients with lower back pain should be mindful of the patient's needs, both physically and mentally, when developing a care plan. Paramedics could use screening tools such as the Patient Health Questionnaire-2 (PHQ-2) to screen patients for symptoms of depression.

In England alone, the annual cost of hip fractures to the UK is estimated at being around £1.1 billion (Office for Health Improvement and Disparities 2022).

> ## Take Home Points
>
> - A solid understanding of the function and features of the musculoskeletal system is key to being able to treat patients that present with injuries and disorders of the musculoskeletal system.
> - The vast majority of low back pain cannot be attributed to a single cause and does not usually have a sinister cause.
> - Injury to the cervical spine is rare in blunt force trauma and cervical spine immobilisation is not a risk-free procedure.
> - Adequate splinting of a musculoskeletal injury can provide significant pain relief to the patient.

Summary

The musculoskeletal system is essential to every aspect of a patient's life. Our fundamental requirements (e.g. breathing, moving, eating) all rely on a healthy MSK system. When the MSK system fails to function normally, daily activities can become painful or impossible; not only will this affect physical health but it could also easily impact mental health. Some patients that paramedics encounter will have chronic musculoskeletal disorders that need managing acutely. Other patients will have serious acute disorders that could be life changing.

This chapter has touched on a small range of MSK-related conditions that paramedics might see. However, in a chapter of this size, it is challenging to address these conditions and the associated assessment and treatment options in depth. It would be prudent for the reader to explore more detailed texts following the completion of this chapter.

References

Armstrong, B.P., Simpson, H.K., Crouch, R., and Deakin, C.D. (2007). Prehospital clearance of the cervical spine: does it need to be a pain in the neck? *Emergency Medicine Journal* 24 (7): 501–503. https://doi.org/10.1136/emj.2006.041897.

Darwood, R. (2022). Acute Limb Ischaemia. London: RCEM Learning. www.rcemlearning.co.uk/reference/acute-limb-ischaemia/#1567523573427-07296499-aef5 (accessed 11 October 2023).

Fennelly, J.T., Gourbault, L., Neal-Smith, G. et al. (2020). A systematic review of pre-hospital shoulder reduction techniques for anterior shoulder dislocation and the effect on patient return to function. *Chinese J Traumatol* 23 (5): 295–301.

Glyn-Jones, S., Palmer, A.J.R., Agricola, R. et al. (2015). Osteoarthritis. *Lancet* 386 (9991): 376–387. https://doi.org/10.1016/S0140-6736(14)60802-3.

Healthcare Quality Improvement Partnership (2021). *National Hip Fracture Database Annual Report 2021*. London: Healthcare Quality Improvement Partnership.

Lord, B. and Nicholls, T. (2014). A brief history of analgesia in paramedic practice. *Journal of Paramedic Practice* 6 (8): 400–406. https://doi.org/10.12968/jpar.2014.6.8.400.

McKelvin, R. (2018). Splinting of injuries: best practice guidance. *Journal of Paramedic Practice* 10 (12): 534–536. https://doi.org/10.12968/jpar.2018.10.12.534.

Nabian, M.H., Zadegan, S.A., Zanjani, L.O. et al. (2017). Epidemiology of joint dislocations and ligamentous/tendinous injuries among 2,700 patients: five-year trend of a tertiary center in Iran. *Archives of Bone and Joint Surgery* 5 (6): 426–434.

National Institute for Health and Care Excellence (2016). Fractures (Non-complex): Assessment and management. NICE Guideline NG38. London: National Institute for Health and Care Excellence.

National Institute for Health and Care Excellence (2020). How should I assess a suspected sprain or strain? Clinical Knowledge Summary. London: National Institute for Health and Care Excellence. https://cks.nice.org.uk/topics/sprains-strains/diagnosis/assessment (accessed 11 October 2023).

National Institute for Health and Care Excellence (2022). *Fractures (Complex): Assessment and management.* NICE Guideline NG37. London: National Institute for Health and Care Excellence.

Office for Health Improvement and Disparities (2022). Falls: Applying all our health. https://www.gov.uk/government/publications/falls-applying-all-our-health/falls-applying-all-our-health (accessed 11 October 2022).

Peate, I. (ed.) (2021). *Fundamentals of Applied Pathophysiology: An Essential Guide for Nursing and Healthcare Students*, 4e. Oxford: Wiley Blackwell.

Peate, I. and Evans, S. (2020). *Fundamentals of Anatomy and Physiology for Nursing and Healthcare Students*, 3e. Oxford: Wiley Blackwell.

Reginato, A.M., Mount, D.B., Yang, I., and Choi, H.K. (2012). The genetics of hyperuricaemia and gout. *Nature Reviews Rheumatology* 8 (10): 610–621. https://doi.org/10.1038/nrrheum.2012.144.

Roddy, E. and Doherty, M. (2010). Gout. epidemiology of gout. *Arthritis Research and Therapy* 12 (6): 223. https://doi.org/10.1186/ar3199.

Rosser, A. (2020). PP16 A review of the annual case epidemiology and clinical exposure of 45 paramedics, in a UK ambulance service: a service evaluation. *Emergency Medicine Journal* 37 (10): e8.3–e9. https://doi.org/10.1136/emermed-2020-999abs.16.

Sebbag, E., Felten, R., Sagez, F. et al. (2019). The world-wide burden of musculoskeletal diseases: a systematic analysis of the World Health Organization burden of diseases database. *Annals of the Rheumatic Diseases* 78 (6): 844–848. https://doi.org/10.1136/annrheumdis-2019-215142.

Swift, A. (2015). The importance of assessing pain in adults. *Nursing Times* 111 (41): 12–14, 16–17.

Turner, J., Siriwardena, A.N., Coster, J. et al. (2019). Developing new ways of measuring the quality and impact of ambulance service care: the PhOEBE mixed-methods research programme. *Programme Grants for Applied Research* 7 (3): 1–90. https://doi.org/10.3310/pgfar07030.

Versus Arthritis. (2023). *The State of Musculoskeletal Health 2023: Arthritis and other musculoskeletal conditions in numbers*. Chesterfield: Versus Arthritis. https://versusarthritis.org/about-arthritis/data-and-statistics/the-state-of-musculoskeletal-health (accessed 14 October 2023).

Wong, J.J., Tricco, A.C., Coté, P., and Rosella, L.C. (2019). The association between depressive symptoms or depression and health outcomes in adults with low back pain with or without radiculopathy: protocol of a systematic review. *Systematic Reviews* 8: 267. https://doi.org/10.1186/s13643-019-1192-4.

World Health Organization (2022). Musculoskeletal conditions. Fact sheet. https://www.who.int/news-room/fact-sheets/detail/musculoskeletal-conditions.

Zhu, Y., Pandya, B.J., and Choi, H.K. (2011). Prevalence of gout and hyperuricemia in the US general population: the National Health and Nutrition Examination Survey 2007–2008: prevalence of gout and hyperuricemia in the US. *Arthritis and Rheumatism* 63 (10): 3136–3141. https://doi.org/10.1002/art.30520.

Further Reading

329

Manna, A., Sarkar, S., and Khanra, L. (2015). PA1 An internal audit into the adequacy of pain assessment in a hospice setting. *BMJ Supportive and Palliative Care* 5 (Suppl. 1): A19.3–A20. https://doi.org/10.1136/bmjspcare-2015-000906.61.

Online Resources

NHS England. Urgent Care for Paramediv Injuries. https://www.e-lfh.org.uk/urgent-care-for-paramedics-injuries-elearning-available/ Office for Health Improvement and Disparities. Musculoskeletal health: applying All Our Health. https://www.gov.uk/government/publications/musculoskeletal-health-applying-all-our-health/musculoskeletal-health-applying-all-our-health

Glossary

Appendicular skeleton	The appendicular skeleton comprises the upper and lower extremities, which include the shoulder girdle and pelvis.
Arthritis	Arthritis is a common condition that causes pain and swelling (inflammation) in the joints.
Axial skeleton	The axial skeleton is made up of the bones in the head, neck, back and chest.

Cartilage	A strong, flexible connective tissue that protects joints and bones.
Fracture	A broken bone, the same as a crack or a break.
Ligament	Ligaments often connect two bones together, particularly in the joints.
Metatarsal	The bones of the forefoot.
Ossification	The process of bone formation.
Osteoarthritis	The most common form of arthritis. It is a chronic condition that causes pain, stiffness and reduced joint function when the cartilage between bones begins to wear down.
Osteoblast	Cells that build bone.
Osteoclast	Cells that break down bone tissue.
Osteocyte	A bone cell.
Phalanges	Bones that are found in the toes.
Tendon	A cord of strong flexible tissue.

Multiple Choice Questions

1. Which of the following is NOT part of the '6 Ps' of vascular compromise?
   a. Pain
   b. Position
   c. Pallor
   d. Paralysis

2. What are some of the risk factors for gout?
   a. Age over 80
   b. Female sex
   c. Poor diet
   d. All of the above

3. Elbow, knee and interphalangeal are all types of which joint?
   a. Hinge
   b. Plane
   c. Pivot
   d. Saddle

4. What are the main functions of the musculoskeletal system?
   a. Support
   b. Storage
   c. Movement
   d. All of the above

5. Blunt force trauma can lead to cervical fractures in what percentages of incidences?
   a. 2–4%
   b. 10%
   c. 6–8%
   d. <1%

6. What is the world's leading cause of disability?
   a. Fractures
   b. Lower back pain
   c. Gout
   d. Arthritis

7. If a patient had stretched or torn a ligament connecting two bones together, they are said to have what condition?
   a. Sprain
   b. Fracture
   c. Strain
   d. Dislocation

8. Which of the following is a symptom of arthritis?
   a. Pain
   b. Swelling
   c. Stiffness
   d. All of the above

9. A fracture that is caused by an excessive axial load is called what?
   a. Spiral
   b. Compression
   c. Displaced
   d. Transverse

10. Which of the following is a factor that influences bone structure?
    a. Exercise
    b. Diet
    c. Gait
    d. All of the above

CHAPTER 16

Fluid, Electrolyte Balance and Associated Disorders

Noleen P. Jones

AIM

The aim of this chapter is to provide the reader with insight and understanding with regards to fluid, electrolyte balance and associated disorders.

LEARNING OUTCOMES

On completion of this chapter, you will be able to:

- Identify the fluid compartments of the body.
- Differentiate between osmosis, diffusion, filtration and active transport, and their roles in the movement of fluid around the body.
- Discuss the roles of different body systems in regulating the body's fluid composition and volume.
- Explain different clinical manifestations of fluid imbalance, including how they may be treated.

Test Your Prior Knowledge
1. Where is most of the body's fluid volume found?
2. Define the function of body fluids and electrolytes.
3. Define the terms hypotonic, hypertonic and isotonic solutions.
4. What are the signs and symptoms of dehydration?

Introduction

Fluid and electrolytes are essential for homeostatic body function. The constant movement of fluid and electrolytes ensures that cells have a steady supply of electrolytes for cellular function, such as sodium, chloride, potassium, magnesium, phosphate, bicarbonate and calcium.

Fundamentals of Applied Pathophysiology for Paramedics, First Edition. Edited by Ian Peate and Simon Sawyer.

Changes in the movement of fluid and electrolytes between compartments can occur because of disease or environmental changes. This chapter considers fluid and electrolyte balance and some conditions that result when there is an imbalance.

Body Fluid Compartments

Fluid forms approximately 60% of the body weight of an adult male, 50% in an adult female and 70% in infants (Rogers 2022). The percentage of fluid distribution varies with age and sex. Women have a lower volume of body fluid compared with men, as women have more body fat and men have more muscle mass (Rogers 2022). Fat cells contain less water than muscle cells.

The two principal body fluid compartments are intracellular and extracellular. The intracellular compartment is the space inside a cell. Fluid inside the cell is called intracellular fluid. The extracellular compartment is outside the cell and consists of extracellular fluid.

The extracellular compartment is divided into the interstitial compartment and the intravascular compartment (Figure 16.1). Two-thirds of body fluid is found inside the cell and one-third is outside. Eighty percent of the extracellular fluid is in the interstitial compartment and 20% in the intravascular compartment as plasma (Figure 16.2).

Composition of Body Fluid

Body fluid is composed of water and dissolved substances such as electrolytes (sodium, potassium and chloride), gases (oxygen and carbon dioxide), nutrients, enzymes and hormones. Total body water constitutes 60% of total body weight. Water plays an important part in body function as it:

- Lubricates.
- Transports nutrients, oxygen, hormones and enzymes to the cells, and waste products of metabolism (e.g. carbon dioxide, urea and uric acid) from the cells for excretion.

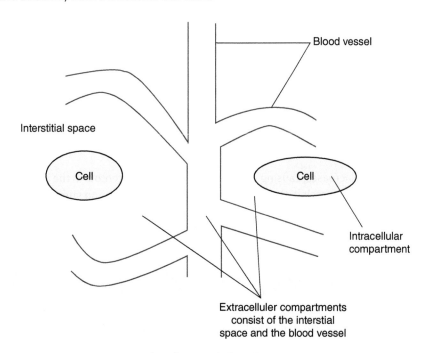

FIGURE 16.1 Fluid compartments. Source: Peate (2021) pg. 485/John Wiley & Sons.

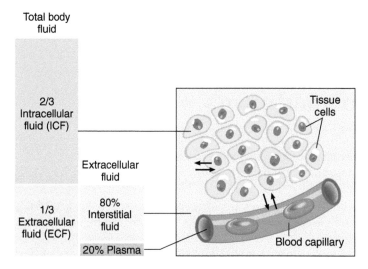

FIGURE 16.2   Fluid distribution. Source: Peate (2021) pg. 485/John Wiley & Sons.

- Helps in the regulation of body temperature.
- Provides a medium for chemical reactions.
- Breaks down food particles in the digestive system.

Body Fluid Balance

The term *fluid balance* indicates that the body's required amount of water is present and distributed proportionally among compartments. Generally, water intake equals water loss, so body fluid remains constant. Fluid intake varies with individuals but the body regulates fluid volume within a narrow range for homeostasis. Most of the water essential for body function comes from drinking, with lesser amounts obtained from food and cellular metabolism.

The kidneys play a vital role in fluid balance, as water excess is excreted through urine. A small amount of water is lost through respiration, skin and in faeces. Table 16.1 gives details of fluid intake and output.

The body regulates body fluid volume via thirst receptors. Body fluid balance disrupts if there is an excess of water loss through sweating that is not replaced through drinking. Dehydration, a state of negative fluid balance, stimulates the thirst reflex in three ways:

- The blood osmotic pressure increases, causing the stimulation of osmoreceptors in the hypothalamus.
- Circulating blood volume decreases, initiating the renin–angiotensin system and stimulating the thirst centre in the hypothalamus.
- The mucosal lining of the mouth dries and the production of saliva decreases, also stimulating the thirst centre.

Red Flag Alert: Fluid Overload

Just as dehydration can be detrimental to a person's health and wellbeing, so too is fluid overload. Fluid overload occurs when circulating volume is more than the heart can effectively manage. This results in heart failure, which causes pulmonary and peripheral oedema.

TABLE 16.1 Fluid intake and output.

Fluid	Amount (ml)
Intake	
Drinking (approximately 60%)	1400–1800
Water from food (approximately 30%)	700–1000
Water of oxidation (approximately 10%)	300–400
Total balance (100%)	2400–3200
Output	
Urine (approximately 60%)	1400–1800
Faeces (approximately 2%)	100
Expiration (lungs approximately 28%)	600–800
Skin (approximately 10%)	300–600
Total balance 100%	2400–3200

Source: Adapted from McCance et al. (2019).

Fluid overload usually presents as acute pulmonary oedema, with the primary symptom of severe dyspnoea. Persistent fluid overload (as occurs in the context of intravascular fluid overload) manifests as chronic heart failure. Nevertheless, the signs and symptoms of heart failure can resemble other respiratory conditions and paramedics must be able to differentiate between these conditions to implement the correct treatment. The main symptoms of chronic heart failure are:

- Fatigue
- Dyspnoea
- Tachycardia
- Pitting oedema.

Osmosis

Water movement between the intracellular and the extracellular compartments takes place through osmosis. Osmosis is a process where water moves from an area of high volume to an area of low volume through a selectively permeable membrane. The movement of water depends on the number of solutes dissolved in the solution and determines its concentration. This is expressed as the osmolality of the solution (Vujovic et al. 2018). The membrane allows water molecules to move across, but it is impermeable to solutes such as sodium, potassium and other substances. Osmotic pressure is the force created by water moving across a membrane due to osmosis: the higher the volume of water, the higher the osmotic pressure.

Tonicity is an alternate term for osmolality. Solutions are termed to be hypertonic, hypotonic or isotonic. A hypertonic solution describes a solution that has a high percentage of solutes dissolved in it (e.g. 5% dextrose). A hypotonic solution is one that has a low concentration of solutes dissolved in it (e.g. 0.45% physiological saline) and an isotonic solution has the same osmolality as body fluids (0.9% physiological saline).

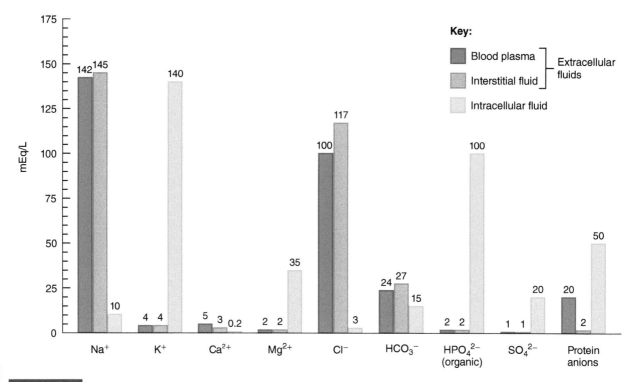

FIGURE 16.3   Electrolytes of intracellular and extracellular compartments. Source: Peate (2021) pg. 571/John Wiley & Sons.

Electrolytes

Fluid balance is linked to electrolyte balance. Electrolytes are chemical compounds that dissociate (separate) in water to form charged particles (ions). They include potassium (K), sodium (Na), chloride (Cl), magnesium (Mg) and hydrogen phosphate (HPO_4; Hseieh 2021). Electrolytes are positively charged *cations* (e.g. Na^+ and K^+) or negatively charged *anions* (e.g. Cl– and HCO_3–). An anion and a cation will combine to form a compound (e.g. potassium, K^+, and chloride, Cl–, will combine to form potassium chloride, KCl). The composition of electrolytes differs between the intracellular and extracellular compartments (Figure 16.3).

Electrolytes have numerous functions in the body:

- Regulation of fluid balance.
- Regulation of acid–base balance.
- Essential in neuromuscular excitability.
- Essential for neuronal function.
- Essential for enzyme reaction.

Table 16.2 Summarises the principal electrolytes and their functions.

Medicines Management: Fluid Mismanagement

Sodium chloride 0.9% is the primary fluid administered by paramedics in the out-of-hospital setting. Fluid administration in the prehospital environment should be administered following careful assessment of the patient's presenting condition and history in conjunction with appropriate clinical practice guidelines. Patients suffering from congestive heart failure, chronic liver or kidney disease and those with swelling due to excess fluid retention are particularly susceptible to the adverse effects of fluid overload.

TABLE 16.2 Principal electrolytes and their functions.

Electrolytes	Normal values in extracellular fluid (mmol/l)	Function	Main distribution
Sodium (Na^+)	135–145	Plays an important role in fluid and electrolyte balance. One of the cations which generate action potentials	Main cation of extracellular fluid
Potassium (K+)	3.5–5	Important cation in establishing resting membrane potential. Regulates pH balance. Sustains intracellular fluid volume	Main cation of intracellular fluid
Calcium (Ca^{2+})	2.1–2.6	Paramount for clotting. Essential in neurotransmitter release in neurons. Maintains muscle tone and excitability of nervous and muscle tissue	Mainly found in the extracellular fluid
Magnesium (Mg^{2+})	0.5–1.0	Helps to maintain normal nerve and muscle function; maintains regular heart rate, regulates blood glucose and blood pressure. Essential for protein synthesis	Mainly distributed in the intracellular fluid
Chloride (Cl^-)	98–117	Maintains a balance of anions in different fluid compartments	Main anion of the extracellular fluid
Hydrocarbons (HCO_3^-)	24–31	Main buffer of hydrogen ions in plasma. Maintains a balance between cations and anions of intracellular and extracellular fluids	Mainly distributed in the extracellular fluid
Phosphate – organic (HPO_4^{2-})	0.8–1.1	Essential for the digestion of proteins, carbohydrates and fats and absorption of calcium. Essential for bone formation	Mainly found in the intracellular fluid
Sulphate (SO_4^{2-})	0.5	Involved in detoxification of phenols, alcohols and amines	Mainly found in the intracellular fluid

Diffusion

Diffusion is a process by which solutes move from an area of high concentration to an area of low concentration. It is subdivided into simple and facilitated diffusion. Liquid-soluble molecules and gases move by simple diffusion through a concentration gradient (Figure 16.4). Larger molecules such as glucose and amino acids are transported across a cell membrane by a carrier protein and concentration gradient (Figure 16.5).

Hormones That Regulate Fluid and Electrolytes

Two principal hormones regulate fluid and electrolyte balance: antidiuretic hormone (ADH) and aldosterone (Ebright 2020). ADH regulates fluid balance in the body. It is produced in the hypothalamus by neurons called osmoreceptors and is stored by the posterior pituitary gland. Osmoreceptors are sensitive to plasma osmolality and a decrease in blood volume. ADH acts on the distal convoluted tubule and the collecting ducts (see Chapter 11) of the kidney, making them more permeable to water, thus increasing reabsorption of water.

Aldosterone is a steroid hormone produced by the cortex of the adrenal glands, situated atop of each kidney (Figure 16.6). The adrenal gland is divided into the cortex and the medulla (Figure 16.7). Aldosterone regulates electrolyte and fluid balance by sodium and water retention.

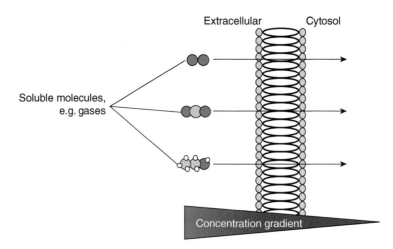

FIGURE 16.4   Simple diffusion. Source: Peate (2021) pg. 572/John Wiley & Sons.

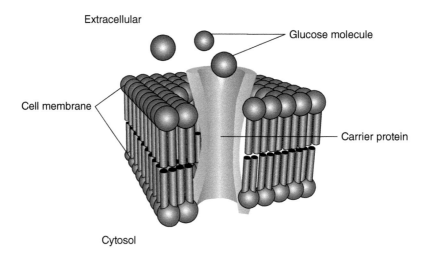

FIGURE 16.5   Carrier protein (facilitated diffusion). Source: Peate (2021) pg. 572/John Wiley & Sons.

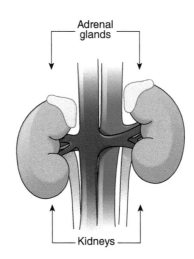

FIGURE 16.6   Adrenal glands. Source: Peate (2021) pg. 573/John Wiley & Sons.

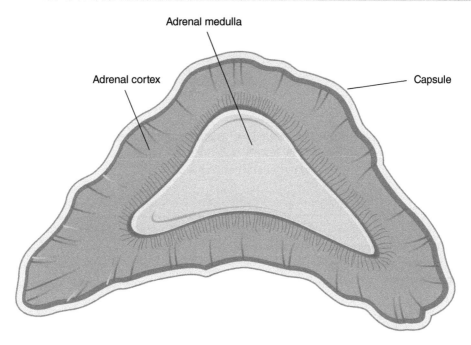

FIGURE 16.7 Cross-section of the adrenal gland. Source: Peate (2021) pg. 574/John Wiley & Sons.

Oedema

Oedema is the abnormal accumulation of fluid, mainly water (Kumar and Clark 2020), in the interstitial space. It is a problem of fluid distribution and does not indicate fluid excess (Rogers 2022). The accumulation of fluid may be localised, as in thrombophlebitis, or generalised, as in heart failure, which affects all body tissue. Localised oedema is normally temporary and resolves without intervention. Generalised oedema is an abnormal condition that requires treatment.

Oedema can either be pitting or non-pitting. If an indentation develops after gently pressing the swollen lower limb with a finger, this is pitting oedema (Wilson 2017). The causes of oedema include:

- Heart failure
- Obesity resulting in increased fluid pressure and salt retention
- Drugs such as calcium antagonists (e.g. verapamil and nifedipine) and prolonged steroid therapy
- Renal conditions such as nephrotic syndrome
- Venous stasis resulting from immobility
- Varicose veins
- Liver cirrhosis causing hypoalbuminaemia.

Pulmonary Oedema

Pulmonary oedema is a condition where there is accumulation of fluid in the lungs, resulting in impaired gas exchange and pulmonary function. Pulmonary oedema can result from:

- Congestive heart failure
- Fluid overload as a result of renal failure
- Myocardial infarction with left ventricular failure
- Chest injury as a result of a road traffic collision or other trauma

- Upper airway obstruction
- Severe chest infection.

Peripheral Oedema

Peripheral oedema describes localised soft-tissue swelling resulting from fluid accumulation in the interstitial space. Fluid accumulates in parts of the body affected by gravity (e.g. the lower limbs in mobile patients or around the sacral region in patients who are immobile). Causes of peripheral oedema include:

- Immobility
- Obesity
- Heart failure
- Pregnancy as a result of fluid retention and venous stasis
- Liver diseases such as cirrhosis of the liver
- Prolonged steroid therapy.

Disorders Associated with Fluid and Electrolyte Imbalance

Maintaining Fluid Balance

Fluid balance occurs where the amount of fluid taken into the body equals the amount of fluid that leaves the body (Marieb and Hoehn 2019). Maintenance of fluid balance is an important activity, essential for optimal health. If a patient has too much fluid and there is an imbalance, this can cause health problems; likewise, if the patient has too little fluid, this too can cause problems. There are some pathophysiological conditions that can result in fluid overloading (e.g. kidney disease and some types of heart disease); when this occurs, the person finds it difficult to rid the body of excess water and can experience oedema (i.e. there is too much fluid in the tissues of the body – care of the patient with oedema is discussed later).

Most people are able to maintain an adequate level of hydration – they are prompted by thirst to seek fluids. However, those who are ill and dependent are unable to do this and may be at risk of becoming dehydrated. Dehydration is a common fluid and electrolyte imbalance in older people (Picetti et al. 2017).

This section considers the healthcare professional's responses to ensure that patients are adequately hydrated. It draws on previous sections of the chapter in respect to fluid and electrolyte balance. Hydration is the state of fluid balance of the body and dehydration occurs when the state of fluid output exceeds intake. Rapid weight loss as a result of dehydration can be the consequence of a lack of fluid intake or hyponatraemia (sodium depletion) with an accompanying loss of water (Giddens 2017).

Benefits of Good Hydration

There are many benefits associated with good hydration. The implications of poor hydration from a pathophysiological perspective can have many ramifications and some are discussed here.

Elderly patients who are poorly hydrated have the potential to develop pressure sores (decubitus ulcers). Dehydration results in a reduction in padding over bony prominences. Additionally, inadequate fluid intake is a common cause of chronic constipation. Improving hydration can increase stool frequency and enhance the beneficial effects of daily dietary fibre intake (Bellini et al. 2021). Optimising hydration can also help to promote renal function, prevents urinary tract infections and gallstone formation.

In relation to heart disease, hydration reduces the risk of coronary heart disease, as adequate hydration decreases blood viscosity, thereby protecting against clot formation. Extracellular volume depletion is the result of a net loss of total body sodium with a reduction in intravascular volume. A well-hydrated patient will also find it easier to expectorate respiratory secretions (Myatt 2016).

Dehydration can worsen diabetic control. Water is an essential aspect of the dietary management of diabetes mellitus. People who have poorly controlled diabetes may experience an increase in urinary output which can, in turn, result in dehydration. Good hydration levels can slow down the development of diabetic ketoacidosis, helping to maintain healthy blood glucose levels (Effective Diabetes Education Now 2018).

Dehydration is a risk factor associated with falls in older people (Hamrick et al. 2020). Disorientation, dizziness, headache and tiredness are symptoms of dehydration, which increases the possibility of fainting and falling. Adequate hydration is therefore part of an effective falls prevention strategy.

Children generate extra metabolic heat, sweat less and produce higher core temperature responses when compared with adults, causing them to overheat rapidly. This means that their bodies are less efficient at handling heat dissipation. Heatstroke can develop quickly in active children who are not drinking properly, or in infants who are overdressed. Symptoms include:

- Confusion
- Seizures
- Flushed, hot, dry skin.

Heatstroke is a medical emergency and should be treated with temperature-lowering techniques, such as the removal of clothing and the application of wrapped chemical cold packs to neck, groin and axillae (Joint Royal College Ambulance Liaison Committee 2021).

There may be instances where paramedics are required to commence an intravenous infusion to replace a patient's fluid loss; for instance, in severe hypovolaemia. Particular caution should be exercised with children and cardiac patients because of the risk of unintentional fluid overload.

Orange Flag Alert: Delerium

Maintaining normal fluid and electrolyte balance can help to prevent delirium (sudden confusion). Dehydration is a modifiable delirium risk factor. Changes in mental status begin with mild dehydration and worsen with each stage, culminating in delirium. In moderate dehydration, short-term memory loss occurs. Failure to recognise signs of dehydration predisposes older people to becoming increasingly and chronically dehydrated, which can lead to delirium.

Snapshot 16.1 Heatstroke

Pre-arrival Information

Six-year-old Aisha is found unconscious inside her father's car during a summer afternoon. She had gone out to play with her neighbour two hours earlier and they had been playing hide and seek. Aisha had found her father's car unlocked in the driveway, hidden in there and fallen asleep. Her friend was called home by her mother and did not return to play. She was discovered when her father went to get some papers from the car. An ambulance was called and control has requested you respond.

Dispatched: 2.15 p.m.
Arrival: 2.30 p.m.

On Arrival with the Patient

Airway: clear.
Breathing: bilateral chest rise, lung sounds clear, fast.
Cardiac: pulses present, weak, fast.
Disability: Not alert or rousable.
Exposure: no immediate life threats found.
Background: age six years, female; weight and height: approx. 25 kg and 117 cm.
Medical history none.
Medications: none.

Paediatric Assessment Triangle

Appearance: unrousable.
Work of breathing: increased work of breathing, bilateral chest rise and fall.
Circulation to skin: flushed dry skin.

Vital Signs

Vital signs taken are:

Vital sign	Observation	Normal ranges
Pulse (beats/min)	130	80–100 regular
Respiration rate (breaths/min)	2	12–20
SpO$_2$ (%)	95 (on air)	94–98
Blood pressure (mmHg)	108/60	120/80
Temperature (°C)	39.4	37
Eyes	1	4 – spontaneously
Verbal	1	5 – orientated
Motor	1	6 – obeys commands
Total GCS score	3	15
ECG	Sinus tachycardia	

Reflective Learning Activity

Considering the details in Snapshot 16.1, how you would proceed:

- What is potentially going on from a pathophysiology perspective?
- What are your priorities of treatment in this case?
- How will your interventions and treatment plan improve the child's condition?

Red Flag Alert: Shivering

Shivering increases endogenous heat production and should therefore be suppressed, particularly in children with heatstroke. Benzodiazepines may be considered to induce muscle relaxation.

Nausea and Vomiting

There are many reasons why a person may feel nauseous and/or vomit. Most patients will experience nausea and/or vomiting during a disease process because of its pathology or the consequence of treatment. Both nausea and vomiting can be particularly upsetting for the patient and can also impact on the person's ability to perform their activities of living.

Nausea

Leslie (2019) describes nausea as an unpleasant sensation of imminent vomiting of the stomach contents through the mouth. The sensation produces a feeling of discomfort in the region of the stomach with a feeling of a need to vomit. Nausea can be short-lived or long-lasting. A person may experience nausea alone, with no vomiting, or they may vomit without any feeling of nausea beforehand. Nausea is a symptom of many conditions. It is not an illness and not all of its causes are related to the stomach (e.g. those patients who are receiving chemotherapy may experience nausea due to adverse drug effects). The following can also cause nausea:

- Diabetes mellitus
- Influenza
- Gastroenteritis
- Renal failure
- Adrenal insufficiency
- Peptic ulcer
- Vertigo
- Pregnancy.

Treatment of nausea will depend on its cause. For instance, the paramedic may opt for an antiemetic more suited to manage the cause.

Medication Management: Antiemetics

Antiemetics are medications given to prevent or stop nausea and vomiting. They work by blocking specific neurotransmitters, thereby addressing different origins of nausea. For instance, the drug ondansetron is a serotonin receptor blocker, which acts on gastrointestinal nerve terminals and alleviates feelings of sickness for people on chemotherapy. Promethazine, another antiemetic, inhibits histamine, which can cause motion sickness.

Vomiting

Vomiting is a complex physiological activity, defined as the forceful expulsion of gastric contents through the mouth and/or nose. Excessive vomiting can have a profound effect on a person's fluid and electrolyte balance (Waugh and Grant 2018). The vomiting centre, situated in the medulla oblongata of the brain, is responsible for the initiation of vomiting. Both physical and psychological impulses can excite the vomiting centre, such as:

- Fear/anxiety
- Odours
- Pain
- Unpleasant sights

343

- Adverse effects of some drugs
- Radiotherapy
- Hypercalcaemia.

It is important to determine, if possible, the cause of vomiting. Removal of the causative factor, if possible, should be the first line of treatment. Caring for the patient who is vomiting will include the following steps:

- Disinfect hands.
- Don personal protective equipment.
- Ask the patient if they have any tried and tested methods of dealing with vomiting and, if appropriate, implement them.
- Ensure the patient is cared for in an upright (unless contraindicated) position.
- Consider the lateral position if the patient is unconscious and unable to protect their own airway.
- Administer an appropriate antiemetic medication.
- Provide easy access to a vomit bowl and tissues.
- Observe, measure, record and report vomitus.
- Provide the patient with the opportunity to use a mouthwash.
- Provide the patient with the opportunity to 'freshen up' after they have finished vomiting.
- Dispose soiled items according to policy and procedure.
- Document type and quantity of vomitus.

The patient may complain of exhaustion or headache, and muscle soreness can also occur with excessive vomiting. An explanation of why the person may feel like this, as well as the administration of an appropriate analgesic, can help to provide comfort. Attention must be paid to the effects of extreme vomiting, as it can lead to electrolyte imbalance and an ensuing acid–base (i.e. acidosis) discrepancy. The management of this imbalance will depend on the extent of vomiting and the patient's overall condition.

344

Snapshot 16.2   Hyperkalaemia

Pre-arrival Information

Brian, who is 67 years of age, was found collapsed by his son on his bathroom floor in an agitated state. His son had spoken to Brian on the phone yesterday evening during which he had complained of nausea, diarrhoea, abdominal cramps and general muscle weakness. Brian lives alone and is regularly visited by his son and two daughters. An ambulance was called and control has requested you respond.

Dispatched: 10:20 a.m.
Arrival: 10:35 a.m.

On Arrival with the Patient

Airway: clear.
Breathing: bilateral chest rise, shallow, fast.
Cardiac: pulses present, weak, regular.
Disability: altered mental status, agitated.
Exposure: no immediate life threats found.
Background: age 67 years, male; weight approx. 75 kg.
Medical history: congestive heart failure, diabetes, osteoarthritis, hypertension.
Medications: amlodipine, ramipril, metoprolol, ibuprofen, metformin.

Vital Signs

His vital signs are:

Vital sign	Observation	80–100 regular
Pulse (beats/min)	72	12–20
Respiration rate (breaths/min)	32	94–98
SpO$_2$ (%)	90	120/80
Blood pressure (mmHg)	80/62	37
Temperature (°C)	37.2	80–100 regular
Blood glucose level (mmol/l)	24.2	
Eyes	4	4 – spontaneously
Verbal	4	5 – orientated
Motor	5	6 – obeys commands
Total GCS score	13	15
ECG	Sinus rhythm with elongated PR interval, wide QRS, depressed ST segment and tall peaked T waves.	

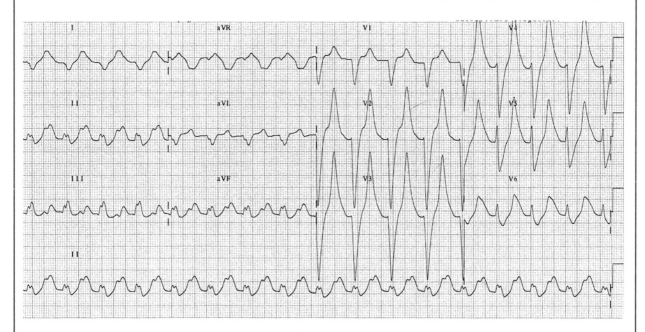

Reflective Learning Activity

Consider how you would manage the patient's condition:

- What is your differential diagnosis here?
- The patient is confirmed to have a potassium level of 9.1 mmol/l; what is going on from a pathophysiology perspective?
- What are your priorities for managing Brian's care?

Reflective Learning Activity

Reflect on the following:

- How can an ECG be beneficial in detecting electrolyte imbalances?
- What additional symptoms could Brian have experienced with hyperkalaemia?
- What treatment is Brian likely to receive in the emergency department?

Medicines Management: Diuretics

Diuretics are commonly referred to by patients as 'water tablets'. They are used to assist with the excretion of excess fluids from the body. The reduction in fluid volume contributes to the reduction in pressure and therefore improves cardiac function. There are different categories of diuretics. Loop diuretics can remove a significant amount of fluid and tend to be used in emergency situations. Potassium-sparing diuretics assist with the retention of potassium while assisting with the excretion of fluid.

Clinical Investigations

A colonoscopy is a type of imaging test that is undertaken to visualise the inner lining of the large intestine. A thin, flexible tube is slowly and gently inserted into the anus and then moved gradually through the rectum and colon. An internal camera inside the scope electronically transmits images to an external video-processing unit. Air is used to inflate the colon to promote visualisation.

The examination helps doctors to determine whether there is any internal trauma from polyps, tumours or areas of inflammation. A biopsy (a tissue sample) is obtained while the procedure is being performed if the examiner notices any abnormal growths. The test takes approximately 30–45 minutes.

In most cases, prior to the test, bowel preparation is usually required; however, in an emergency this test may be negated. Bowel preparation is normally started one to two days before the examination, depending on local policy and procedure. During the test, local preference may be to administer intravenous analgesia and a sedative. These preparations help the patient to relax during the procedure and often they remember very little about it. Instructions are given to the patient after the test, depending on what procedure was carried out, what was found and whether any treatment was given. This must be documented in the patient's notes.

Red Flag Alert: Colonoscopy Damage

There is a possibility that a colonoscopy may cause damage to the colon. This may result in bleeding, infection and perforation (rare). The paramedic should be vigilant to the following if the patient has undergone a colonoscopy within the last 48 hours:

- Abdominal pain, in particular if this becomes gradually worse and is different or more intense to any 'usual' pains the patient may have.
- Pyrexia (fever).
- Excessive bleeding from the rectum. A small amount of bleeding is not unusual after colonoscopy, and is acceptable for a couple of days. People should seek help if the bleeding is heavy and accompanied by severe abdominal pain or fever.

Caring for the Patient with Oedema

The abnormal collection of fluid in the interstitial spaces is known as oedema (Kumar and Clark 2020). This section of the chapter provides an overview of the care required for the patient with oedema to maintain a safe environment and provide comfort. The causes of pulmonary and peripheral oedema are discussed above.

Pulmonary Oedema

Many patients who are diagnosed with pulmonary oedema will be acutely ill and they (and their families) may be highly anxious and afraid. The paramedic must provide care that takes both the physical and psychological aspects of the condition into account for both the patient and family.

The first line of treatment should be to determine the cause of pulmonary oedema and to take steps to eliminate or reduce it; attempts should be made to reverse the specific cause(s). For example, if the cause is left-sided heart failure, then measures should be taken to improve the pumping action of the left side of the heart.

Signs and Symptoms

The signs and symptoms of pulmonary oedema can include some or all of the following:

- Dyspnoea/orthopnoea
- Wheeze
- Tachycardia and tachypnoea
- Hypotension
- Cardiogenic shock
- Sweating
- Pallor/cyanosis
- Nausea
- Anxiety
- Dry or productive cough (pink frothy sputum).

Clinical Investigations

It is important to remember that pulmonary oedema can result in mild to severe dyspnoea; therefore, when obtaining a history from the patient to make a diagnosis, this must be borne in mind; questioning of the patient should be kept to an absolute minimum. The paramedic should ask questions that are only absolutely necessary and framed in such a way that the patient need only nod or shake their head to make a response. After a detailed history has been taken from the primary source (the patient) or secondary sources (i.e. other healthcare professionals, the patient's partner, family or friends), the following investigations may be required once in hospital:

- Chest x-ray
- Blood gas analysis
- Estimation of cardiac enzymes
- Liver function tests
- Estimation of urea and electrolytes
- Electrocardiogram.

Care and Management

Treatment of the specific cause of pulmonary oedema should continue and the patient's airway must also be managed, if dyspnoea becomes so severe that this is in danger; in the acute phase, the patient may need to be resuscitated. The key aim should be to improve oxygenation, and this can be done by the administration of oxygen therapy. As pulmonary oedema indicates that there is an abnormal collection of fluid in the interstitial spaces, it is imperative that there is strict control of fluid balance and, in some cases, a urinary catheter may need to be necessary to provide close monitoring of urinary output.

Below is an overview of the management of the patient with pulmonary oedema in the prehospital period. This is not a comprehensive list and care will be dictated by the patient's condition and response to the therapeutic interventions possible during this time:

- Provide reassurance, psychological and physical support and explanations (for the patient and family) for care interventions.
- Provide a sputum receptacle and tissues.
- Care for the patient in an upright position (unless this is contraindicated), supported by pillows.
- Administer prescribed humidified oxygen via a face mask.
- Administer prescribed medication (e.g. diuretics such as furosemide) with appropriate analgesia to alleviate anxiety, pain and distress.
- Monitor, measure and report oxygen saturation, blood pressure, respiratory rate, depth and rhythm; also monitor pulse frequency, dictated by the patient's condition.

Peripheral Oedema

Peripheral oedema presents as a collection of excessive fluid that pools within the tissues in the dependent regions (e.g. the legs, ankles, feet and sacral region; Waugh and Grant 2018). Pitting oedema is the more serious type of oedema. Goyal et al. (2021) suggest that peripheral oedema does not appear or become visible until the body has retained up to 3 litres of fluid. If, for example, a patient retains 5.5 litres of fluid, this is equivalent to 5.5 kg of weight; hence, one way of determining whether the patient is retaining fluid is to record daily weight, together with meticulous fluid balance monitoring when in hospital.

Snapshot 16.3   Lymphoedema

Pre-arrival Information

Dispatched: 8.16 a.m.
Arrival: 8.43 a.m.

Background

Leon Radcliffe is 72 years of age. He lives alone with his wife, who is blind. He is her main carer. They have no children. Leon has metastatic prostate cancer. He developed severe scrotal oedema while he was receiving palliative chemotherapy. The swelling has caused him much distress, anxiety and fear. He cannot wear underpants and has to be very selective with the style of trousers he wears. He rarely goes out because of the scrotal oedema, which causes him pain and embarrassment. He relies on neighbours to help with shopping and odd jobs around the house.

Leon's scrotal oedema makes standing and sitting very difficult. He finds it difficult to get comfortable, he struggles to have a good night's sleep and there is now fluid seepage in the scrotum.

Leon wakes one morning after a restless night to find his scrotum more painful than usual as well as hot and red. He feels feverish and lethargic and although he has called for an ambulance, he is anxious to remain at home to care for his wife.

Primary Survey

Airway: Airway clear. Patient able to talk.
Breathing: Patient noted to be short of breath. End-tidal carbon dioxide 30 mmHg. Clear, bilateral air entry. 3 l O_2 administered via nasal cannula.
Circulation: Radial pulse 108 beats/minute, regular.
Blood pressure: 101/55 mmHg.
Capillary refill time: 2.5 seconds.

Disability: Alert.
Medications: has taken paracetamol 1 g 2 hours ago for pain.
Exposure: Gross oedema and pustules noted on scrotum.

Vital Signs

Vital signs are:

Vital sign	Observation	Normal range
Pulse (beats/min)	108	12–20
Respiration rate (breaths/min)	24	94–98
SpO$_2$ (%)	93 (on air)	120/80
Blood pressure (mmHg)	101/55	37
Temperature (°C)	38.4	80–100 regular
Eyes	4	4 – spontaneously
Verbal	5	5 – orientated
Motor	6	6 – obeys commands
Total GCS score	15	15
Pain	7	
ECG	Sinus tachycardia	

Background: age 72 years, male; weight/height 76 kg.
Medical history: metastatic cancer of the prostate.
Medication: fentanyl transdermal patch 50 µg/minute.

Reflective Learning Activity

Reflect on the information in Snapshot 16.3, then consider the following questions:

- What indicates that Leon may have an infection?
- It is clear that Mr Radcliffe is distressed. How can paramedics, working in an integrated way, assist him from a psychosocial perspective?
- What is your proposed treatment to manage Leon?

Skin that has become oedematous predisposes the patient to the development of pressure sores (decubitus ulcers) and infection, particularly when the skin over the oedematous area has broken down (Jaul et al. 2018). This risk can become more evident when healthcare professionals who handle patients with oedema have long or sharp fingernails, watches, pens, badges and scissors that can potentially catch the patient's skin and cause more trauma; hence, the importance of short nails and the covering of items of equipment in the healthcare professional's pockets. The principles of care for the patient who has peripheral oedema include:

- A clear explanation of the condition to the patient and, if appropriate, their family.
- Assessment of skin condition in association with local policy for skin assessment.

349

- Fluid balance monitoring/ daily weight measurement.
- Administration of prescribed diuretics (e.g. furosemide).
- Elevation of oedematous ankles when sitting out of bed to aid drainage of the pooled fluid.

Medicines Management: Furosemide

Furosemide is a diuretic often used to reduce oedema due to heart failure, hepatic impairment or renal disease and to treat hypertension. The drug works by inhibiting the reabsorption of sodium and chloride from the loop of Henle and distal renal tubule. It increases renal excretion of water, sodium, chloride, magnesium, potassium and calcium. Therapeutically, the medication causes diuresis and subsequent mobilisation of excess fluid (oedema, pleural effusions). It can decrease blood pressure. The drug can be administered orally, intramuscularly or intravenously. It should be used cautiously in:

- Severe hepatic disease (may cause hepatic coma; concurrent use with potassium-sparing diuretics may be necessary)
- Electrolyte depletion
- Diabetes mellitus
- Hypoproteinaemia
- Severe renal impairment.

Orange Flag Alert:Diuretics

A major anxiety for people taking diuretics is the fear of wetting themselves (Meraz 2020). This may lead to non-adherence with treatment. The paramedic who suspects that a stable patient is not taking their medication should allow for discussion about their concerns but still reinforce the importance of treatment adherence. They should also suggest that the patient consult their doctor or practice nurse about their fears.

Take Home Points

- Body fluid balance is essential to maintain homeostasis.
- Imbalances in the levels of fluid and electrolyte can result in severe illness.
- Unrecognised circulatory overload and dehydration can have series repercussions for individuals.
- Vulnerable groups such as the very young and the elderly are particular susceptible to serious illness from fluid imbalances.
- Paramedics are required to understand the pathophysiology of body fluid balance to identify and treat related disorders.

Summary

Understanding the complex concepts and processes of fluid and electrolyte balance is vital if safe and effective care is to be provided to patients who may sometimes be critically ill as a result of fluid and electrolyte imbalance. Healthcare professionals have a pivotal role to play when helping people who are experiencing pathophysiological changes associated with fluid and electrolyte imbalance.

The dynamics of fluid balance can have a profound effect on an individual's health and wellbeing. The subtle changes associated with fluid balance have to be recognised quickly by the healthcare professional to avert harm; this can be done in many ways, using all the senses as well as implementing the fundamentals of science.

It is not possible in a chapter of this size to address in depth all concerns associated with fluid and electrolyte balance and its associated disorders. The reader is advised to access more detailed texts and other forms of information related to fluid and electrolytes with the key aim of providing care that is safe, effective and founded on a sound evidence base.

References

Bellini, M., Tonarelli, S., Barracca, F. et al. (2021). Chronic constipation: is a nutritional approach reasonable? *Nutrients* 13: 3386. https://doi.org/10.3390/nu13103386.

Ebright, C. (2020). *Back to Basics: Perfusion*. Limmer Education. https://limmereducation.com/article/back-to-basics-perfusion. (accessed 11 October 2023).

Effective Diabetes Education Now (2018). *Sick Day Rules: Type 1 Diabetes*. Leicester: Leicester Diabetes Centre. https://static1.squarespace.com/static/5a6439bab7411c94f2ebe216/t/5dcd223fc05f010766bd0bf6/1573724736814/Sick_Day_Rules_Infographic_V2.pdf. (accessed 11 October 2023).

Giddens, J.F. (2017). *Concepts for Nursing Practice*, 2e. Philadelphia, PA: Elsevier.

Goyal, A., Cusick, A.S., and Bhutta, B.S. (2021). *Peripheral Edema*. Treasure Island, FL: StatPearls Publishing. https://www.ncbi.nlm.nih.gov/books/NBK554452 (accessed 11 October 2023).

Hamrick, I., Norton, D., and Birstler, J. (2020). Association between dehydration and falls. *Mayo Clinic Proceedings: Innovations, Quality Outcomes* 4 (3): 259–265.

Hseieh, A. (2021). *What EMS providers need to know about electrolyte disorders*. EMS1. https://www.ems1.com/patient-assessment/articles/what-ems-providers-need-to-know-about-electrolyte-disorders-GqF3TECwDcimTslV (accessed 111 October 2023).

Jaul, E., Barron, J., Rosenzweig, J.P. et al. (2018). An overview of co-morbidities and the development of pressure ulcers among older adults. *BMC Geriatrics* 18: 305. https://doi.org/10.1186/s12877-018-0997-7.

Joint Royal College Ambulance Liaison Committee (2021). Heat illness. In: *JRCALC Clinical Guidelines*, 250–255. Bridgewater: Class Professional Publishing.

Kumar, P. and Clark, M. (2020). *Clinical Medicine*, 10e. Edinburgh: Elsevier.

Leslie, T. (2019). Nausea and vomiting. In: *Patient Assessment in Clinical Pharmacy* (ed. S. Mahmoud), 79–89. Cham, Switzerland: Springer.

Marieb, E.N. and Hoehn, K. (2019). *Human Anatomy and Physiology*, 11e. Boston, MA: Pearson.

Rogers, J. (2022). *McCance and Huether's Pathophysiology: The Biologic Basis for Disease in Adults and Children,* 9e. St Louis, MO: Mosby.

Meraz, R. (2020). Medication nonadherence or self-care? Understanding the medication decision-making process and experiences of older adults with heart failure. *Journal of Cardiovascular Nursing* 5 (1): 26–34.

Myatt, R. (2016). Sputum collection and analysis: what the nurse needs to know. *Nursing Standard* 31 (27): 40–43. https://doi.org/10.7748/ns.2017.e10228.

Peate, I. (ed.) (2021). *Fundamentals of Applied Pathophysiology: An essential guide for nursing and healthcare students*, 4e. Oxford: Wiley Blackwell.

Picetti, D., Foster, S., Pangle, A.K. et al. (2017). Hydration health literacy in the elderly. *Nutrition and Healthy Aging* 4 (3): 227–237. https://doi.org/10.3233/NHA-170026.

Vujovic, P., Chirillo, M., and Silverthorn, D.U. (2018). Learning (by) osmosis: approach to teaching osmolarity and tonicity. *Advances in Physiology Education* 42 (4): 626–635.

Waugh, A. and Grant, A. (2018). *Ross and Wilson Anatomy and Physiology in Health and Illness*, 13e. Edinburgh: Elsevier.

Wilson, S.F. (2017). Perfusion. In: *Concepts for Nursing Practice* (ed. J.F. Giddens), 148–160. St Louis, MO: Elsevier.

Further Reading

Institute for Safe Medication Practices. (2021) *Administration of Concentrated Potassium Chloride for Injection During a Code: Still Deadly!* https://www.ismp.org/resources/administration-concentrated-potassium-chloride-injection-during-code-still-deadly (accessed 11 October 2023).

Online Resources

National Institute for Health and Care Excellence (NICE): www.nice.org.uk

NICE provides guidance, sets quality standards and manages a national database to improve people's health and prevent and treat ill health. There are many excellent resources on this website that can help guide and inform practice.

Lymphoedema Support Network: http://www.lymphoedema.org

The Lymphoedema Support Network is the only national patient-led organisation offering information and support to people with this condition and has a unique understanding of the patients' experience. It provides a high standard of information as well as promoting self-help.

Water UK: www.water.org.uk

This website includes a section called Water for Health and it describes the Water for Health initiative that was launched to guide and inform health professionals and health authorities, to stimulate interest and research in hydration, and to help move water up the public health agenda. This is a user-friendly, helpful site.

Office for Health Improvement and Disparities: https://www.gov.uk/government/organisations/office-for-health-improvement-and-disparities

Focuses on improving the nation's health so that everyone can expect to live more of life in good health, and on levelling up health disparities to break the link between background and prospects for a healthy life. Responsible for publishing health statistics.

Age UK: www.ageuk.org.uk

This national website is packed with information for the general public and healthcare professionals concerning the older population. It includes a section called professional resources; this contains links to (among other things) policy and research.

Glossary of Terms

Adrenal insufficiency	
Amine	An organic compound that contains nitrogen.
Anion	A negatively charged ion.
Anti-emetic	A drug that reduces nausea and vomiting.
Anuria	Failure of the kidneys to produce urine.
Cation	A positively charged ion.
Decubitus ulcers	Pressure sores.
Electrolyte	A chemical element or compound which carries a positive or negative electrical charge, such as sodium, potassium, calcium, chloride and bicarbonate.
Heatstroke	A serious condition caused by the rise of body temperature above 40° Celsius.
Obesity	Disproportionate fat accumulation that presents a risk to health.
Oedema	Excess fluid accumulation in the body tissues characterised by swelling.
Osmolality	Also known as tonicity; a measure of the concentration of dissolved particles in a specific unit of water.

Multiple Choice Questions

1. The highest potassium levels are found in which fluid?
   a. Interstitial fluid
   b. Intracellular fluid
   c. Intravascular fluid
   d. Cerebrospinal fluid

2. Extracellular fluid has what content in relation to intracellular fluid?
   a. Higher protein content
   b. Higher potassium content
   c. Higher sodium content
   d. Higher nutrient content

3. The movement of fluid between compartments is regulated by what?
   a. osmotic and hydrostatic pressure
   b. ADH
   c. the kidneys
   d. the hypothalamus

4. Which of these is NOT a sign of fluid overload?
   a. Tachycardia
   b. Weight gain
   c. Thick and viscous saliva
   d. Oedematous skin

5. What stimulates the release of ADH from the posterior pituitary gland?
   a. Increased blood levels of sodium
   b. Decreased blood levels of sodium
   c. Increased blood levels of potassium
   d. Decreased blood levels of potassium

6. Which of the following statements is true of someone is said to be in a 'positive fluid balance'?
   a. The fluid output has exceeded the input.
   b. The balance of body fluid is even
   c. The fluid input has exceeded the output.
   d. 'Positive' means 'good'.

7. Which of the following is NOT a symptom of heatstroke?
   a. Confusion/loss of consciousness
   b. Hallucinations
   c. Dry lips
   d. Pale skin

8. How does pulmonary oedema usually manifest?
   a. Slow pulse and breathing
   b. Shortness of breath and fast pulse
   c. High blood pressure and chesty cough
   d. Fast pulse and high blood pressure

9. Peripheral oedema may result from what?
   a. Lymphatic blockage
   b. Hypertension
   c. Drinking large amount of beer
   d. Diabetes insipidus

10. What type of intravenous fluid has a low osmolality?
    a. Isotonic
    b. Colloid
    c. Hypertonic
    d. Hypotonic

CHAPTER 17

The Skin and Associated Disorders

Melanie Stephens and Derek Fox

AIM

The aim of this chapter is to increase knowledge of the skin and associated disorders.

LEARNING OUTCOMES

On completion of this chapter, you will be able to:

- Classify and describe the structures and functions of the skin, hair and nails.
- Identify the phases of wound healing.
- Describe the functions of the skin.
- Recognise common skin disorders and wounds.
- Explain the process of a holistic skin and wound assessment.
- Describe initial emergency management of common skin disorders and wounds.
- Identify referral to other care pathways and members of the interdisciplinary team.

Test Your Prior Knowledge

1. What are the three layers of the skin?
2. What are the four phases of wound healing?
3. Wounds can be classified on the length of time they have been present; what are two main classifications?
4. Name five causative factors of burn injuries?

Fundamentals of Applied Pathophysiology for Paramedics, First Edition. Edited by Ian Peate and Simon Sawyer.
© 2024 John Wiley & Sons Ltd. Published 2024 by John Wiley & Sons Ltd.

Introduction

The physical and psychosocial impact of a skin disorder cannot be ignored. When patients are managed holistically from the start of their injury or illness through to the delivery of longer-term care, this impact can be greatly reduced. Paramedics will often only see people with skin disorders at their worst, so to assist in decreasing patient suffering and the recurrence of skin disorders, paramedics require the appropriate level of knowledge and skills in this speciality (National Wound Care Strategy Programme 2021).

Anatomy and Physiology

Hair, nails and skin make up the 'integumentary system' which supplies the body with an external cover and a divider between the organs of the body and the external environment. Weighing 2.7–3.6 kg with an average surface area of 1.9 m², the skin is the largest organ of the body and has many functions related to the structures and layers contained within it.

The Hair

Situated in the dermis of the skin, the hair protects the skin from ultraviolet rays, heat loss and injury (Figure 17.1).

The Nails

Nails are made up of dead cells and aid the development of fine motor skills such as grasping, scratching and manipulation. They also provide protection against trauma to the fingers and toes.

The Skin

Figure 17.2 shows a cross section of the skin.

The Epidermis
The epidermis is slightly acidic (pH 4.5–6) and is made up of four to five layers of epithelial cells (Figure 17.3). It contains melanin, keratinocytes, Langerhans cells and tactile cells.

The Dermis
The two layers of the dermis are the *papillary* layer and *reticular* layer. The dermis contains capillaries, sweat and sebaceous glands and receptors for touch, pressure and pain. 'Cleavage lines' are formed in the dermis and create ridges around the body. Surgical incisions should run parallel to the cleavage lines to promote healing with less scarring (Figure 17.4).

Hair Follicles

A hair follicle comprises a papilla, matrix, root sheath, hair fibre and bulge (Figure 17.5) and can create 'goose bumps', when very small muscles flex in the skin, making the hair follicles rise up. Sebum and sweat are secreted on to the hair follicle for protection, lubrication and pliability. Melanin produces hair colours: dark hair contains

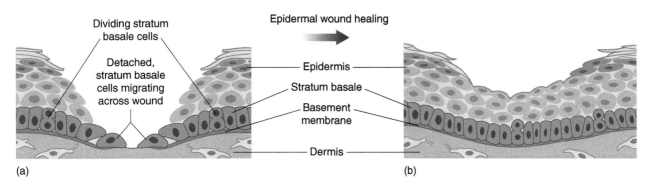

Dividing stratum basale cells

Detached, stratum basale cells migrating across wound

Epidermal wound healing

Epidermis

Stratum basale

Basement membrane

Dermis

(a)

(b)

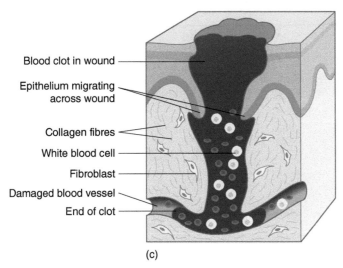

Blood clot in wound

Epithelium migrating across wound

Collagen fibres

White blood cell

Fibroblast

Damaged blood vessel

End of clot

(c)

Deep wound healing

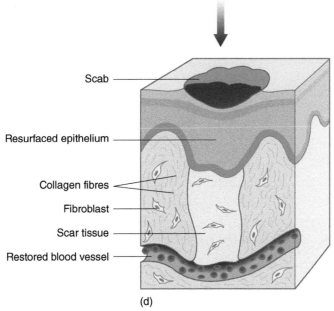

Scab

Resurfaced epithelium

Collagen fibres

Fibroblast

Scar tissue

Restored blood vessel

(d)

Source: Peate I, Wild K & Nair M (eds) Nursing Practice: Knowledge and Care (2014)

FIGURE 17.1 Cross section of a hair.

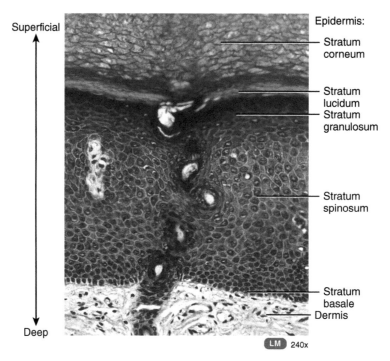

Superficial

Epidermis:

Stratum corneum

Stratum lucidum

Stratum granulosum

Stratum spinosum

Stratum basale

Dermis

Deep

LM 240x

FIGURE 17.2 Cross-section of the skin.

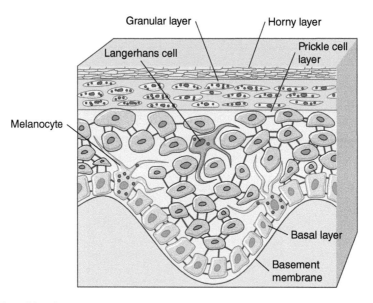

Granular layer

Horny layer

Langerhans cell

Prickle cell layer

Melanocyte

Basal layer

Basement membrane

FIGURE 17.3 Layers of the epidermis.

true melanin; blonde and red hair contain variants of melanin; grey hair contains less melanin and white hair lacks melanin and contains air bubbles.

Blood Vessels

Arterioles, capillary networks and venules assist with the flow of blood through the skin, controlled by hormones and the nervous system. Their role is transport and distribution of oxygen, nutrients and hormones and removal of waste products.

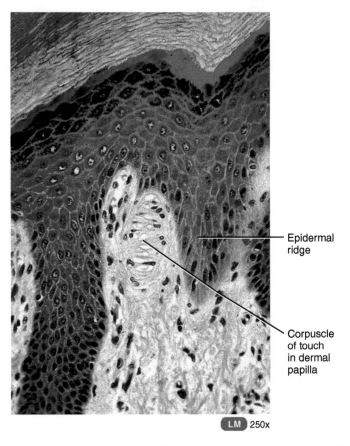

LM 250x

FIGURE 17.4 Epidermal ridges and sweat pores. Source: Jenkins and Tortora (2013); reproduced with permission of Wiley.

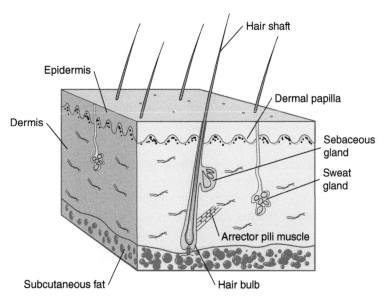

FIGURE 17.5 Structure of the hair.

Nerve Fibres

Sensory and motor nerves are found in the dermis. Sensitivity to touch, or signals such as warmth, coolness, pain, pressure, vibration, tickling and itching are initiated by sensory receptors. Motor nerves assist vasodilation and vasoconstriction of blood vessels and glands and the contraction and relaxation of muscle tissues.

Lymphatic Vessels

The lymphatic system absorbs proteins, lipids and interstitial fluid, when pressure is greater in the interstitial fluid than in the lymph. Its role is to transport lymphatic fluid, to aid in circulating body fluids and to help guard against disease-triggering agents.

Subcutaneous Tissue

Subcutaneous tissue is primarily adipose tissue (fat) that lies under the dermis and helps the skin to adhere to underlying structures.

Glands of the Skin

There are many glands of the skin: *ceruminous glands* produce earwax, *sebaceous glands* secrete sebum and *sudoriferous glands* produce perspiration.

Skin Pigmentation

Haemoglobin, carotene and melanin affect the colour of the skin. A golden skin tone (in people of Asian ancestry) has large amounts of carotene (a yellow–orange pigment) and melanin (a yellow–brown pigment). People born with brown or black skin have greater levels of melanin; however, sun exposure can cause an accumulation of melanin, resulting in darkening or tanning of the skin. A pink skin tone is due to lack of melanin. Regardless of racial origin, carotene is found in the stratum corneum, and all scar tissue heals pink.

Clinical Investigation: Oxygenation of the Skin

A clinical investigation used to measure the oxygenation of a person's haemoglobin (oxygen saturation or SpO_2) may be necessary. A lack of oxygen can lead to cell death and tissue breakdown in patients susceptible to pressure ulcers.

Skin colour may change due to embarrassment, a fever, hypertension or inflammation. Other causes include reaction to a a drug, sunburn or rosacea. Blue colour to the lips, ears and nose (cyanosis) may suggest poor oxygenation and a lack of haemoglobin. Those patients presenting with pallor may appear shocked; a yellow to orange colour of the skin may indicate jaundice and pink may appear in the healing of skin in black patients.

Clinical Investigations: Skin Tone Assessment

Cultural awareness of differences in skin tone assessment should be acknowledged. Classification tools for objectively assessing human skin colour include the Munsell skin tone chart (Konishi et al. 2007), which can assist with predicting pressure ulcer risk, the six Fitzpatrick (1988) skin types for assessing risk of damage from ultraviolet light and the neonatal skin colour scale (Maya-Enero et al. 2020).

Function of the Skin

The skin, hair and nails each have many functions:

- Protection against mechanical, thermal and physical injury, and hazardous substances.
- Sensation detects touch, pain, heat and pressure.
- Synthesis of vitamin D to reduce harmful effects of ultraviolet radiation.
- Excretion of water, salts and toxins.
- Absorption of medications and creams.
- A storage reservoir for adipose tissue.
- Regulation of body temperature by sweating and shivering.

Wound Healing

When there is skin loss, a sequence of four phases called wound healing is signalled to return the skin to near normal structure and function.

- *Haemostasis*: on injury, bleeding occurs and circulating platelets become sticky, connecting with fibrin and red blood cells to form a plug, and haemostasis occurs. Once haemostasis is completed, fibrinolysis (the breaking down of the clot) commences.
- *Inflammation*: cells, substances, hormones and growth factors are released in the inflammatory phase. At this stage, patients often complain of pain, heat, swelling and redness/hyperpigmentation at the wound bed.
- *Proliferation*: formation of granulation tissue occurs, and a red and granular wound bed is visible in all skin tones. Wound edges come together and pink epithelial sites are seen.
- *Maturation*: a reduction in blood supply and cellular activity occurs and normally a scar forms. Keloid and hypertrophic scarring may occur in people under 30 years and in those who have darker pigmented skin.

Snapshot 17.1

Pre-arrival Information

Control has requested that you respond to Blake, a 57-year-old man with leg pain. There is no additional pre-arrival information.
Dispatched: 9:30 a.m.
Arrival: 9:45 a.m.

Assessment

Airway: clear.
Breathing: bilateral chest rise, lung sounds clear, no extra effort required.
Cardiac: pulses present, regular and bounding.
Disability: Patient is alert and orientated.
Exposure: no immediate life threats found.
Background: age 57 years, male; weight/height: approximately 85 kg and 178 cm.
Medical history: diabetes type 2 (non-insulin dependent).
Medications: metformin.

Examination

On specific examination of Blake, you observe a poorly demarcated, warm, erythematous area with associated oedema and tenderness to palpation of the right leg below the knee. Blake informs you he cut his leg at the beach three days ago and this swelling and redness has progressed quickly over the past two days.

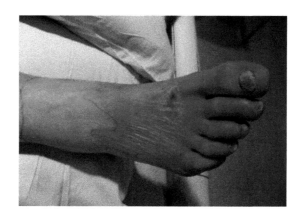

Vital Signs

Vital signs taken are:

Vital sign	Observation	Normal range
Pulse (beats/min)	90	80–100 regular
Respiration rate (breaths/min)	18	12–20
SpO$_2$ (%)	98	94–98
Blood pressure (mmHg)	108/60	120/80
Eyes	4	4 – spontaneously
Verbal	5	5 – orientated
Motor	6	6 – obeys commands
Total GCS score	15	15
Temperature (°C)	37.3	37
ECG	Normal sinus rhythm	
Pain score	6/10	

Reflective Learning Event

Take some time to reflect on Snapshot 17.1, then consider the following questions:

1. What is your differential and working diagnosis here?
2. What would be your initial management in this case?
3. What is the worst-case scenario here, which may not be apparent?

Assessment

Assessment of the skin includes the collection of a detailed history of the patient's skin condition, a general assessment of the patient, an assessment of the patient's knowledge and a physical assessment (Lawton 2001).

Patient Assessment Interview

On first meeting a patient with a skin disorder, the paramedic may carry out a health assessment using the DRABCDE approach. Other skin-related data should include:

- When the patient noticed the skin disorder.
- How long it has been present.
- How often it occurs or recurs.
- Characteristics of the skin disorder.
- What route the disorder has taken.
- Whether it is affected by seasonal changes.
- The severity of the skin disorder.

Any precipitating or predisposing factors (e.g. family history of the condition).
What relieves the disorder (pharmacological and non-pharmacological).
Any related symptoms.

Questioning a patient's knowledge of the disorder can assist if health promotion and education is required at the end of the assessment. Questions should focus on past medical and surgical history to explore symptoms linked to other disorders, current and past medication and treatments, and how the condition affects current activities of living.

Skin cancer and malignant melanoma may be explored, including factors such as the presence and number of moles on the skin, and prior exposure to radiation, x-rays, coal, tar or petroleum-based products.

Reflective Learning Activity

According to the National Institute for Health and Care Excellence (NICE 2023b), the Eron classification of cellulitis is a useful tool to aid clinical decision making:

Class I   There are no signs of systemic toxicity or uncontrolled comorbidities.

Class II   The person is either systemically unwell or systemically well but with a comorbidity (for example peripheral arterial disease, chronic venous insufficiency, or morbid obesity) which may complicate or delay resolution of infection.

Class III   The person has significant systemic upset (such as acute confusion, tachycardia, hypotension) or unstable comorbidities that may interfere with a response to treatment, or a limb-threatening infection due to vascular compromise.

Class IV   The person has sepsis or a severe life-threatening infection, such as necrotising fasciitis.

Reflect on Snapshot 17.1 and the above guidance. What would you expect the paramedics to do differently next time, if anything, when called to assess a patient with suspected cellulitis?

363

Examination of the Skin

Holistic assessment has two parts: a general assessment and a physical skin assessment. Some lesions/wounds may need visualising; equipment such as torches and tape measures may be needed.

General Assessment
Health status is often reflected in the skin; for example, general appearance indicates the patient's self-caring abilities, state of mind and existence of support.

Physical Assessment
A physical assessment should ideally occur in an area with bright natural light, with consent, and you should be mindful of any distress and discomfort for the patient. Vital information includes the colour of the skin, including race, and the

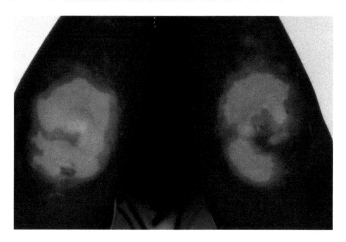

FIGURE 17.6   Vitiligo. Source: Buxton and Morris-Jones (2013); reproduced with permission of Wiley.

skin disorder, skin texture and temperature, moisture, turgor and the presence of oedema. Document findings, such as scars, missing fingers, toes and limbs, and the presence of any open wounds and their aetiology. The skin tells a story: assess the distribution, character and shape of any lesions, their site and location. For example, chicken pox would be documented as a variable polymorphic rash (character), with small fluid-filled lesions (shape), covering the entire body with some in the mouth and around the eyes of the patient (distribution).

In patients with darkly pigmented skin, some skin disorders will present differently (Lang 2000). For example, lesions may often present as black or purple on dark skin. Compare an unaffected area of skin with the skin disorder and document abnormalities. Use touch to detect heat on an area of skin as mild inflammatory reactions may not be visible. Look for changes in pigmentation normal variant (i.e. pigmentary demarcation) and midline primary conditions (e.g. vitiligo; Figure 17.6), and secondary conditions such as post-inflammatory hypopigmentation and hyperpigmentation (darkening of the pigment of the skin) in atopic eczema. People with darker skins also show reaction patterns such as follicular (affecting hair follicles), papular (elevations of the skin) and annular (ring-like skin conditions), and keloid scarring.

Red Flag Alert: Inflammatory Response

A localised area of heat to the touch can be an indicator of an inflammatory response caused by infection.

Documenting Lesions

Lesions can be described as primary (i.e. they occur at commencement of a skin disorder) and secondary (i.e. they occur over time) from manipulation (scratching, rubbing, picking). Using your finger and thumb, palpate the lesions (unless extensive) so you can assess whether the lesion is soft, firm, hard, raised or irregular, and its texture. Then document the colour (e.g. pink, red, purple and mauve – due to blood; brown, black and blue – due to pigment; white – due to lack of blood or pigment; or yellow and orange – due to bilirubin levels).

Consider whether the lesions are solitary (a single lesion), satellite (a single lesion in close proximity to a larger group), grouped (a cluster of lesions), generalised (total body area) or localised (a limited area of involvement that is clearly defined). Assess and document any itching, pain and discomfort felt by the patient.

Assessment of the Nails, Hair and Mucous Membranes

Complete the assessment with an examination of the nails, hair and mucous membranes. Look for blistering, scarring and erosions of the mucous membranes, including colour, shape, capillary refill and pigment changes of the nails. Remember to note any recent hair loss, erythema and scales on the scalp.

Snapshot 17.2

Pre-arrival Information

Control has requested you to respond to Emily, a five-year-old female patient with a 'severe rash' as per her mother who called.
Dispatched: 11:20 a.m.
Arrival: 12:15 p.m.

Assessment

Appearance: good tone, interacting with parent playing with blocks, is consolable, no fixed gaze and minimally distressed.
Work of breathing: no signs of abnormal posturing, retractions or nasal flaring; no audible abnormal breath sounds.
Circulation to skin: skin pink with no signs of pallor, mottling or cyanosis. Red rash observed to elbows and back of the patient's knees; she was scratching both and seems uncomfortable.
Disability: patient is alert and orientated.
Exposure: no immediate threats to life found.
Background: age five years, female; weight approx. 20 kg.
Medical history: none known.
Medications: no regular medications taken.

Examination

On specific examination of Emily, you observe a red, dry and itchy rash to the back of both of Emily's knees and elbows approximately 4 cm × 3 cm. Emily says that they are very itchy and uncomfortable. Emily's mother advises that the rash has developed over the past three days and she is worried that Emily might have meningitis.

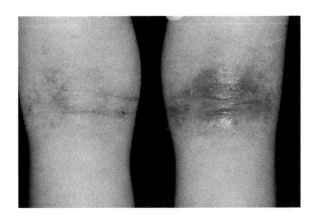

Vital Signs

Vital signs taken are:

Vital sign	Observation	Normal range
Pulse (beats/min)	104 regular	80–135 regular
Respiration rate (breaths/min)	22	20–30
SpO$_2$ (%)	99	94–98
Blood pressure (mmHg)	108/60	120/80
Temperature (°C)	36.6	37
Pain score	2/10	

Reflective Learning Activity

Take some time to reflect on the information in Snapshot 17.2, then consider the following questions:

1. What is your differential diagnosis here?
2. How would you perform a skin rash assessment for Emily and what factors would you be looking for?
3. How would you manage this situation?

Wound Assessment

Wound assessment includes collection of data to diagnose the underlying cause of a wound to aid decision making (Benbow 2016). The assessment should include the minimum data set (Coleman et al. 2017):

- *Cause of the wound* – how did the wound develop, has the aetiology been determined and addressed, is the wound acute, chronic or palliative and what previous interventions (if any) have been used.
- *Wound size* – measure for length, width and depth, creating an initial baseline for assessment and wound progression. In care homes or patients cared by community nurses, you may find a wound assessment chart in the patient's notes.
- *Wound site* – correctly name and document the site(s) of the wound.
- *Colour and type of tissue at the wound bed* – can often indicate the stage of wound healing or the presence of a complication. This can be necrotic, infected, sloughy, granulating or epithelialising tissue.
- *Level of exudate* – review the colour, consistency, odour and amount (e.g. clear, amber coloured and no odour).
- *Signs and symptoms of infection* –include pyrexia, oedema, pain, inflammation or hypo/hyperpigmentation and an increase in exudate. Additional signs include delayed healing, increased watery exudate rather than pus, pocketing at the wound base, bridging, increased pain, malodour, friability of tissues, a change in the colour of granulation tissue and wound breakdown.
- *Pain at the wound bed* – can be caused by neuropathy (diabetic), anticipatory (before dressing removal) or can be iatrogenic (self-harm).
- *Surrounding skin* – the wound margins alter as a wound heals or deteriorates. Changes can include colour or appearance (e.g. macerated or excoriated from too much wound exudate).
- *Other clinical data* – document the type of wound, the phase of wound healing, any grading, staging or classification for the wound, factors affecting wound healing, diagnostic tests and any current management.

Red Flag Alert: Patients with Diabetes

Patients with diabetes who have skin disorders or wounds may fail to present with any wound/skin infection symptoms apart from a delay in wound healing or exacerbation of their skin disorder (Patel 2010).

Orange Flag Alert: Wounds and Pain

Pain does not always correlate with the size and depth of wound and can often be psychological rather than physical; both pharmacological and non-pharmacological approaches should be explored.

Skin Infections: Viral, Bacterial and Fungal

Viral Skin Infections

A virus is a microorganism smaller than a bacterium and consists of an RNA or DNA core surrounded by a protein coat. In a living cell, the virus can grow and reproduce and skin lesions can have numerous causes: antibiotics, contraceptive medication, corticosteroids, any medication that causes immunosuppression and the COVID-19 coronavirus. Common viral skin infections include warts, herpes zoster (shingles), and varicella zoster (chickenpox). COVID-19 skin manifestations include acral areas of erythema (named 'COVID toes' – pseudo-chilblains), urticarial lesions (hives and wheals rash), maculopapular eruptions, a skin rash that contains flat discoloured areas and raised bumps in adults, vesicular eruptions (chickenpox-like rash) and livedo (mottling of the skin).

Medicines Management: Ibuprofen

Using ibuprofen in children who have chickenpox may lead to a masking of symptoms and an increased risk of necrotising fasciitis.

Bacterial Skin Infections

Gram-positive *Staphylococcus aureus* and beta-haemolytic streptococci are the most common cause of bacterial skin infections, with infections caused by a single pathogen from the skin, or secondarily, occurring in diseased or traumatised skin. Contributing factors include no apparent cause, poor hygiene, poor nutrition, prolonged skin moisture or excessive moisture from perspiration, trauma to the skin (including trauma from shaving), systemic diseases such as diabetes mellitus and haematological malignancies, and heavy fabrics on the upper legs. Common bacterial skin infections are included in Table 17.1. Patients who present with bacterial infections should be monitored carefully, noting the spread of inflammation and marking and measuring it clearly on a body map.

Medicines Management: Antibiotics

Patients who present to paramedics in the situations discussed above often live in a care home setting. The paramedic should always consider current or recent antibiotic use and recent blood cultures, if available, before starting the patient on broad-spectrum intravenous antibiotics.

Candidiasis

Candida albicans is a yeast-like infection found on mucous membranes, the skin, vagina and gastrointestinal tract. Candidal intertrigo (sweat rash) arises from perspiration being trapped in skin folds or tight clothes and not being able to evaporate.

Red Flag Alert: Erysipelas

Erysipelas is a medical emergency. The patient will receive antibiotics for the first seven days and needs to be hospitalised.

TABLE 17.1   Common types of bacterial skin infections.

Bacterial infection of the skin	Most common causative bacteria	Signs, symptoms and complications	Site
Folliculitis: bacterial infection of the hair follicle	*Staphylococcus aureus* and *Pseudomonas aeruginosa*	Inflammation, pustules and lesions at the hair follicle. Discomfort ranging from slight burning to intense itching. Complication of abscess formation	Scalp, face of bearded men (sycosis barbae), eye (stye) and the legs of women who shave
Furuncles (boils): inflammation of the hair follicle	*Staphylococcus aureus*	Deep, firm, red, painful nodule 1–5 cm in diameter. The nodule changes to large painful cystic nodule draining infected, purulent pus	Any part of the body that has hair (neck, face, flexures and buttocks)
Carbuncles: group of infected hair follicles	*Staphylococcus aureus*	Firm mass located in the subcutaneous tissue and lower dermis. Painful and swollen mass with multiple openings to the skin surface. Chills, fever and malaise may follow.	Neck, back and lateral thighs
Cellulitis: localised infection of the dermis and subcutaneous tissue	*Streptococcus pyogenes*	Red, swollen and painful area. Vesicles may form over the cellulitic area, accompanied by chills, fever, malaise, headache and swollen lymph glands	Anywhere on the body. Most common on lower legs in adults and eye and perianal area in children
Erysipelas: infection of the skin	*Streptococcus pyogenes*	Chills, fever and malaise (4–20 hours) precede a skin lesion appearing. Lesion(s) appear as firm red spots enlarging to form a circumscribed, bright red, raised, hot lesion. Petechiae, necrosis and blistering can occur if not treated early	Face, ears and lower legs

368

Infestations

Infestations can affect anyone but are often connected to crowded or unsanitary conditions. Common infestations are lice, scabies, fleas and bedbugs.

Acne Fulminans

Acne fulminans is a rare and severe form of acne conglobate. It presents with a sudden onset of systemic symptoms such as inflammatory, ulcerated and painful nodular acne on the chest and back. The upper trunk may also present with bleeding crusts and is accompanied by a fever, complaints of painful joints and generally feeling unwell. Appetite and weight loss may be accompanied by assessment of an enlarged liver and spleen. NICE (2023a) recommend a same-day referral for urgent dermatological assessment.

Medicines Management: Entonox

Paramedics should consider the therapeutic effects of nitrous oxide and oxygen (Entonox®) when treating patients with painful skin disorders. You can read more about pain management in Chapter 14.

Generalised Pustular Psoriasis

Generalised pustular psoriasis is a rare form of psoriasis which presents as inflamed skin with clusters of pustules that join together. This type of psoriasis is a medical emergency, and the patient may appear toxic with severe pain. This skin disorder is often precipitated by a course of high-dose steroids (topical or systemic).

Erythroderma

Erythroderma (generalised exfoliative dermatitis) is a rare but severe and potentially life-threatening inflammation of most of the body's skin surface. It is often caused by a reaction to a medicine, another skin condition or cancer. The patient presents with inflamed skin with clusters of pustules that amalgamate. Erythrodermic atopic dermatitis mostly affects children and young adults, but other forms of erythroderma are more common in middle-aged and elderly people.

Fungating Tumours

Fungating wounds are more frequently found in head and neck, breast and skin cancers. They develop either at the primary site of the cancer or at lymph nodes (groin or axillae) and occur when the tumour has invaded the epithelial layer of the skin and breaks through the surface, forming an ulcerative area (crater) or proliferative area (cauliflower-like nodules; Dealey 2005). Significant blood loss and, in some instances, major haemorrhage and ultimately death can occur if the tumour erodes a blood vessel. Where erosion into a major artery is a potential complication, patients and their families should be prepared for such a catastrophic event (Sood et al. 2020).

Medicines Management: Fungating Wounds

Patients with fungating wounds that potentially will erode a major artery should be provided with an emergency pack by the primary care team. This usually contains an appropriate medication for emergency administration (rectal diazepam 10 mg, intramuscular/subcutaneous midazolam 10 mg, or intravenous/subcutaneous diamorphine), information for the patient and their relatives, and red or dark coloured blankets/sheets.

Wounds

Wounds can be categorised according to their aetiology, morphology, tissue damage, tissue colour and by the process by which they heal:

- *Primary intention* is where there is no tissue loss and the edges of the wound are brought together for suturing, gluing or taping (surgical or traumatic wounds).

TABLE 17.2   Classification of wound types.

Classification	Types
Acute	Surgical incisions, traumatic injuries: lacerations, bites, abrasions, burns and avulsions
Chronic	Pressure ulcers, leg ulcers, burns, dehisced surgical wounds, diabetic foot ulcers
Palliative	Malignant skin lesions, epidermolysis bullosa and progressive arterial disease

- *Secondary intention* is when the wound needs to fill with granulation tissue before epithelialisation occurs.
- When a wound is initially left open to allow drainage of exudate or infected pus before closing it is termed *tertiary intention*.

Wounds can also be *acute* wounds, healing in a timely manner following the normal phases of wound healing. *Chronic* wounds last longer than four to six weeks; they take longer to heal and may not fully regain functional and anatomical integrity. A *palliative* wound however, will not heal and care is based on symptom management such as exudate, pain and odour. Table 17.2 highlights wounds that can be termed 'acute', 'chronic' or 'palliative'.

Types of Wounds

Minor Injuries

Many wounds are minor and can include:

- *Avulsions* usually occur when skin of the digits or limbs has been pulled off with or without the involvement of bone by an external device or machine. These wounds are present in patients with friable skin or following trauma (e.g. a motorcycle accident).
- *Contusions* (or bruises) are trauma to the skin where bleeding has occurred in the tissue spaces. Contusions are graded from 0 to 5, with 5 being a critical bruise from bleeding into the brain or compartment of a muscle and 0 being a light bruise with very little damage. Underlying medical conditions should be considered (e.g. leukaemia, coagulation problems and physical abuse).
- *Cuts* are wounds with well-defined edges, little bruising and usually straight in alignment. Sharp implements are the usual cause.
- *Abrasions* are caused by friction and shear between a blunt item and the skin. Abrasions dry out, scab over and heal without scarring; however, embedded gravel should be removed to prevent tattooing.
- *Bites* can cause heavily contaminated wounds, which require assessment for toxins and bacteria and antibiotics.
- *Skin tears* involve shear and friction forces separating the epidermis from the dermis or dermis from the subcutaneous layers. Fragility of the skin increases susceptibility. Skin tears can be classified by the amount of skin loss and the ability to reposition the flap of skin post injury. The most common classification system is that developed by the International Skin Tear Advisory Panel (LeBlanc et al. 2013):
  - Type 1 skin tears involve no skin loss with a linear or flap tear in which the skin flap can be used to cover the wound bed.
  - Type 2 skin tears involve partial flap loss in which the skin flap cannot be repositioned to cover the entire wound bed.
  - Type 3 skin tears involve total flap loss with exposure of the entire wound bed.
  - Skin closure strips are no longer advocated.
- *Lacerations* are breaks in the skin with an irregular wound edge caused by blunt trauma.

TABLE 17.3 Description of types of surgical wound.

Type	Description
Clean	An incision in which no inflammation is encountered in a surgical procedure, without a break in sterile technique and during which the respiratory tract, alimentary or genitourinary tracts are not entered
Clean contaminated	An incision through which the respiratory, alimentary or genitourinary tract is entered under controlled conditions but with no contamination encountered
Contaminated	An incision in which there is a major break in sterile technique, or gross spillage from the gastrointestinal tract, or an incision in which acute, non-purulent inflammation is encountered as well as open traumatic wounds that are more than 12–24 hours old
Dirty or infected	An incision in which the viscera (internal organs) are perforated or when acute inflammation with pus is encountered (e.g. emergency surgery for faecal peritonitis) and for traumatic wounds where treatment is delayed, there is faecal contamination or devitalised tissue

Surgical Wounds

Post-surgery wounds can be classified as clean, clean contaminated, contaminated, and dirty or infected (NICE 2020; Table 17.3). Complications can include fistulas, where a passage is formed between two organs, such as the bowel and the vagina (rectovaginal), and faeces from the bowel will pass out of the vagina. Common fistulas occur between the bowel and skin (enterocutaneous).

- A *cavity* or *bursa* lined with epithelial cells that leads from the outside of the body inside is known as a sinus and is caused by infection, a foreign body or breakdown of dead tissue.
- *Dehiscence* or unplanned opening of the wound is often caused by poor surgical technique, haematoma formation, insufficient number of sutures, infection, age, diabetes and trauma to the wound.
- *Evisceration* is when the gastrointestinal tract protrudes through the wound opening (Figure 17.7). Observe for signs of shock, cover the open wound and bowel with moist sterile dressings. Lie the patient down with the foot of the stretcher elevated 20 degrees, and transport to an appropriate facility as soon as possible.

371

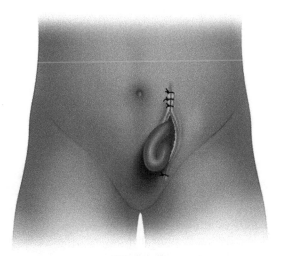

Evisceration

FIGURE 17.7 Evisceration of a wound can be frightening for the patient.

Factitious/Iatrogenic/Self-Harm Wounds

Self-harm wounds present as unusual injuries to easily accessible areas of the skin, reached by the patient's dominant hand, presenting with sharp geometric margins surrounded by normal-looking skin (Gupta et al. 1987). Tourniquets, excoriation or chemical injuries can present as blisters, purpura, ulcers, erythema, oedema, sinuses or nodules. At times, skin loss can be so significant that the person requires immediate hospitalisation and timely management to avoid surgery and morbidity (Tantam and Huband 2009). Self-harm is classified as pathological and non-pathological. Patients may have underlying dermatological conditions (Harth et al. 2010) and no suicidal intent. NICE (2022) guidance is available for details of further management.

Red Flag Alert: Self-Harm

Paramedics may visualise previous attempts of self-harm when conducting an assessment of a patient's condition. This may be observed in the condition of the skin at self-harm sites. While this is to be considered, it should not distract the paramedic from their assessment and treatment of presenting complaint.

Leg Ulcers

The prevalence of leg ulcers in the UK is 0.1–0.3% (NICE 2023c). Leg ulcers are open lesions between the knee and the ankle joint that occur in the presence of venous disease and take more than two weeks to heal (NICE 2023c). The causes can be venous hypertension (60–80%), arterial disease (22%), rheumatoid arthritis and systemic vasculitis (9%), diabetes (5%), and iatrogenic (induced by patient, treatment or physician). A holistic examination of the patient's past medical and surgical history, examination of the leg, the ulcer and ankle brachial pressure indices is required to exclude peripheral arterial disease.

372

Pressure Ulcers

Defined as 'localised damage to the skin and/or underlying tissue, usually over a bony prominence (or related to a medical or other device), resulting from sustained pressure (including pressure associated with shear). The damage can be present as intact skin or an open ulcer and may be painful' (NHS Improvement 2018). The causes of pressure ulcers are either from direct or indirect forces:

- *Indirect forces* include nutrition, body temperature, dehydration, age, medication, immobility, sleeping, elimination, anxiety and depression (this list is not exhaustive).
- *Direct forces* include the impact of pressure, friction and shear.

All susceptible patients should have initial and continuing assessment of their risk of developing pressure ulcers and regular skin assessment (NICE 2014). Any damage should be assessed using a pressure ulcer classification system (National Pressure Ulcer Advisory Panel et al. 2014).

Reflective Learning Activity

Elderly patients are at increased risk of pressure ulcers because of direct and indirect forces. NICE (2014) guidance recommends a risk assessment and skin assessment for those at risk of developing pressure ulcers.

Access the NICE (2014) guidance on pressure ulcers: prevention and management and the National Pressure Ulcer Advisory Panel et al. (2014) pressure ulcer classification, and the pressure ulcer risk assessment instrument PURPOSE T (Coleman et al. 2018). What would you expect the paramedics to do when caring for an elderly patient identified at risk of pressure ulcers who will remain on the ambulance stretcher for more than two hours?

Burns

A burn is an injury to the skin caused by heat, electricity, chemicals, radiation or friction. Most are accidental and many involve children, the elderly and adults who are obese or have cardiovascular and neurological conditions. Classification of burns is in accordance with the depth of tissue damage (Table 17.4).

Relevant information specific to burns includes history of the burn, time of injury, causative agent, early treatment, age and body weight. Most questions are asked quickly, as initially on arrival burns patients are awake, but conscious states can alter rapidly in major burn injuries. Assessment may include the use of the Lund and Browder tool for children and rule of nines in adults; only partial- or full-thickness bums are included in the estimation (Figure 17.8).

TABLE 17.4   Classification of burns.

Classification of burn	Appearance	Pain	Healing techniques and times
Full thickness	Pale, waxy, yellow, brown, mottled, charred or non-blanching red. Surface is dry, leathery and firm to touch, thrombosed blood vessels are visible	No sensation of pain or light touch	Require excision and skin grafting and are hard to heal. Often require initial fasciotomy and escharotomy. Often have contractures and hypertrophic scarring
Deep partial thickness	Pale and waxy, moist or dry, ruptured blister may occur that appear as tissue paper	Less pain than superficial thickness as areas of decreased sensation	Excision and grafting. More than 21 days' healing time often with contractures and hypertrophic scarring
Superficial partial thickness	Bright red, moist glistening appearance with blisters. Blanches on pressure	Pain is severe in response to air and temperature. Pain and touch response intact	Dressing products and skin substitutes. Healing within 21 days with minimal or no scar formation
Superficial	Pink to bright red in colour	Stinging sensation	Water-soluble lotions and dressings. Healing in 3–6 days; no scar

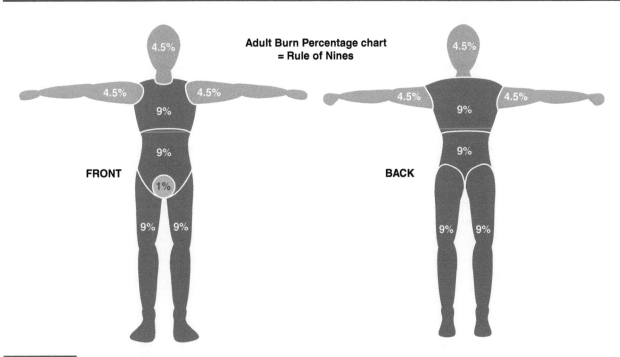

FIGURE 17.8   Lund and Browder and 'rule of nines' tools.

The following patients should be referred to a specialist burns unit for further management (National Network for Burn Care 2012):

- Patients with burns to the face, hands or feet
- Children aged 5 years and under
- Patients aged 60 years and over
- Any patient with a circumferential burn to a joint or chemical and electrical burns
- Inhalation injuries
- A burn covering more than 5% total body surface in children or 10% in an adult
- A burn not healed in 14 days.

Snapshot 17.3

Pre-arrival Information

Control has requested you respond to Tanveer, a two-year-old boy with burns to his face, chest and arm following the spill of a cup of coffee.
Dispatched: 1:20 p.m.
Arrival: 1:29 p.m.

Assessment

Appearance: good tone, not interacting with parent, not consolable, no fixed gaze and very distressed. He is being held by mother on kitchen chair with wet towel on his chest and arm.
Work of breathing: no signs of abnormal posturing, retractions or nasal flaring, no audible abnormal breath sounds.
Circulation to skin: skin dark redness to face chest and arm.
Disability: patient is alert and orientated.
Exposure: patient wearing only a nappy, which does not appear to be wet.
Background: age two years, male; weight approximately 12 kg.
Medical history: none known.
Medications: no regular medications taken.

Background

Tanveer's mother advises she had made a cup of coffee and he had knocked the cup from the table on to himself. She immediately took him to the sink to apply running water but he would not tolerate it so she soaked a towel in cold water and placed it on him.

Vital Signs

Vital signs taken are:

Vital sign	Observation	Normal range
Pulse (beats/min)	154	100–150 regular
Respiration rate (breaths/min)	34	20–30
SpO$_2$ (%)	99 (room air)	94–98
Blood pressure (mmHg)	108/60	70/120
Temperature (°C)	37.3	37
Pain score	10/10	/10
Burns (%)	27	

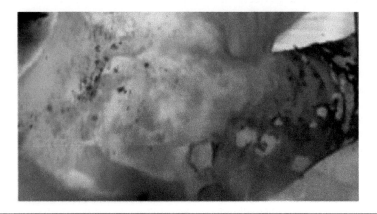

Reflective Learning Activity

Take some time to reflect on Snapshot 17.3, then consider the following:

1. What is your primary concern here?
2. What is your initial management of this case?
3. Are there any additional factors to consider in this case?

The Diabetic Foot

A diabetic foot ulcer is defined as a 'foot ulcer in a person with current or previously diagnosed diabetes mellitus, and usually accompanied by peripheral neuropathy and/or peripheral artery disease in the lower extremity' (van Netten et al. 2023). This type of ulcer includes a variety of pathological changes, such as loss of sensation (neuropathy), reduced blood flow (ischaemia and calcification), deformities of the foot (Charcot) and uneven distribution of pressure.

Take Home Points

- The skin is the largest organ of the body and patients who present with skin disorder cannot be overlooked.
- Wound healing is a sequence of four phases, which occurs to return the skin to near- normal structure and function.
- Holistic assessment has two parts: a general assessment and a physical skin assessment. Some lesions/wounds may need visualising; and equipment such as torches and tape measures may be needed.
- Skin disorders/wounds can range from infestations, infections, fungating wounds, minor injuries, surgical wounds, factitious, iatrogenic, and self-harm wounds, leg ulcers, pressure ulcers, diabetic foot ulcers and burns.
- Management of skin disorders require pharmacological and wound management practices, with transport to hospital in emergency situations.

Summary

The incidence of skin disorder and wounds is increasing. Management has advanced from a simple wound assessment to assessment using tools and examining the biological, psychological and economic impact of the skin disorder and wound on the patient. It is essential that as patient-facing practitioners, paramedics acquire the necessary knowledge, skills and attitudes to assess, plan, implement and evaluate evidence-based care delivered to this group of patients.

References

Benbow, M. (2016). Best practice in wound assessment. *Nursing Standard* 30 (27): 40–47.

Buxton, P.K. and Morris-Jones, R. (2013). *ABC of Dermatology*, 5e. Chichester: Wiley.

Coleman, S., Nelson, E.A., Vowden, P. et al. (2017). Development of a generic wound care assessment minimum data set. *Journal of Tissue Viability* 26 (4): 226–240.

Coleman, S., Smith, I.L., McGinnis, E. et al. (2018). Clinical evaluation of a new pressure ulcer risk assessment instrument, the Pressure Ulcer Risk Primary or Secondary Evaluation Tool (PURPOSE T). *Journal of Advanced Nursing* 74 (2): 407–424.

Dealey, C. (2005). *The Care of Wounds*. Oxford: Wiley Blackwell.

Fitzpatrick, T.B. (1988). The validity and practicality of sun-reactive skin types through VI. *Archives of Dermatology* 124: 869–871.

Gupta, M., Gupta, A., and Haberman, H. (1987). The self-inflicted dermatoses: a critical review. *General Hospital Psychiatry* 9 (1): 45–52.

Harth, W., Taube, K.M., and Gieler, U. (2010). Factitious disorders in dermatology. *Journal der Deutschen Dermatologischen Gesellschaft* 8 (5): 361–373.

Jenkins, G. and Tortora, G.J. (2013). *Anatomy and Physiology: From science to Life*, 3e. Chichester: Wiley.

Konishi, N., Kawada, A., Morimoto, Y. et al. (2007). New approach to the evaluation of skin color of pigmentary lesions using skin tone color scale. *Journal of Dermatology* 34 (7): 441–446.

Lang, P.G. (2000). Dermatoses in African-Americans. *Dermatology Nursing* 12 (2): 87–98.

Lawton, S. (2001). Assessing the patient with a skin condition. *Journal of Tissue Viability* 11 (3): 113–115.

LeBlanc, K., Baranoski, S., Christensen, D. et al. (2013). International Skin Tear Advisory Panel: a tool kit to aid in the prevention, assessment, and treatment of skin tears using a simplified classification system. *Adv Skin Wound Care* 26: 459–476.

Maya-Enero, S., Candel-Pau, J., Garcia-Garcia, J. et al. (2020). Validation of a neonatal skin color scale. *European Journal of Pediatrics* 179: 1403–1411.

National Institute for Health and Care Excellence. (2014). *Pressure Ulcers: Prevention and management*. Clinical Guideline CG179. London: National Institute for Health and Care Excellence.

National Institute for Health and Care Excellence. (2020). *Surgical Site Infections: Prevention and treatment*. NICE Guideline NG125. London: National Institute for Health and Care Excellence.

National Institute for Health and Care Excellence. (2023a). Acne vulgaris: Management. NICE Guideline NG198. London: National Institute for Health and Care Excellence.

National Institute for Health and Care Excellence. (2023b). Cellulitis – acute. Clinical Knowledge Summary. https://cks.nice.org.uk/topics/cellulitis-acute (accessed 13 October 2023).

National Institute for Health and Care Excellence. (2023c). Leg ulcer – venous. Clinical Knowedge Summary. https://cks.nice.org.uk/topics/leg-ulcer-venous (accessed 13 October 2023).

National Institute for Health and Care Excellence. (2022). Self-harm: Assessment, management and preventing recurrence. NICE Guideline NG225. London: National Institute for Health and Care Excellence.

National Network for Burn Care (2012). *National Burn Care Referral Guidance*. London: British Burn Association.

National Pressure Ulcer Advisory Panel, European Pressure Ulcer Advisory Panel (2014). *Prevention and Treatment of Pressure Ulcers: Quick Reference Guide*, 2e. Perth, Australia: Cambridge Media.

National Wound Care Strategy Programme (2021). *National Wound Care Core Capabilities Framework for England*. Bristol: Skills for Health.

van Netten, J.J., Bus, S.A., Apelvist, J. et al. (2023). Definitions and criteria for diabetic foot disease. Diabetes Metab Res Rev e3654. [online ahead of print] https://doi.org/10.1002/dmrr.3654

NHS Improvement. (2018). *Pressure Ulcers: Revised Definition and Measurement. Summary and recommendations*. London: NHS Improvement.

Patel, S. (2010). Investigating wound infection. *Wound Essentials* 5: 40–47.

Sood, R., Mancinetti, M., Betticher, D. et al. (2020). Management of bleeding in palliative care patients in the general internal medicine ward: a systematic review. *Ann Med Surg* 50: 14–23.

Tantam, D. and Huband, N. (2009). *Understanding Repeated Self-Injury: A Multidisciplinary Approach*. Basingstoke: Palgrave Macmillan.

Further Reading

Peate, I. and Stephens, M. (2020). *Wound Care at a Glance*. Chichester: Wiley.
Ryan, S. (2008). Psoriasis: characteristics, psychosocial effects and treatment options. *British Journal of Nursing* 17 (5): 284–290.

Online Resources

National Wound Care Strategy Programme: https://www.nationalwoundcarestrategy.net.
Stop the Pressure: www.stopthepressure.co.uk
Legs Matter: https://legsmatter.org
British Association of Dermatologists: www.bad.org.uk
Northern Burn Care Network: https://www.northern-burncare-network.nhs.uk

Glossary

Erythema	A superficial redness of the skin.
Extrinsic	Originates externally.
Fissure	A groove or tear.
Histology	The study of a tissue's microscopic anatomy.
Hyperkeratosis	Excess keratins are produced resulting in thickening of the skin.
Integument	The external covering of the body – the skin.
Intrinsic	Originates internally.
Keratin	A tough insoluble protein.
Keratinise	To convert into keratin.
Lichenification	Thickening of the skin as a result of chronic scratching.
Naevus	A pigmented lesion of the skin.
Pheromone	A chemical that triggers an innate behavioural response in another.
Prognosis	A prediction about how a person's disease will progress.
Pruritus	Itchy sensation on the skin.
Radiotherapy	The medical use of radiation to treat cancer.
Relapse	When the person is again affected by a condition that has occurred in the past.
Sebum	An oily substance made of fat and the debris of fat-producing cells.
Suture	A stitch.
Topical	A medication applied to the body surface.
Vesiculation	Collection of fluid in the skin.
Viscous	Relating to the thickness of a fluid.
Xerosis	Dry skin.

Multiple Choice Questions

1. What is the integumentary system made up of?
   a. Skin, hair and nails
   b. Skin, hair and kidneys
   c. Skin, hair and heart
   d. Skin, hair and liver

2. What are the most common bacterial skin infections caused by?
   a. *Escherichia coli*
   b. Skin flora
   c. Pseudomonas
   d. Staphyloco*ccus aureus* and beta-haemolytic streptococci

3. Which speciality is associated with skin disorders?
   a. Dermatology
   b. Plastic surgery
   c. Neurology
   d. Allergy and immunology

4. What is the common description of hyperpigmentation?
   a. Lightening of the skin
   b. Darkening of the skin
   c. Excess growth of the skin
   d. Poor blood supply of the skin

5. What three things should you assess when examining a patient who presents with lesions on a part of their body?
   a. Distribution, site and shape
   b. Distribution, location and shape
   c. Distribution, size and shape
   d. Distribution, character and shape

6. What are the signs of infection?
   a. Pyrexia, oedema, pain, inflammation and an increase in exudate production
   b. Pyrexia, hypotension, pain, inflammation and an increase in exudate production
   c. Hypothermia, oedema, pain, inflammation and an increase in exudate production
   d. Pyrexia, oedema, pain, inflammation and reduced exudate

7. What is a furuncle?
   a. Inflammation of the hair follicle
   b. A bacterial infection of the hair follicle
   c. A group of infected hair follicles
   d. Localised infection of the dermis and subcutaneous tissue

8. What direct forces contribute to the development of pressure ulcers?
   a. Pressure, friction and shear
   b. Pressure, moisture and temperature
   c. Pressure, shear and nutrition
   d. Pressure, nutrition and ageing

9. What are the two main causes of leg ulcers?
   a. Diabetic and arterial
   b. Iatrogenic and arterial
   c. Venous and arterial
   d. Rheumatoid arthritis and venous

10. Self-harm wounds are categorised into two types; what are they called?
    a. Acute and chronic
    b. Primary and secondary
    c. Tertiary and palliaitve
    d. Pathological and non-pathological.

CHAPTER **18**

The Ears and Eyes

Carl Clare

AIM

The aim of this chapter is to introduce the reader to the anatomy and physiology of the ears and eyes along with associated disorders.

LEARNING OUTCOMES

After reading this chapter you will be able to:

- Describe the way in which human beings maintain a sense of balance.
- Describe the symptoms of a rupture of the tympanic membrane.
- Describe the structure of the eye.
- Explain how a visual image is focused on the retina.

Test Your Prior Knowledge

1. What is the purpose of the Eustachian tube?
2. Name the main parts of the ear involved in the sense of balance.
3. Name the two substances that fill the eye chambers and help to maintain the shape of the eye.
4. What is the name used to describe short-sightedness?

Introduction

The senses are usually thought of as the five senses of smell, taste, hearing, vision and touch. However, in physiology, the sense of touch is excluded from the senses as it is considered a somatic sense. As disorders of the senses of smell and taste are not normally associated with the use of paramedic services, this chapter focuses on the senses of hearing and sight.

This chapter explores the senses in two sections:

- The senses associated with the ear: those of equilibrium and hearing.
- The sense of sight.

Fundamentals of Applied Pathophysiology for Paramedics, First Edition. Edited by Ian Peate and Simon Sawyer.
© 2024 John Wiley & Sons Ltd. Published 2024 by John Wiley & Sons Ltd.

In both these sections, there is a review of the anatomy of the organs involved, followed by a discussion of the physiology of how these senses are monitored and create action potentials to be transmitted to the brain. Finally, the pathways these action potentials take to the brain are reviewed, together with a brief discussion of the processing of this information in the brain itself.

The Senses of Equilibrium and Hearing

The ear is divided into three sections: external, middle and inner (Figure 18.1). Each of these three sections is integral in the process of hearing. The inner ear is also essential in the maintenance of the sense of balance.

The Structure of the Ear

The Outer Ear

The outer ear consists of the:

- Auricle (also known as the pinna)
- External auditory canal
- Tympanic membrane.

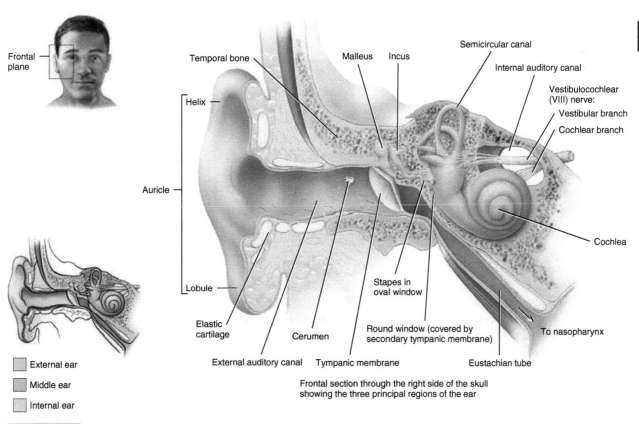

FIGURE 18.1 Structure of the ear. Source: Tortora (2016). Reproduced with permission of Wiley.

The auricle is the shaped projection surrounding the exit of the external auditory canal. Made up of elastic cartilage covered with skin, the auricle can be further delineated into the rim, known as the helix, and the earlobe. The earlobe lacks supporting cartilage and so is soft and lacking in structure. The function of the auricle is to direct sound waves into the external auditory canal.

The external auditory canal (meatus) is an S-shaped passage about 2.5 cm long and 0.6 cm wide. Extending from the auricle to the tympanic membrane, the channel is lined with skin and fine hair. The majority of the canal is channelled through the temporal bone and thus needs no supporting cartilage; however, near the opening of the canal (at the auricle), the structure of the tube is supported by elastic cartilage. The skin of the external canal is lined with sebaceous (oil) glands and modified sweat glands called ceruminous glands. The ceruminous glands secrete a yellow-brown waxy cerumen (ear wax). The purpose of the oils and the wax is to lubricate the ear canal, to kill bacteria and, in conjunction with the hairs, to keep the canal free of debris.

Medications Management: Routes of Administration

- Medications applied to the eye are administered ocularly.
- Medications applied to the ear are known as otic medications.
- Medications sprayed into the nose and absorbed through the nasal membranes are administered nasally.
- Those medication that are breathed into the lungs, through the mouth are administered by inhalation or by the mouth and nose by nebulisation.

Sound waves entering the external auditory canal are channelled through the tube until they reach the tympanic membrane (ear drum), a membrane made of thin translucent connective tissue covered by skin on its external surface and internally by mucosa. It is shaped like a flattened cone protruding into the middle ear. When sound waves reach the tympanic membrane, they make it vibrate, and this vibration is transmitted to the bones of the middle ear.

Middle Ear

Otherwise known as the tympanic cavity, the middle ear is an air-filled cavity lined with mucosa; it is contained within the temporal bone. The middle ear is enclosed at both ends, by the ear drum at the lateral end and medially by a bony wall with two openings:

- The oval (vestibular) window
- The round (cochlear) window.

The middle ear is connected to the nasopharynx by the Eustachian (auditory) tube, a 4-cm long tube that consists of two portions.

When open, the Eustachian tube allows the passage of air, and thus ensures the equalisation of the pressures on both sides of the tympanic membrane so both are subject to the same atmospheric pressure. The Eustachian tube is normally closed at the end nearest the nasopharynx but opens during yawning and swallowing, hence the effect of swallowing during take-off and landing during flight which allows equalisation of pressures either side of the eardrum. If equalisation of pressures does not happen, then the difference in pressures between the two sides can lead to reduced hearing as the tympanic membrane cannot move freely.

Within the middle ear, there are three bones known as the ossicles or ossicular chain. These three bones connect the tympanic membrane with the receptor complexes of the inner ear:

- The malleus (hammer) attaches to the inner surface of the tympanic membrane.
- The incus (anvil) attaches the malleus to the stapes.
- The stapes (stirrup) – the base of the stapes are bound to the edge of the oval window.

Vibration in the tympanic membrane converts the sound waves into mechanical movement. The ossicles collect the force applied to the tympanic membrane, amplify it and transmit it to the oval window. This amplification helps to explain why humans can hear even very quiet noises but can also be a problem in very noisy environments. To protect the tympanic membrane and the ossicular chain from violent movement resulting from extreme noises, they are supported by two small muscles, the tensor tympani and stapedius muscles.

Inner Ear

The senses of equilibrium (part of the sense of balance) and hearing are provided by the receptors in the inner ear. The inner ear is also known as the labyrinth, owing to the complicated series of canals it contains. The inner ear is composed of two main, fluid-filled parts:

- The bony labyrinth – a series of cavities within the temporal bone that contain the main organs of balance (the semicircular canals and the vestibule) and the main organ of hearing (the cochlea).
- The membranous labyrinth – a series of fluid-filled sacs and tubes that are contained within the bony labyrinth.

As noted above, the bony labyrinth can be divided into three parts (Figure 18.2):

- The vestibule consists of a pair of membranous sacs: the saccule and the utricle. Receptors in these two sacs provide the sensations of gravity and linear acceleration.
- The semicircular canals enclose slender semicircular ducts. Receptors in these ducts are stimulated by the rotation of the head. The combination of the vestibule and the semicircular canals is known as the vestibular complex.
- The cochlea is a spiral-shaped, bony chamber that contains the cochlear duct of the membranous labyrinth. Receptors within this duct give us the sense of hearing.

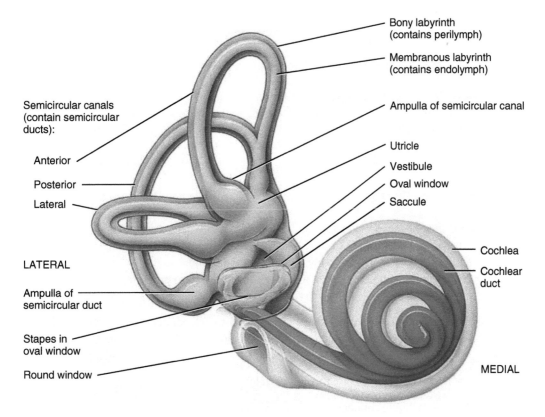

Components of the right internal ear

FIGURE 18.2 Inner ear. Source: Tortora (2016). Reproduced with permission of John Wiley & Sons.

Equilibrium

The sense of equilibrium is part of the sense of balance and is controlled by receptors in the semicircular ducts, the utricle and the saccule of the inner ear. The sensory receptors in the semicircular ducts are active during movement but inactive when the body is motionless. These receptors respond to rotational movements of the head. There are three of these ducts: lateral, posterior and anterior.

Each semicircular duct contains an ampulla, an expanded region that contains the majority of the receptors. Hair cells (the receptors) are surrounded by supporting cells and are monitored by the sensory neurones.

The free surfaces of the hair cells are covered with stereocilia, which resemble very long microvilli. Together with the fine stereocilia, the hair cell will also have one kinocilium – a single, large and thick cilium. When an external force pushes against the cilia, the distortion of the plasma membrane of the hair cell alters the rate that the cell releases chemical transmitters. Any movement of the head can be perceived by varying combinations of stimulation of the three ducts and their receptors (Figure 18.3).

In contrast to the semicircular canals, the utricle and the saccule provide equilibrium information about whether the body is moving or stationary. The two chambers are connected by a narrow passageway that is also connected to the endolymphatic duct. As with the hair cells of the ampullae, the cilia of the hair cells in the utricle and saccule are embedded in a gelatine-like substance. However, the surface of this substance contains densely packed calcium carbonate crystals called statoconia. This combination of gelatine-like substance and calcium carbonate crystals is known as an otolith (Figure 18.4).

When the head is in a neutral position, the statoconia sit on top of the hairs. Thus, the pressure they generate is downwards and the hairs are pushed down. When the head is tilted, the pull of gravity on the statoconia shifts and the hairs are moved to one side or the other. This distorts the cell membrane and triggers altered neurotransmitter release (Figure 18.5).

A similar type of activity happens when the body is subject to linear acceleration; for example, as a car speeds up, the otolith lags behind due to inertia. The brain would normally differentiate between the action of gravity and the action of acceleration by integrating the information from the receptors with visual information.

Pathways for the Equilibrium Sensations

The hair cells in the semicircular canals, the vestibule and the saccule are monitored by sensory neurones located in the vestibular ganglia. Sensory fibres from these ganglia form the vestibular branch of the vestibulocochlear nerve (cranial nerve VIII).

Hearing

The sense of hearing is provided by receptors in the cochlear duct; they are hair cells similar to those of the semicircular canals and vestibule. However, their positioning within the cochlear duct and the organisation of the surrounding structures protect them from stimuli generated by anything other than sound waves.

The ossicular chains transmit and amplify pressure waves from the air into pressure waves in the perilymph of the cochlea. These waves stimulate the hair cells along the cochlear spiral:

- The frequency of the perceived sound is detected by the part of the cochlear duct that is stimulated.
- The intensity (volume) of the sound is detected by the number of hair cells that are stimulated at the particular point in the cochlea.

Within the bony labyrinth of the cochlea there are three ducts (Figure 18.6):

- The vestibular duct (scala vestibuli) connects to the oval window.
- The tympanic duct (scala tympani) connects to the round window.
- The cochlear duct (scala media) is separated from the tympanic duct by the basilar membrane.

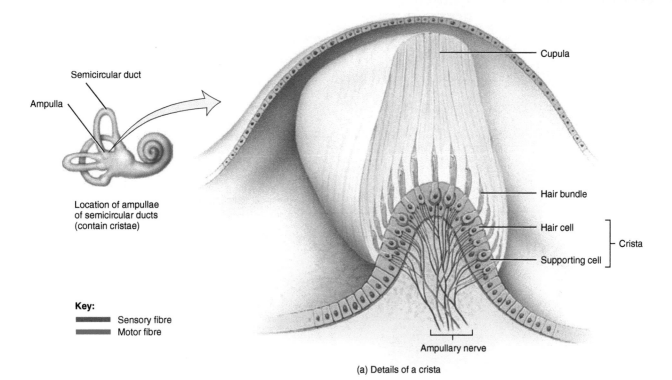

Semicircular duct

Ampulla

Location of ampullae
of semicircular ducts
(contain cristae)

Cupula

Hair bundle

Hair cell

Crista

Supporting cell

Ampullary nerve

(a) Details of a crista

Key:

Sensory fibre
Motor fibre

Cupula

Ampulla

Ampullary nerve

As the head rotates
in one direction, cupula
is dragged through
endolymph and bent
in opposite direction

Head in still position

Head rotating

(b) Position of a cupula with the head in the still position (left)
and when the head rotates (right)

FIGURE 18.3 (a, b) Ampulla at rest and in response to movement. Source: Tortora (2016). Reproduced with permission of
John Wiley & Sons.

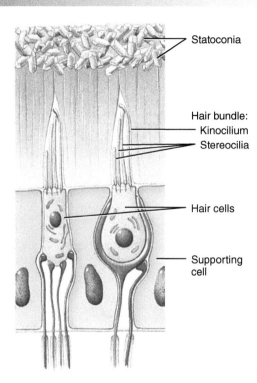

Details of two hair cells

FIGURE 18.4 Hair cells and otolith. Source: Tortora (2016). Reproduced with permission of John Wiley & Sons.

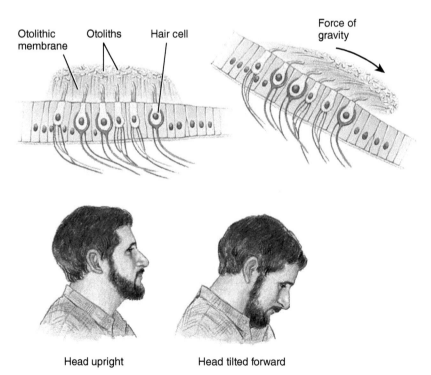

Position of macula with head upright (left) and tilted forward (right)

FIGURE 18.5 Action of gravity on the otolith. Source: Tortora (2016). Reproduced with permission of John Wiley & Sons.

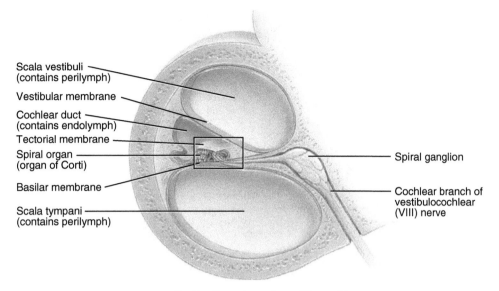

Section through one turn of the cochlea

FIGURE 18.6 Cross-section of the cochlea. Source: Tortora (2016). Reproduced with permission of John Wiley & Sons.

Red Flag Alert: Ototoxicity

Ototoxicity is the property of being toxic to the ear. There are over 200 drugs that can lead to ototoxicity, tinnitus and associated hearing loss. Many of these drugs are used in common practice, such as:

- furosemide
- gentamicin
- metropolol
- ramipril
- sodium valproate.

Paramedics should inform patients that if they do experience any suspected tinnitus or hearing loss with a drug, it is important that they do not stop taking the drug until they have talked to their doctor.

Avoiding Ototoxicity

Many ototoxic drugs are excreted in the urine, and thus it is best to avoid ototoxic drugs in patients with renal impairment, and they should be used with caution in the elderly. Furosemide toxicity is related to the speed of administration and, therefore, it is essential that the instructions for the speed of delivery of intravenous furosemide are followed.

Red Flag Alert: Noise Exposure and Ear Damage

As noise levels increase, the chance of damage to the ear increases. The table gives examples of the types of noise levels at certain decibel (dB) levels and the exposure time at which damage may occur:

dB level	Maximum exposure per day (hours)	Examples
10		Breathing
20		Rustling leaves
60		Conversation

dB level	Maximum exposure per day (hours)	Examples
75		Typical car interior on motorway
85	16	City traffic (inside car)
90	9	Power drill, food blender
97	3	French horn at 3 m (10 ft)
100	2	Farm tractor, outboard motor, jet take-off at 304 m (1000 ft)
110	0.5	Chainsaw, pneumatic drill, car horn at 1 m (3 ft)
120	0	Typical rock concert, loud thunderclap
125	Hearing damage occurring	Pneumatic riveter at 1.2 m (4 ft)
132–140	Permanent hearing damage	Gunshot, very loud rock concert 15.2 m (50 ft) in front of speakers
150–160	Eardrum rupture	Jet take off at 29 m (75 ft), gunshot at 30 cm (1 ft)
190	Immediate death of tissue	Jet engine at 30 cm (1 ft)
194		Loudest sound in air, air particle distortion (sonic boom)

Disorders of the Ear

Tympanic Membrane Rupture

Signs and Symptoms

Rupture of the tympanic membrane can be caused by blows to the side of the head or blast injuries. Symptoms include:

- Ear pain that may subside quickly.
- Clear, pus-filled or bloody drainage from the ear.
- Hearing loss.
- Ringing in the ear (tinnitus).
- Spinning sensations (vertigo).
- Nausea or vomiting that can result from vertigo.

Diagnosis

Diagnosis is based on taking a patient history and the paramedic should undertake a physical examination of the tympanic membrane if trained to do so.

Care and Treatment

Tympanic membrane rupture often heals without intervention as long as there is no infection present. While natural healing occurs, patients should be advised to avoid the entry of water into the ear and introducing foreign objects such as cotton buds into the ear. If there is persistent deafness this may be due to damage or displacement of the ossicular chain and may require surgery to repair.

Otitis Media

Signs and Symptoms

Acute otitis media is a condition that is often a complication of upper respiratory tract infections or sinusitis. The infection travels up into the middle ear via the Eustachian tube, leading to infection and the collection of pus. The infection and the pressure resulting from the collection of pus may lead to a range of potential symptoms including (Gopen 2010):

- Pain
- High temperature
- A generalised feeling of being unwell
- Headache
- Nausea and vomiting
- Tinnitus
- Reduction in hearing.

Diagnosis

The paramedic takes a patient history and physical examination of the ear to enable them to make a diagnosis.

Care and Treatment

The treatment for otitis media includes:

- Antibiotics
- Pain relief
- Antipyretics
- Application of warmth to the affected ear in order to reduce pain
- Avoiding water entering the ear canal.

389

Orange Flag Alert: Hearing Loss

The paramedic should bear in mind that hearing loss is not only associated with not being able to hear sounds clearly. Hearing loss has also been associated with brain atrophy, cognitive decline and dementia. The effects of hearing loss may also be linked to feelings of depression, loneliness, and anxiety.

Untreated or repeated episodes of acute otitis media may lead to chronic infection of the middle ear. In chronic infection, tympanic membrane rupture is common and destruction of the bones of the ossicular chain is also possible. Symptoms include:

- Pus-filled discharge
- Pain – may be associated with redness and swelling of the bone behind the pinna
- High temperature
- Hearing loss
- Nausea and vomiting
- Vertigo.

Snapshot 18.1   Ear Pain Following a Surfing Accident

Pre-arrival Information

You are dispatched to a 13 year old female, who is complaining of ear pain. The patient is located at the local surf beach.

On Arrival with the Patient

On arrival, you notice that the swell of the waves is larger than normal today. You are taken to the patient by the local lifeguards, who tell you that she had a wipeout (fell off her board and then hit by the wave) on a larger wave. The patient left the water on their own and sought care from the lifeguards.

The lifeguards have performed a thorough assessment and confirm that the patient is negative on the NEXUS (National Emergency X-Radiography Utilisation Study) criteria (no altered level of consciousness or head strike, no neck pain), and all their vital signs are in normal ranges.

You approach the patient and introduce yourself. The patient's name is Michelle.

Michelle explains that she fell while riding a wave. You ask for specific details of what happened and she tells you that she fell on her right side, and as she struck the water and the wave passed over her, she felt a sudden intense pain in her right ear, which she describes as 8/10. She tells you it feels like the pain is inside her ear, rather than on the auricle.

You ask about other symptoms. Michelle also tells you that she feels dizzy and nauseous.

You perform a quick examination of the right ear. You see no discharge or other obvious injuries. You perform a quick hearing test, first asking Michelle to cover her right ear, and then asking her to cover her left ear. You discover that Michelle has significantly diminished hearing in her right ear, and that she can hear a faint ringing sound in that ear.

Michelle has no significant medical history, although she does state that she gets a lot of ear infections. She is not on any medications and has no allergies.

What is Your Diagnosis?

Before reading on, think about this patient's presentation and try to determine what you think has happened and what you should do.

In this case, the patient's story is the key to determining their diagnosis. Initially, Michelle did not give you much information, but by asking targeted questions you were able to determine that the pain occurred right after a water force to the right ear, followed by a pressure change as the wave passed over. This has made you suspect a perforated eardrum.

Michelle's symptoms match this suspicion, with her experiencing intense inner ear pain, hearing loss, tinnitus, dizziness and nausea.

You inform Michelle what you think is happening and she appears worried, she asks you if this means she will be deaf in that ear permanently. You reassure her that permanent deafness is a highly unlikely outcome, and that the eardrum can actually heal by itself, although she will need to see a doctor to ensure the best outcome.

Michelle contacts her mother and you all agree that Michelle should go to the hospital emergency department with you and her mother will meet you there.

You ask Michelle if she would like pain relief and she says that she thinks she will be OK, so you tell her to let you know if she changes her mind.

Clinical Investigations: Basic Hearing Test

Hearing can be conductive and sensorineural, both should be tested if testing hearing. A simple 'Can you hear me?' would be suffice. There are other simple additional tests that the paramedic can perform to come to a diagnosis.

- Whisper test (conductive): cover each ear in turn and whisper '123' and 'ABC'. Ask the patient what they heard.
- Rhomberg test (sensorineural): ask the patient to stand up, eyes closed, feet together. Assess for swaying.

Ménière's Disease

Symptoms

Ménière's disease is a disorder of the inner ear. Symptoms include:

- Vertigo
- Nausea and vomiting
- Tinnitus
- Varying hearing loss
- 'Drop attacks' – a feeling of being pulled to the ground; alternatively, some patients feel as though they are whirling through space.

Diagnosis

The diagnosis of Ménière's disease is based on taking a patient history and the presence of symptoms suggestive of Ménière's disease in the absence of any other cause.

Care and Treatment

The duration of an episode can last for hours or days. When caring for patients having an acute episode of Ménière's disease, the paramedic needs to:

- Provide reassurance
- A quiet, darkened, environment
- A comfortable position (often semi-recumbent)
- Avoid sudden head movements
- Avoid fluorescent and flickering lights, and watching television.

Treatment of the disease requires lifestyle changes and long-term medication, which may include diuretics to reduce fluid retention, vestibular suppressants to manage dizziness and anti-nausea medications to alleviate associated symptoms. The choice of medication may vary based on the individual's specific symptoms and needs. Table 18.1 gives an overview of betahistine dihydrochloride, an H1 receptor agonist and H3 receptor antagonist, which means that it acts on histamine receptors in the inner ear and central nervous system to help regulate the flow of signals related to balance and dizziness. Patients who do not respond to medical treatment may require surgery.

Medication Management: Prescribed Medications and Vertigo

There are several medications associated with dizziness and vertigo. The assessment of the drug history of any patient with episodes of vertigo should give special consideration to polypharmacy (Muncie et al. 2017). The causal mechanisms range from cardiovascular effects to central anticholinergic effects and cerebral toxicity. Medications known to be associated with dizziness/vertigo include:

- Antiepileptics
- Antiarrhythmics
- Antihypertensives
- Nitrates
- Urinary and gastrointestinal antispasmodics
- Aminoglycosides.

This list is in no way exhaustive, and it is always preferable to refer to an appropriate text if there is any suspicion regarding the cause of vertigo/dizziness.

TABLE 18.1   Medications associated with Ménière's disease.

Drug	Drug classification	Reason for administration	Route of administration	Dose	Adverse effects	Contraindications
Betahistine dihydrochloride	Anti-vertigo medication	Vertigo associated with Ménière's disease	Oral	16 mg three times a day increasing to 24–48 mg daily	Gastrointestinal disturbances, headache, rash	Phaeochromocytoma

Clinical Investigations: Examination of the Patient with Dizziness

A useful diagnostic approach to the assessment of dizziness can be found in the acronym TiTrATE (Pfieffer et al. 2019):

Timing of the symptoms

Triggers that provoke the symptoms

And a

Targeted **E**xamination

For instance, *timing* can refer to the time of day (e.g. early morning dizziness may be associated with postural hypotension) or the length of the episodes of dizziness.

Triggers include rapid rotation of the head (possible vestibular problems), straining at stool (possible parasympathetic activity leading to reduced heart rate) among others.

Targeted examination includes several potential detailed examinations, including vital signs, ears, eyes, and other physical assessments. A full drug history should also be taken.

Reflective Learning Activity

Many conditions of the ear are non-specific and do not have external signs that are easy to see. It is therefore likely that carers would not notice many ear conditions in their everyday interactions with the people they care for. Pain from an ear infection or loss of hearing may lead to changes in behaviour or the worsening of behaviours that are already present. Often, these changes are put down to the learning disability and paramedics and other healthcare professionals will fail to look for physical causes that may be treatable. This is known as *diagnostic overshadowing*.

Diagnostic overshadowing is a common problem for patients with learning disabilities and can be made worse when the patient is not compliant with diagnostic examinations and has difficulty communicating their symptoms.

Avoiding diagnostic overshadowing takes time and requires the paramedic to create a bond of trust and a rapport with the patient. Often this is not possible for paramedic staff and therefore it necessitates the paramedic to ensure a full handover including the impressions gained by care staff.

Take some time to think about diagnostic overshadowing and reflect on your own practice. Think about the impact on overshadowing for the person with a learning disability.

The Sense of Sight

Vision is usually considered the sense that we value the most; we learn more about the world around us through sight than we do with any of the other senses. Without sight, many of our daily tasks and pleasures would be impossible and many others would become more difficult. The sense of sight is based on the eyes, and around the eyes there are accessory structures that help to keep the eyes safe and working well (Figure 18.7):

- Eyelids (palpebrae) – a continuation of the skin (epithelium). Continual blinking keeps the surface of the eye lubricated and removes dirt. The gap between them is known as the palpebral fissure.

- Eyelashes – robust hairs that help to keep foreign matter out of the eyes. They are associated with the tarsal glands, which produce a lipid-rich secretion that helps to prevent the eyelids from sticking together.
- Lacrimal caruncle – a small collection of soft tissue that contains accessory glands.
- Commissure – the point where the eyelids meet; there are two: the lateral and the medial.
- Conjunctiva – the epithelial cell layer that lines the inside of the eyelids and the outer surface of the eye.

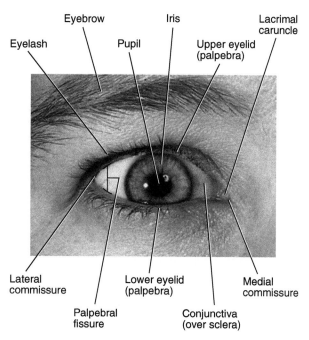

FIGURE 18.7   Accessory structures of the eye. Source: Tortora (2016). Reproduced with permission of Wiley.

Snapshot 18.2   Foreign Body in Eye

Pre-arrival Information

You are dispatched to a 32 year-old woman who was working on a building site when she suffered an eye injury. Dispatch was unable to ascertain the nature of the injury.

On Arrival with the Patient

On arrival, you are met by another tradesperson who takes you to the patient. On the way, they tell you that the patient was cutting wood and a splinter went in her eye.

The patient is sitting and holding her eye and is in significant pain and distress. You do not see any evidence of haemorrhage at this point.

You introduce yourself, and the patient, who is named Beatrix, tells you that she has something big in her eye. She was wearing safety glasses, but the splinter came through the bottom of the frame. She describes the pain as 10/10.

Beatrix is in significant distress and while she will move her hand she says it is too painful to open her eye. At this point, you can see a splinter protruding from between her top and bottom eyelids, but you cannot visualise the eye itself.

You perform a quick assessment and find she has no allergies, is not on any medications, has no significant medical history, and all her vital signs are within normal ranges.

You offer Beatrix pain relief and she allows you to cannulate her and administer intravenous morphine. After five minutes, Beatrix is feeling the effects of the morphine and opens her eye briefly. You can see that the splinter is protruding from the centre of her pupil at a 90-degree angle.

Beatrix closes her eye again and you tell her to keep her eye closed. She asks if you are going to pull the splinter out and you tell her that you can't do that, and she will have to see an eye specialist in the emergency department. You tell her that you are going to cover her eye and provide her with enough pain relief to keep her calm during transport to hospital.

You take an eye patch and cut a hole in the centre and carefully place it over the eye with the splinter protruding out through the hole in the centre. You tape the patch to Beatrix's face to hold it in place.

You tell Beatrix that she is best to keep both eyes closed during transport, as her eyes will move together and you want her to keep her eyes still.

You tell Beatrix that you will stay with her throughout the transport, and you want to make sure that her eye does not hurt at all, so she should tell you if she feels any discomfort and you will provide her with more pain relief.

During the journey, you continually check in with Beatrix and keep her calm and relaxed. You call ahead to a specialist hospital for receiving patients with serious eye injuries and provide a summary of the case. On arrival you are met in the emergency department and taken straight to a specialist team, who take over the patient's care and successfully remove the splinter.

Lacrimal Apparatus

A constant flow of tears washes over the eyes to keep the conjunctiva moist and clean. Tears have several functions; they:

- Reduce friction
- Remove debris
- Prevent bacterial infection
- Provide nutrients and oxygen to parts of the conjunctiva.

The lacrimal gland (tear gland) creates most of the content of tears (about 1 ml/day). Once the lacrimal secretions reach the eye, they mix with the products of other glands. This results in a mixture that lubricates the eye and reduces evaporation. The nutrient and oxygen requirements of the corneal cells are supplied by diffusion from the lacrimal secretions. The secretions also contain antibacterial enzymes and antibodies to attack pathogens before they enter the body.

The Eye

The Wall of the Eye

The wall of the eye has three layers (Figure 18.8):

- Fibrous tunic
- Vascular tunic
- Neural tunic.

Fibrous Tunic

The fibrous tunic is the outermost layer of the eye and consists of the sclera and the cornea; it has three main functions:

- Provides support and some protection
- Is the attachment site for the extrinsic muscles
- Contains structures that assist in the focusing process.

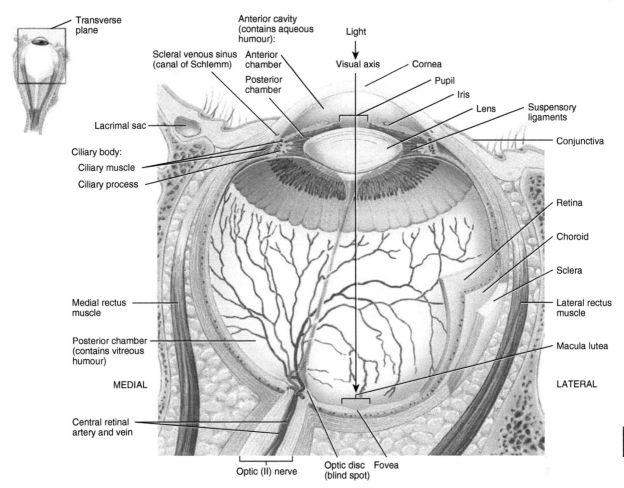

Superior view of transverse section of right eyeball

FIGURE 18.8 Anatomy of the eye. Source: Tortora (2016). Reproduced with permission of John Wiley & Sons.

Most of the ocular surface is covered by the sclera (the 'white' of the eye), which is made up of dense fibrous connective tissue containing collagen and elastic fibres. The surface of the sclera contains small blood vessels and nerves. The transparent cornea is continuous with the sclera and is made up of a dense matrix of fibres laid down in such a way that they do not interfere with the passage of light.

Vascular Tunic (Uvea)

The vascular tunic is the middle of the three layers of the eye and contains numerous blood vessels, lymph vessels and the smooth muscles involved in eye functioning. The vascular tunic is made up of:

- The iris
- The ciliary body
- The choroid.

Iris

The iris is the central, coloured portion of the eye and regulates the amount of light entering the eye by adjusting the size of the central opening (the pupil). It is formed of two layers of pigmented cells and fibres and two layers of smooth muscle (the pupillary muscles). Both sets of muscles are controlled by the autonomic nervous system; activation of the parasympathetic nervous system leads to constriction of the pupil in response to bright light. Activation of the sympathetic nervous system leads to the dilation of the pupil in response to dim light levels.

Ciliary Body

The greater part of the ciliary body is made up of the ciliary muscle, a smooth muscular ring that projects into the interior of the eye. The epithelial covering of this muscle has many folds called ciliary processes. The suspensory ligaments of the lens attach to the tips of these processes.

Choroid

The choroid is a vascular layer that separates the fibrous and neural tunics. It is covered by the sclera and attached to the outermost layer of the retina. The choroid contains an extensive capillary network that delivers oxygen and nutrients to the retina.

Neural Tunic (Retina)

This is the innermost layer of the eye, consisting of a thin outer layer called the pigmented part and a thicker inner layer called the neural part. The pigmented part of the retina absorbs the light that passes through the neural part; this prevents light bouncing back through the neural part and causing 'visual echoes'. The neural part of the retina contains light receptors, support cells and is responsible for the preliminary processing and integration of visual information.

Organisation of the Retina

Two types of receptor cells are contained within the outermost layer of the retina (closest to the pigmented part). These receptor cells are the cells that detect light (photoreceptors).

- *Rods* – these photoreceptors do not discriminate between colours. They are very sensitive and enable us to see in very low light levels.
- *Cones* – these photoreceptors provide colour vision and give sharper, clearer images than the rods do, but they require more intense light.

There are three types of cones (red, blue and green) and colour discrimination is based on the integration of information received from the three types of cones. For instance, yellow is shown by highly stimulated green cones, less strongly stimulated red cones and a relative lack of stimulation of the blue cones.

The rods and cones synapse with neurons called bipolar cells, which in turn synapse within a layer of neurons called ganglion cells. At both these synapse areas, there are associated cells that can stimulate or inhibit the communication between the two cells, and therefore alter the sensitivity of the retina (for instance, in response to very bright, or dim, light levels).

Axons from the ganglion cells converge on the optic disc, at which point they turn and penetrate the wall of the eye and proceed to the diencephalon of the brain as the optic nerve. The central retinal artery and vein pass through the centre of the optic nerve. The optic disc contains no photoreceptors, and thus this area is known as the blind spot; however, we do not notice the blind spot in our vision as involuntary eye movements keep the visual image moving and the brain can thus supply the missing information.

The Chambers of the Eye

The eye is divided into two main cavities: a large posterior cavity and a smaller anterior cavity. The anterior cavity is further divided into the anterior chamber and the posterior chamber.

- The *anterior cavity* is filled with a substance called aqueous humour that circulates between the anterior and posterior chambers by passing through the pupil and performing a vital role as a transport medium for nutrients and waste products. The fluid pressure created by the aqueous humour in the anterior cavity helps to maintain the shape of the eye.

- The *posterior cavity* is the larger of the two cavities of the eye and is filled with a gelatinous mass known as vitreous humour. The vitreous humour helps to stabilise the shape of the eye, as the activity of the extraocular muscles would otherwise distort the shape of the eye. The pressure it creates also helps to keep the neural part of the retina against the pigmented part; although the two are close together, they are not fixed to each other, and thus this external pressure is required.

Focusing Images onto the Retina

For a visual image to be useful, it must be focused on to the retina; this is the purpose of the lens of the eye. First, the light entering the eye is subject to refraction, and the lens provides the additional, adjustable refraction required to focus the image onto the retina.

Refraction

Light is refracted (bent) when it passes from one medium to another medium with a different density (Figure 18.9). The majority of the refraction in the eye happens when light enters the cornea from the air; additional refraction occurs when light passes from the aqueous humour into the lens. The lens provides the extra refraction to focus the light on to the retina and can adjust this refraction according to the focal length.

Focal length is the distance between the focal point (e.g. on the retina) and the centre of the lens (Figure 18.10). It is dependent on:

- The distance from the object to the lens. The further away an object is, the shorter the focal length.
- The shape of the lens. The rounder the lens the more refraction occurs. A very round lens has a shorter focal length than a flatter lens.

The lens lies behind the cornea and is held in place by ligaments that are attached to the ciliary body. The process of changing the shape of the lens to focus an image on to the retina is known as accommodation. The shape of the lens is altered by tension being applied to or relaxed on the suspensory ligaments by smooth muscles within the ciliary body (Figure 18.11).

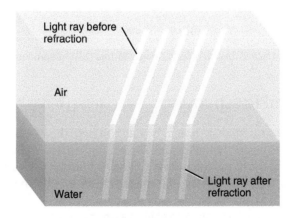

Refraction of light rays

FIGURE 18.9 Refraction of light passing from air (less dense) to water (dense). Source: Tortora (2016). Reproduced with permission of John Wiley & Sons.

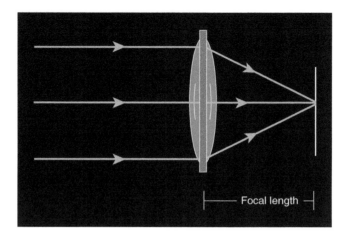

FIGURE 18.10   Focal length.

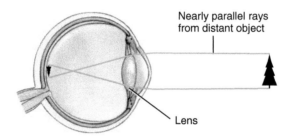

(a) Viewing distant object

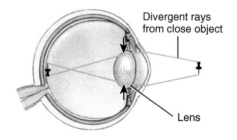

(b) Accommodation close object

FIGURE 18.11   Accommodation to (a) far and (b) near objects. Source: Tortora (2016). Reproduced with permission of John Wiley & Sons.

Myopia, Hyperopia and Presbyopia

In a person who has myopia (short-sightedness), the lens is unable to focus the image on to the retina and the focus of the image falls short (Figure 18.12). With myopia, people can see objects close to them but those that are far away are blurred. Myopia is easily corrected for by the use of corrective lenses, either in the form of glasses or contact lenses.

In the person with hyperopia (long-sightedness), the image is focused on to a point behind the retina (Figure 18.13); thus, these people can see things at a distance but not near to them.

Presbyopia is the loss of the ability to focus on close objects as the person ages; the most common theory for this is the loss of elasticity in the lens. The loss of the ability to focus on near objects occurs in everyone, but at different rates and with different effects on vision. The onset of presbyopia is most commonly noticed at 40–50 years of age. Presbyopia is treatable with corrective glasses (usually known as reading glasses, although they are corrective for all tasks that require near vision).

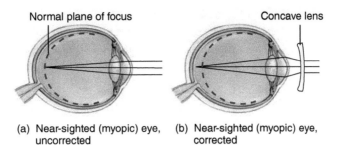

(a) Near-sighted (myopic) eye, uncorrected

(b) Near-sighted (myopic) eye, corrected

FIGURE 18.12 (a) Myopic eye uncorrected and (b) corrected by a concave lens. Source: Tortora (2016). Reproduced with permission of John Wiley & Sons.

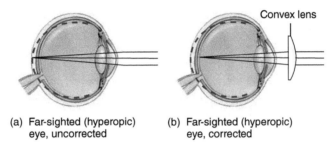

(a) Far-sighted (hyperopic) eye, uncorrected

(b) Far-sighted (hyperopic) eye, corrected

FIGURE 18.13 (a) Hyperopic eye uncorrected and (b) corrected by a convex lens. Source: Tortora (2016). Reproduced with permission of John Wiley & Sons.

The Processing of Visual Information

Once axons from the ganglion cells have exited the eye through the optic disc, they proceed to the diencephalon as the optic nerves (cranial nerve II). Involuntary eye control (such as pupillary reflexes) is processed in the diencephalon and the brainstem.

Reflective Learning Activity

A person can be fined if they do not tell the Driver and Vehicle Licensing Agency (DVLA) about a medical condition that affects their driving. If a person with an eye condition is involved in an accident as a result, they may be prosecuted. Go to the GOV.UK web site (https://www.gov.uk/driving-eyesight-rules) and find out more information about the eye conditions that need to be reported.

Disorders of the Eye

Retinal Detachment

Retinal detachment is the detachment of the neural layer from the rest of the retina. Patients may experience:

- Flashing lights
- Floaters – small dark particles in the vision caused by small haemorrhages
- Loss of vision – related to the area of detachment.

Orange Flag Alert: Loss of Vision

Loss of vision can not only affect a person's physical health by increasing the risk of falls and impacting negatively on quality of life, but can also have a big impact on an individual's mental health. Loss of vision has been linked to loneliness, social isolation as well as feelings of worry, anxiety, and fear.

Treatment is with surgery:

- *Laser therapy* or photocoagulation is used to seal tears or holes in the retina and prevent the further accumulation of subretinal fluid, which would otherwise make the detachment worse.
- *Plombage* (scleral buckling) – a small square of material is sutured to the sclera over the site of the hole, thus pushing the retinal layers back together.
- *Encirclement* – a silicone band is placed around the eyeball. This is used where there is a large area of detachment or multiple holes.
- *Vitrectomy* (pars plana vitrectomy) – removal of the vitreous humour allows the surgeon better access to the tear. Cryotherapy or laser therapy is then used to heal the break. The vitreous is then replaced with gas or fluid to splint the retina in place. Postoperative positioning is vital to ensure that the gas or fluid remains in the correct place. If a gas is used, the patient must not fly until given permission by a doctor, as changes in pressure can cause increased intraorbital pressure. The most commonly used gas is air but other gases are used (such as perfluoropropane). The gas will remain in place for 2–12 weeks and will be gradually replaced by vitreous humour over that time. If fluid (such as silicone-based oil) is used, then it will need to be removed at a later date.
- *Pneumatic retinopexy* – a gas is injected into the vitreous humour. The gas expands in place pushing the retina back in place. The break is treated with cryotherapy before the gas is injected or laser therapy after the retina has flattened in place.

Subretinal fluid is drained during all these procedures to allow the separated layers to come into contact again.

Post discharge patient care includes:

- Analgesia – patients will experience eye pain after surgery.
- Eye care – the eyelids and conjunctiva are usually swollen after surgery.

Medication Management: Gas in the Eye

Other than air, the most commonly used gases in vitrectomy and pneumatic retinopexy can interact with nitrous oxide (used as pain relief in childbirth and for pain relief in emergency situations). It is important that any paramedics/emergency healthcare practitioners are informed of the gas in the eye so that they avoid the use of nitrous oxide. If the patient requires a general anaesthetic, it is important that the anaesthetist is informed.

Snapshot 18.3   Sudden Vision Loss

Pre-arrival Information

You are dispatched to a 67 year old man who is complaining of sudden vision loss.

On Arrival with the Patient

On arrival, you are met at the door by the patient, who introduces himself as Gary. You ask Gary what has happened.

Gary tells you that he was watching TV when he started to see dark squiggly lines floating across his eyes. He said he was rubbing his eyes to make them go away and that was working until he started to see flashes of light in his left eye. All of a sudden he noticed that his sight became 'weird'. He says it feels like someone has closed a curtain on either side of his eyes and he can only see in the middle. He says it feels like he has lost his peripheral vision.

You ask when his symptoms started and he said about an hour ago.

You perform a quick assessment and learn that Gary's vital signs are all within normal ranges and that Gary has high blood pressure and diabetes. You also learn that Gary had cataract surgery last year.

What is your diagnosis?

Before reading on, think about this patient's presentation and try and determine what you think has happened and how you would manage this case.

In this case, you can see that Gary is showing symptoms consistent with retinal detachment. The squiggly lines, flashes of light and 'curtains' on peripheral vision are all classic symptoms.

Gary also has risk factors of recent eye surgery and diabetes. You ask Gary if he has ever heard of retinal detachment, and Gary says he thinks he remembers his mother had that before she went blind. Knowing that a family history is another risk factor, you feel comfortable concluding that this is the mostly likely diagnosis.

You tell Gary that he should be transported to the hospital emergency department and he says that he doesn't want to go. He says that he hates the emergency department and would prefer to see his general practitioner (GP) tomorrow. You tell Gary that he has to see a specialist doctor in the emergency department straight away. Gary says that he is not in any pain and he is sure his own GP can handle this tomorrow.

You explain to Gary that while his GP may be an excellent healthcare provider, they will not be able to treat him for this problem. You explain that retinal detachment is an emergency, even if there is no pain, and if he does not get treatment right way he may lose his sight altogether. Gary reluctantly agrees to go with you.

Retinopathy

The leading cause of retinopathy in the UK is diabetes mellitus (Khan et al. 2017). It can be divided into two types:

1. *Non-proliferative retinopathy* – aneurysms of the capillaries of the eyes, retinal haemorrhages and hardened exudates of lipids.

2. *Proliferative retinopathy* – the retina has become ischaemic and, in response, there is a development of new blood vessels in the eye; however, new blood vessels are fragile and have a tendency to bleed. These blood vessels also grow into the vitreous humour. Eventually, fibrous bands develop, which pull on the retina and cause retinal detachment.

Treatment of retinopathy includes:

- Control of cholesterol levels.
- Advice on diet and glycaemic control.
- Laser therapy to the retina – dead retinal tissue does not encourage new blood vessel formation. A laser beam is therefore used to create multiple small areas of dead retinal tissue (scotomas), which will not have an effect on vision but will reduce the growth of new blood vessels.
- Vitrectomy – removal of the vitreous humour; this removes blood vessels and haemorrhages. Vitreous humour is not naturally replaced by the body; however, replacement with aqueous humour will occur.

Clinical Investigations: Examination Using the Glasgow Coma Scale

Best Eye Opening Response

If a patient's eyes are closed due to swelling or facial fractures, this is recorded as 'C' on the chart. Under these circumstances, eye opening is then meaningless.

a. *Spontaneous eye opening*: it is important to exclude the fact that a patient is asleep prior to proceeding to assess eye opening. This is recorded when a patient is observed to be awake with eyes open. This observation is made without any speech or touch. Spontaneous eye opening is allocated a score of 4.

b. *Eye opening to speech*: where there is no spontaneous eye opening, this is recorded when a patient opens their eyes to loud, clear commands. Eye opening to speech is allocated a score of 3.

c. *Eye opening to pain*: there is no eye opening to loud, clear commands. Eye opening to pain is recorded when a patient opens their eyes to a painful stimulus: fingertip pressure and supraorbital ridge pressure are the two most commonly used methods of applying a painful stimulus with caution. These guidelines recommend that eye opening to pain is assessed by applying supraorbital ridge pressure to stimulate the supraorbital nerve, increasing the pressure until a response is obtained. It could be suggested that supraorbital ridge pressure could cause the patient to grimace and keep the eyes closed. Fingertip pressure could lead to misinterpretation of the eye opening response due to other complicating factors such as hemiparesis and high spinal cord injury. Further, the response caused by fingertip pressure can also be misinterpreted as a motor response, particularly when the problems associated with 'localising' and 'withdrawing' to pain are taken into account. Eye opening to pain is allocated a score of 2.

d. *None*: this is recorded when there is no response to a painful stimulus observed. No eye opening is allocated a score of 1. A patient with flaccid ocular muscles may lie with their eyes open all the time. This is not a true arousal response and should be recorded as a 'no eye opening' response and allocated a score of 1. It should not be documented as spontaneous eye opening.

Take Home Points

- It is considered that there are five senses of smell, taste, hearing, vision and touch. The sense of touch is excluded from the senses as it is considered a somatic sense.
- Paramedics play a critical role in providing initial care and stabilisation for patients with ear and eye emergencies.
- Proper assessment, protection and transport are key to ensuring the best possible outcomes for patients with ear and eye complaints.
- Effective paramedic care for the ears and eyes is essential to maintain the health and functionality of these sensory organs.
- The provision of high-quality care involves a combination of assessment, education, preventive measures and, when necessary, treatment and intervention.

Summary

This chapter has provided an exploration of the anatomy of the ears and eyes including details of:

- Equilibrium, which is a part of the sense of balance and is based in the hair cells of the semicircular canals and the vestibule.
- Hearing, which is based in the hair cells in the organ of Corti in the cochlea of the inner ear.
- Sight, which is based in the photoreceptors of the eye.

Details have also been provided on some common disorders of the ears:

- Tympanic membrane rupture
- Otitis media
- Ménière's disease.

And disorders of the eyes:

- Retinal detachment
- Retinopathy.

References

Gopen, Q. (2010). Pathology and clinical course: inflammatory diseases of the middle ear. In: *Glassock–Shambaugh Surgery of the Ear*, 6e (ed. A.J. Gulya, L.B. Minar, and D.S. Poe), 425–436. Beijing: Peoples Medical Publishing House.

Khan, A., Petropoulos, I.N., Ponirakis, G., and Malik, R.A. (2017). Visual complications in diabetes mellitus: beyond retinopathy. *Diabetic Medicine* 34 (4): 478–484.

Muncie, H.L., Sirmans, S.M., and James, E. (2017). Dizziness: approach to evaluation and management. *American Family Physician* 93 (3): 154–162.

Pfieffer, M.L., Anthamatten, A., and Glassford, M. (2019). Assessment and treatment of dizziness and vertigo. *The Nurse Practitioner* 44 (10): 29–36.

Tortora, G.J. (2016). *Principles of Anatomy and Physiology*, 15e. Hoboken, NJ: Wiley.

Further Reading

Kaur, S., Larsen, H., and Nattis, A. (2019). Primary care approach to eye conditions. *Osteopathic Family Physician* 11 (2): 28–34.

Muncie, H.L. Jr., Sirmans, S.M., and James, E. (2017). Dizziness: approach to evaluation and management. *American Family Physician* 95 (3): 154–162.

Online Resources

Royal National Institute of Blind People (RNIB): www.rnib.org.uk
The RNIB is a UK-based charity offering information, support and advice to people experiencing sight loss. The website is a useful source of information, including sections on eye conditions, tests and coping with sight loss.

National Institute on Deafness and Other Communication Disorders: http://www.nidcd.nih.gov/health/Pages/Default.aspx
A useful website maintained by the United States National Institutes of Health detailing various disorders of the ear and mouth, including taste disorders, balance disorders and disorders of the ear.

ENT UK: https://entuk.org
The website of the British Association of Otorhinolaryngologists and the British Academic Conference in Otolaryngology. This group states its aims as including promoting care, professional education and information for the public. The site has useful information on a variety of conditions of the ear and the nose.

eyeSmart: http://www.geteyesmart.org/eyesmart/index.cfm
This is a website created and maintained by the American Association of Ophthalmology (eye doctors). It contains useful sections on eye conditions, symptoms and lifestyle advice related to eye health.

Glossary

Ampulla	A sac-like enlargement of a canal or duct.
Autonomic nervous system	The part of the nervous system that controls involuntary functions, made up of the parasympathetic and sympathetic nervous systems.
Balance	The ability to control equilibrium.
Cartilage	A supporting connective tissue made up of various cells and fibres.
Cilia	Small, hair-like processes on the outer surface of some cells.
Connective tissue	Tissue that supports and binds other body tissue.
Convergence	The movement of the eyes inwards to see an object close to the face.
Endolymph	The fluid in the membranous labyrinth of the inner ear.
Equilibrium	Stability at rest or when moving.
Focal length	The distance between the focal point (e.g. on the retina) and the centre of the lens of the eye.
Fovea (fovea centralis)	A small depression in the retina containing cones and where vision is the most acute.
Ganglion	A mass, or group, of nerve cells.
Hyperopia	Long-sightedness.
Iris	The central, coloured portion of the eye.
Lacrimal	Relating to tears.
Ligament	Fibrous tissue that binds joints together and connects bones and cartilage.
Myopia	Short-sightedness.
Parasympathetic nervous system	Part of the autonomic nervous system.
Perilymph	The clear fluid found between the bony labyrinth and the membranous labyrinth in the inner ear.
Photoreceptor	Light-sensing neuron.
Presbyopia	The loss of the ability to focus on close objects as the person ages.
Refraction	The change of direction of light as it passes from one medium to another with a different density.

404

Multiple Choice Questions

1. What is the purpose of the Eustachian tube?
   a. to equalise the pressure between the outer ear and the nasopharynx
   b. to equalise the pressure between the inner ear and the nasopharynx
   c. to equalise the pressure between the middle ear and the nasopharynx
   d. to equalise the pressure between the inner ear and middle ear

2. The utricle and saccule of the ear are stimulated by:
   a. gravity
   b. speed
   c. rotation of the head
   d. vertical acceleration

3. The organ of Corti is found in:
   a. the vestibulocochlear duct
   b. the tympanic duct
   c. the vestibular duct
   d. the cochlear duct

4. Information about equilibrium is transmitted to the brain via a branch of which cranial nerve?
   a. VI
   b. VIII
   c. IX
   d. X

5. The eyelids are made of:
   a. elastic cartilage
   b. connective tissue
   c. muscle tissue
   d. epithelial tissue

6. The coloured part of the eye is known as:
   a. the uvea
   b. the cornea
   c. the iris
   d. the choroid body

7. Photoreceptors are found in:
   a. the innermost part of the retina
   b. the outermost part of the retina
   c. the optic disc
   d. the pigmented part of the neural tunic

8. The majority of the refraction of light in the eye happens at what time?
   a. when the light enters the lens of the eye
   b. when the light enters the pupil
   c. when the light enters the posterior cavity
   d. when the light enters the cornea of the eye

9. What does the shape of the lens change?
   a. The refraction of light
   b. The wavelength of light
   c. The production of tears
   d. The amount of light entering the eye

10. Which of the following terms means 'short sighted'?
    a. Presbyopia
    b. Myopia
    c. Hypopia
    d. Hyperopia

CHAPTER 19

Death and Dying

Sarah Lumley and Simon Sawyer

AIM

This chapter aims to review the physiological signs of the dying process, discuss the grieving process, introduce advance care decisions and explore palliative care and what it means in paramedic practice.

LEARNING OUTCOMES

After reading this chapter you will be able to:

- Define death and explore the physiological process of dying.
- Discuss the five stages of grief and the common stages encountered in paramedic practice.
- Understand common terms, legal definitions and their implications.
- Discuss common treatment options that paramedics can offer to palliative care patients.
- Learn how to perform a death notification.

Test Your Prior Knowledge

1. What are the three stages of dying and the signs and symptoms that will be present in each stage?
2. What are the five commonly accepted stages of grieving?
3. What is the definition of an advance decision to refuse treatment?
4. Are you required to start resuscitation in every circumstance where there is no 'do not attempt CPR' recommendation or advance decision to refuse treatment available?

Introduction

The role of a paramedic will inevitably involve interactions with patients who have died or who are nearing the end of their lives. Understanding the complex nature of death and dying is essential for providing compassionate and comprehensive care to these individuals and their families. While this can be confronting for some, the right knowledge and perspective on the end-of-life experience can help you to navigate this profound aspect of the paramedic's role with sensitivity and professionalism.

Fundamentals of Applied Pathophysiology for Paramedics, First Edition. Edited by Ian Peate and Simon Sawyer.
© 2024 John Wiley & Sons Ltd. Published 2024 by John Wiley & Sons Ltd.

Understanding death and dying is not solely about recognising the physiological processes that occur when life comes to an end. It also involves recognising the impact it has on patients, their families and healthcare providers alike. Through this chapter, we aim to help you develop the knowledge and skills necessary to address the unique needs and challenges that arise during the end-of-life journey, while providing comfort and support to those affected by it.

There is no single best definition of death; it can be defined in a number of ways, for example we may need a definition for legal purposes, which will differ from the definition we use for cultural purposes. For medical purposes, we can define death as either:

- The irreversible cessation of circulatory and respiratory functions, or
- The irreversible cessation of all functions of the entire brain, including the brain stem (Sarbey 2016).

How we actually measure death can vary somewhat with different organisations. Essentially, we look at a lack of vital signs which indicate life.

Clinical Investigations: Verification of Death

Any patient who has the following findings may be declared dead:

- No palpable carotid pulse.
- No heart sounds heard for two minutes.
- No breath sounds heard for two minutes.
- Fixed (non-responsive to light) and dilated pupils (may be varied from underlying eye illness).
- No response to centralised stimulus (supraorbital pressure, mandibular pressure or sternal pressure).
- No motor (withdrawal) response or facial grimace to painful stimulus (pinching inner aspect of elbow or nail bed pressure).

The Process of Dying

Death may be sudden and unexpected; for example, when death occurs as an outcome of injury, such as exsanguination from a wound following a car accident. Alternatively, death may occur over a longer period and be expected; for example, when death occurs as an outcome from cancer.

Whether sudden or expected, as an individual approaches death, the body undergoes a series of changes that lead to the eventual cessation of vital functions. There are three distinct stages of dying, usually termed preactive, active and terminal.

The preactive dying phase typically occurs days to weeks before death (so this phase does not apply to sudden, unexpected deaths). During this stage, the body undergoes physiological and psychological changes that indicate the approaching end of life. Patients may experience decreased energy levels, increased fatigue and a gradual decline in overall functioning. They may withdraw socially and may exhibit decreased interest in food and fluids. Physical symptoms such as weakness, weight loss and changes in vital signs may also become more pronounced. Emotional and psychological changes, including introspection, reflection and the desire for solitude may be observed.

The active dying phase is characterised by more evident and pronounced changes. Typically, this stage occurs within days or hours of death. As death approaches, you will see cardiovascular changes; for example, the heart's pumping ability may weaken, leading to a decrease in blood pressure and reduced pulse rate. As a result, there may be reduced blood flow to vital organs, which can manifest as cool extremities, cyanosis and diminished peripheral pulses. Irregular heart rhythms, such as bradycardia, and eventually ventricular tachycardia or ventricular fibrillation, usually also occur.

Respiratory changes also occur. Respiratory rate may fluctuate and become irregular. Breathing patterns may include periods of rapid, shallow or deep breaths interspersed with apnoea or prolonged pauses. This irregularity stems from a decrease in respiratory drive and altered control mechanisms in the brain. Secretions may accumulate in the airways, leading to rattling or gurgling sounds known as the death rattle.

Neurologically, you will see changes in consciousness and sensory perception. Patients may become increasingly drowsy, disoriented or unresponsive. The level of consciousness can fluctuate, ranging from periods of wakefulness to profound sedation. Sensory perception may also be affected, leading to decreased ability to respond to external stimuli such as touch, sound and light. Seizures or myoclonic jerks (involuntary muscle twitches) may occur in some individuals.

The terminal phase refers to the final moments before death. During this stage, the body's vital functions continue to decline. Breathing becomes slower and shallower, eventually ceasing altogether. The heart rate may become irregular (again ventricular tachycardia or ventricular fibrillation are common) and or weak before stopping altogether (asystole). Skin tone may change, appearing pale or mottled due to reduced blood circulation. At this stage, the patient is generally unresponsive and may not exhibit any purposeful movements or sensory responses. The exact moment of death is often marked by the absence of a detectable pulse, breathing and any signs of brain activity. This time should be noted on the patient's records.

It is important to remember that the stages of dying are general patterns and may not be linear or experienced in the same way by every individual. Each person's journey is unique, and factors such as underlying illness, treatment interventions and personal circumstances can influence the progression and manifestation of these stages. Healthcare professionals should therefore approach each patient with empathy, flexibility and individualised care, recognising and respecting their unique experiences and preferences.

Red and Orange Flags Alert: Death

It is often very difficult to know if a patient is *actively* dying. Patient's may be expected to die, and it may appear that they are dying, but there is no reliable way to say how long it will take or exactly what to expect. Here are some common orange flags that may indicate that a death is expected, and red flags that death may be imminent:

Orange Flags

- The patient has a written advance decision to refuse treatment (ADRT or living will) in place or is in palliative care.
- The patient starts the interaction by telling you they have an ADRT or are in palliative care (often they are very clear with you that they do not want resuscitation).
- The patient is in palliative care and has a history of reduced energy or food intake over the past few days with no attributable cause.

Red Flags (With or Without Orange Flags)

- The patient may state to you 'I think I'm dying'.
- The patient is in a reduced conscious state.
- The patient has indicative vital signs such as hypotension, bradypnea, bradycardia, or arrythmias.
- The patient is cold and cyanotic.

The Grieving Process

The grieving process is a natural response to the loss of a loved one or a significant life change. It is a complex and individual experience that encompasses a range of emotions, thoughts and behaviours as individuals come to terms with their loss. While the grieving process can vary widely from person to person, it generally involves several common stages, which are summarised and described in the Kübler-Ross five stages of grief model (Kübler-Ross et al. 1972; Box 19.1).

It is important to note that these stages are not linear or fixed, and people may move back and forth between them or experience them in different ways. Grief is a highly individual process, and everyone grieves in their own time and manner.

It is also essential to recognise that the grieving process is not a linear journey with a definitive endpoint. Rather, it is a continuing process that evolves and changes over time. Healing from grief does not mean forgetting or completely moving on from the loss but rather finding ways to integrate the loss into one's life and continue living while honouring the memory of the person who was lost.

BOX 19.1 **The Kübler-Ross Five Stages of Grief**

1. *Denial and Shock*: initially, individuals may have difficulty accepting the reality of the loss. They may feel a sense of disbelief, numbness, or shock, as if it has not fully sunk in.
2. *Anger and guilt*: as the reality of the loss sets in, individuals may experience anger and frustration. They may direct their anger at themselves, others, or even the person they lost. Feelings of guilt and remorse may also arise, as individuals question what they could have done differently.
3. *Bargaining*: in this stage, individuals may attempt to negotiate or bargain with a higher power or with themselves. They may make promises or seek ways to change the outcome, hoping to alleviate their pain or bring back what was lost.
4. *Depression*: grief often brings a deep sense of sadness, emptiness, and despair. Individuals may withdraw from others, lose interest in activities they once enjoyed, and struggle with feelings of hopelessness and loneliness.
5. *Acceptance*: over time, individuals begin to come to terms with the loss and accept the new reality. They may find ways to adjust to life without the person they have lost and start to regain a sense of stability and purpose.

Palliative Care

Palliative care is a specialised approach to healthcare that focuses on improving the quality of life for individuals facing serious illnesses, especially illnesses that are life-threatening or incurable. The primary goal of palliative care is to provide relief from the symptoms, pain and stress associated with the illness, rather than attempting to cure the disease itself.

For a patient to be *palliated*, a medical doctors must confirm that no available treatment will likely benefit the patient's condition and their longevity is limited.

Palliative care aims to prevent and relieve suffering through a multifaceted approach including early identification, correct assessment, continuing support and awareness, treatment of pain and other symptoms, and concerns of physical, psychosocial or spiritual in nature (World Health Organization 2020). The overall goal is to ensure that the patient's symptoms are effectively managed and care is individualised to their needs (Palliative Care Australia 2015).

Palliative care is typically provided by a team of healthcare professionals, including doctors, nurses, social workers and other specialists who work together to address the physical, emotional, social and spiritual needs of the patient. This multidisciplinary team takes a holistic approach, considering the patient's overall wellbeing and tailoring the care plan to their individual circumstances and preferences.

The demand for paramedics to be able to provide palliative care services is increasing, as the paramedic scope shifts from emergency medicine to community-based care due to an ageing population and an increase in chronic diseases. Furthermore, many patients prefer to palliate at home, and often rely on paramedics to provide care or transport to the hospital emergency department.

Research shows that including paramedics in multidisciplinary palliative care teams can reduce avoidable hospital admissions and better facilitate patient wishes (Juhrmann et al. 2022). Paramedics are often the first point of contact when patients and families are overwhelmed with how to proceed with decisions based on care and are therefore a valued asset to palliative care. Likewise, paramedics are usually capable of providing comprehensive care that places emphasis on the patient's comfort and quality of life. Paramedics can provide pain management, medication administration, emotional support and comfort to patients and family, and other treatments that alleviate symptoms and improve overall wellbeing (Kirk et al. 2017).

Advance Decision to Refuse Treatment

An *advance decision to refuse treatment* (ADRT), also known as an *advance decision* or *living will* (called an advance care directive in the United States) is a legally binding decision that allows an individual to express their healthcare preferences and make decisions about their medical treatment in advance, particularly in the event they become unable to communicate or make decisions for themselves.

An advance decision is legally binding as long as it fulfils certain criteria (NHS England 2023):

- It must comply with the Mental Capacity Act
- It must be valid
- It must apply to the situation.

An ADRT provides guidance to healthcare providers, family members, and caregivers regarding the individual's desired medical interventions and treatment options.

By having an ADRT in place, individuals can ensure that their healthcare decisions align with their personal values, beliefs and wishes, even if they are unable to communicate or make decisions at the time. These decisions provide peace of mind and assist healthcare professionals and loved ones in making informed decisions about medical treatment and end-of-life care.

The Mental Capacity Act exists to protect and empower people over the age of 16 years who may not have the mental capacity required to make their own decisions regarding their care and treatment. It allows people to appoint a trusted person to make a decision on their behalf should they lack capacity in the future. It also allows for people to be provided with an independent advocate who will support them to make decisions in the event when they might have significant restrictions placed on their freedom and rights. If someone lacks the capacity to make a decision, the Mental Capacity Act states that the decision must be made in the person's best interests. It is vital to consult with other people about the person's best interests, including anyone previously named by the individual, anyone engaged in caring for them, close relatives and friends, enduring power of attorney or any deputy appointed by the Court of Protection to make decisions for the person.

If the person who will receive care cannot provide consent or no longer has capacity to form an ADRT, a *substitute decision maker* can make decisions on behalf of the patient. If the patient has not appointed a substitute decision maker, the law generally automatically grants power to somebody to make health decisions for you. A statutory health attorney must maintain or promote the patient's health and wellbeing and treatment must be in the patient's best interests and take into consideration the patient's likely wants and wishes. By law, a statutory health attorney is the first in listed order of people readily available and appropriate to act, for example a spouse or de facto partner, a person responsible for your primary care over the age of 18 or a person who is a close friend or relative who is over 18.

A health and welfare *lasting power of attorney* (LPA) is a legal document that allows individuals to appoint a trusted person to make decisions about their health and welfare on their behalf if they are unable to do so. The designated person should be someone who understands the individual's values, beliefs and healthcare preferences. The appointed proxy can consult with healthcare professionals and make decisions based on the individual's wishes as stated in the LPA or based on their best interests.

A DNACPR order is a specific type of advanced care directive that instructs healthcare providers *not* to perform CPR in the event of cardiac arrest. This order is typically used when a person's health has declined and resuscitation could cause unnecessary suffering. A DNACPR is typically discussed with healthcare professionals and is often used by individuals with terminal illnesses or those who have made a clear decision not to undergo resuscitation measures. A DNACPR does not provide guidance on other healthcare decisions if the patient is still alive.

It is important to note that the availability and specific regulations surrounding advanced care directives can vary depending on the jurisdiction or country. Consulting with legal professionals, healthcare providers or organisations specialising in end-of-life care can help individuals understand the legal requirements and options available to them when making advance care decisions.

It is generally acknowledged that if a paramedic cannot visualise a physical DNACPR or ADRT, they are obligated to provide care or resuscitation to a patient in cardiac arrest, due to their legal and ethical obligations to provide life-sustaining treatments (Waldrop et al. 2020). However, it is also common for legislation to allow paramedics to withhold resuscitation in the event that a DNACPR cannot be sighted, when a trusted person, such as a family member, is on scene and verbally confirms there is a DNACPR in place. It is important to consider that resuscitation may not be appropriate for patients with terminal illness, especially if it would likely be ineffective or would cause unnecessary suffering. In these situations, paramedics are encouraged to discuss with the family ceasing or not commencing resuscitation.

Clinical Investigations: Resuscitation

When encountering a patient that you suspect may have an ADRT or DNACPR in place, it is best practice to ask a direct question: 'Do you have an ADRT (or 'do not resuscitate' order)?' If you encounter an elderly patient who does not have a DNACPR but has a high chance of cardiac arrest, you might ask, 'Have you thought about your wishes should your heart stop? Do you want me to resuscitate you?' It is best to ask direct questions and clarify their wishes with the patient. If they seem unsure or unwilling to answer, you can assume that they want a full resuscitation.

Assisted Dying

The role of a paramedic in assisted dying can vary depending on state or country. Paramedics may be called to provide assistance to a patient who has chosen to end their life, and this may involve providing medication or other interventions to assist a patient in ending their life peacefully with dignity and minimal pain. Specific procedures and protocols will vary depending on location. It is not the role of a paramedic to provide information or suggest access to this type of treatment. It is best to refer the patient to their treating medical team for access to this information (Boughey 2021).

Snapshot 19.1   Assisted Dying in a Legal Jurisdiction

In a jurisdiction where assisted dying is legal, a patient named Robert has been battling terminal cancer for several years. He has discussed his wish to die peacefully with dignity surrounding by his wife and on his own terms with his doctor, oncologist and a psychiatrist. After meeting the legal criteria and obtaining the necessary approvals from medical professionals, Robert has expressed his desire to end his suffering through assisted dying.

Robert's condition rapidly deteriorated one evening and has decided he wants to proceed with the medical regimen to end his life. Robert's wife is quite concerned as she thinks its too soon and she cannot get in contact with any family members to be with her to support her through the process. She has called an ambulance as she is scared to be alone and worried about how much pain Robert appears to be in.

The paramedics are able to provide an important role in assisting both Robert and his wife during this process. They are able to administer necessary medications within their scope to assist with Robert's symptoms, such as pain relief, and can also assist with the delivery of the medication prescribed by the physician to induce a peaceful death. They can provide emotional support to Robert and his wife, who may be experiencing a range of emotions including relief, sadness and anxiety. Paramedics can thoroughly document the situation which can be used for medical and legal records. Paramedics can also provide post-procedure care including grief support and assisting with the organisation of an undertaker.

411

Sudden Unexpected Death in Paediatrics

The unexpected death of children, also known as sudden unexpected death in paediatrics, refers to the sudden and unexpected death of an apparently healthy child. Obviously, this occurrence can be extremely distressing for parents, families and communities.

There are several medical conditions and factors that may contribute to unexpected death in children, but in many cases, the exact cause remains unknown. Some of the potential causes and contributing factors that are often considered in such cases include:

- Sudden infant death syndrome (SIDS) is a diagnosis given when the death of an infant (usually under one year of age) remains unexplained even after a comprehensive postmortem examination. It is believed to be a combination of factors, including an underlying vulnerability, an immature respiratory control centre in the brain and certain environmental stressors.

- Some children may have undiagnosed heart conditions or structural abnormalities in the heart, which can lead to sudden cardiac arrest or arrhythmias. These conditions can be genetic or develop during fetal development.
- Certain infections, such as severe respiratory infections, meningitis or sepsis, can cause a sudden deterioration in a child's health, leading to unexpected death.
- Accidental injuries or trauma, including suffocation, choking or head injuries, can result in sudden death.
- Some rare metabolic disorders, such as certain inborn errors of metabolism, can present with sudden and unexpected symptoms, including death. These disorders often affect the body's ability to break down or use specific substances.
- Accidental ingestion or exposure to toxic substances, medications or household chemicals can result in sudden death in children.
- Certain neurological disorders, such as epilepsy or brain malformations, can predispose children to sudden death due to seizures or other complications.
- Child abuse or neglect can also result in unexpected death in some cases. It is crucial to investigate any suspicious circumstances surrounding a child's death and ensure that appropriate legal action is taken, if necessary.

When a child experiences unexpected death, a comprehensive investigation is typically conducted by the appropriate authorities, which may include police and the coroner. This may involve a thorough medical examination, review of the child's medical history, interviews with family members, and sometimes additional laboratory tests or imaging studies. In some cases, genetic testing may also be recommended to identify underlying genetic abnormalities or predispositions. In such cases, the patient care records completed by the paramedic will be viewed and scrutinised, so it is essential that you complete thorough and accurate records.

Unexpected deaths in children are relatively rare events. Many efforts have been made to raise awareness about safe sleep practices, provide education on reducing risk factors for SIDS, and improve early detection and treatment of various medical conditions. Medical professionals and public health authorities work together to understand these tragedies and implement preventive measures to reduce the occurrence of unexpected deaths in children.

Paramedic Management of Death and Dying

Paramedics have a key role to play in the management of death and dying. Patients receiving palliative care are probably receiving care from a range of health providers; paramedics are expected to communicate effectively and collaborate with other members of their team (Boughey 2021). This includes sharing information about the patient's condition, medications and treatment plan. Paramedics are expected to respect their patients' dignity and autonomy and involve them in decisions about their care, including respecting their cultural and religious beliefs (Anderson et al. 2021).

While paramedics traditionally cannot prescribe for patients, there is a range of supportive treatments that might be required when called to terminally ill or palliated patient, including:

- *Pain management*: pain is the most common symptom recorded by terminally ill patients. While patients will typically be on an individualised pain management plan, sometimes additional support is required, whether it be difficulty accessing the prescribed pain management, assistance with breakthrough pain, or the prescribed amounts have not met the patient's needs.
- *Oxygen therapy*: in the disease progression of terminally ill patients, they will often develop lung and/ or breathing problems requiring oxygen therapy.
- *Fluid therapy*: symptoms such as vomiting, nausea, diarrhoea and nausea are common in terminally ill patients and fluid therapy is sometimes necessary.
- *Symptom management*: paramedics can provide interventions to manage symptoms of pain, nausea, vomiting, anxiety or agitation.

- *Emotional support*: this is often a terrifying time for patients and their families as they navigate uncharted territory. Family members may have initially agreed to provide the care for the patient and, when the disease progresses, they may find that they can no longer provide the care necessary (Waldrop et al. 2020).

Medication Management: Palliation

Common medications used in palliative care include (Good et al. 2006):

- Analgesics:
  - *Opioids* (e.g. morphine, fentanyl, oxycodone, tramadol) are used for moderate to severe pain and can be administered in a range of routes including subcutaneously, orally, intravenously, intramuscularly, intranasally.
  - *Non-steroidal anti-inflammatory drugs* (e.g. ibuprofen, naproxen) are used for mild to moderate pain relief.
  - *Non-opioid analgesics such as* paracetamol are used for mild to moderate pain relief.
  - *Adjuvant analgesics* (e.g. sodium valproate, lyrica, tricyclic antidepressants) are used to enhance pain relief or to manage neuropathic pain.
- Antiemetics are used for the management of nausea and vomiting:
  - Serotonin receptor antagonists (e.g. ondansetron)
  - Phenothiazines (e.g. prochlorperazine)
  - Corticosteroids (e.g. dexamethasone) – also used to improve appetite.
- Anxiolytics and sedatives:
  - Benzodiazepines (e.g. lorazepam, diazepam) are used for anxiety, restlessness and agitation.
  - Antipsychotics (e.g. haloperidol) are used for delirium, agitation and psychosis.
  - Barbiturates (e.g. phenobarbital) are used for severe agitation or intractable symptoms.
- Antidepressants:
  - Selective serotonin reuptake inhibitors (e.g. fluoxetine, sertraline) are used for managing depression and anxiety.
- Bronchodilators:
  - Beta-agonists (e.g. salbutamol) are used for relieving bronchospasm and dyspnoea in patients with respiratory conditions:
- Anticholinergics (e.g. hyoscine) are used for the management of end-stage respiratory reflexes (e.g. grunting, secretions).
- Laxatives (e.g. docusate) are stool softeners, used to treat constipation.

413

While palliated patients have an uncurable underlying condition, they may still develop reversible conditions including sepsis, hyperkalaemia and exacerbations of their conditions requiring acute care (Blackmore 2022). Determining whether the patient's presentation is due to the progression of their incurable medical condition as part of the disease process or a treatable complication, or an entirely separate medical complaint can be difficult to determine, especially as paramedics in the prehospital field with limited access to information.

To assist you in determining whether the patient's current symptoms are related to their terminal illness or are the result of a separate and treatable disease process, you should perform a thorough review of the patient's medical history, assess their current and previous symptoms, perform a thorough physical assessment and, most importantly, consult with other healthcare professionals involved in the patient's care (remember that the patient will probably be managed by a broad team of health professionals with expertise in palliative care).

A patient's general practitioner is also a good source of information. Most ambulance services also have a consultation line that can be used when a higher level of medical knowledge and expertise is needed to assist in the clinical decision-making process.

Remember that the patient may not wish to be transported to hospital, even if you believe that not going will be detrimental to their health. Consider alternatives such as alternative destinations or not transporting the patient altogether. Determine what treatment the patient is probably going to require for their presentation and whether that can be initiated outside the hospital environment.

BOX 19.2   **Cultural Differences**

Cultural beliefs and practices can strongly influence how patient and families approach end-of-life care. For example (Martin and Barkley 2017; Searight and Gafford 2005):

- *Belief about death and dying*: some culture believes in the importance of keeping the body intact and may resist interventions that involve invasive procedures while other cultures may see death as a natural progression in life and wish to prioritise comfort and pain relief.
- *Beliefs about medical treatments*: some cultures may prioritise the use of natural remedies or spiritual healing practices over Western medical treatments.
- *Communication styles and language barriers*: communication styles may differ based on cultural norms and language barriers may make it difficult for paramedics to understand patients' needs and preference.
- *Religious practices and customs*: A family's religion can impact how a patient and their family approach end-of-life care, including decisions about treatments, pain management and spiritual care. Paramedics should be aware of these practices and work with patients and their families to provide care that honours their beliefs.

Overall, cultural differences can have a significant impact on how paramedics deliver palliative care. To provide culturally competent care, paramedics should be aware of cultural differences and work with patients and families to understand their beliefs and preferences and provide care that is respectful and responsive to their needs.

Keep in mind that a key goal in palliative care medicine is to allow the patient to die at place of their choice. Therefore, generally, transportation of the patient to a hospital facility is to be avoided; however, there are some circumstances where the patient will request or agree to transport.

Finally, and above all else, always take the patient's wishes into consideration and do your utmost to seek, listen to and abide by their decisions. Palliative care is patient-centred care. Talk to your patient. Explain to them what currently wrong and the available treatment options are. Advise them what this could mean for their underlying condition. And do whatever you can to meet their expectations (Rome et al. 2011; Blackmore 2022). Also remember that there may be cultural differences that you need to consider (Box 19.2).

Paramedic Conversations

Paramedics perform crucial clinical roles during the death of a patient, but equally important is their role of emotional supporter and caregiver within the same incident. This requires an intricate balance of attending to the patient's needs while also providing calm and compassionate support (Myall et al. 2020). These interactions have the potential to form significant and powerful memories that can remain with individuals on scene for years to come. Thus, the ability to navigate these complex dynamics with carefully considered dialogue and actions all while maintaining empathy and sensitivity, is a crucial aspect of a paramedic's job (Brown 2016; Walker 2018).

It is important to remember that, often, terminally ill patients still have capacity and a good level of comprehension and ability to participate in conversation and decision making, especially earlier on in their disease state. When their disease is more progressed, they can display some difficulties with understanding, or they might be cognitively affected by the medications they are prescribed to manage the symptoms of their condition. Here are some simple techniques to use when communicating to terminally ill patients and their families.

- Approach the conversation with empathy and respect for the patient's decisions, even if they do not align with your own personal values. Let the patient and family know you are there to support them. Use clear, simple and concise language. Avoid using medical terminology but avoid talking in a way that would be deemed condescending or patronising.
- Use active listening. Use both verbal and non-verbal communication techniques and allow the patient to express their thoughts and feelings. Clarify the patient's wants and wishes and endeavour to meet their expectations.

- Be honest. It is important for the patient and family to understand their situation and that paramedics cannot necessarily provide all the answers they are seeking. If a paramedic suspects the patient is likely going to die, it is important to remain professional and continue providing the best care available. Do not try to lighten their situation with false hope. Remember to be honest and respectful and to clarify the patient's wants and wishes.
- Offer emotional support to the patient and their family or carers. Remember, once the patient dies, your new patient becomes their family.

Talking to Family During an Active Resuscitation

It can be difficult to talk to family members throughout a resuscitation effort on their loved one. By making short but frequent contact moments with the family, you can help to prepare them for the potential for a negative outcome and give time for them to process the situation they are being presented with. This is ideally performed by the most competent member of the resuscitation team. This should not be done at the expense of the resuscitation efforts, and discussions with family should only be performed when time and resources enable it. As a general guide:

- Initial encounter: introduce yourself and your role to the family present on scene. Explain to them that the patient is currently not breathing for themselves and that their heart is not beating. Tell them the patient is critically unwell and that resuscitation does not necessarily result in a successful outcome, but by trying to resuscitate them you are giving the patient the best chance for survival. Excuse yourself to return to the resuscitation and tell them you will endeavour to provide them updates when possible.
- Subsequent encounter(s): if time allows, touch base with the family to update them on the progress of the resuscitation at regular intervals (e.g. 5–10 minutes).
- Penultimate encounter: if you are nearing the end of your resuscitation efforts with no indication of gaining spontaneous circulation, make contact with the family and advise them you have not been successful in your attempts. Tell them that your plan is to provide one more round of resuscitation, and if this does not have a positive result then you will cease resuscitation.
- Final encounter: after ceasing resuscitation and performing end-of-life checks to declare the patient deceased (including recording the time of death), return to speak to the family. Gather everybody present on scene so they can hear the death notification at first hand. Advise them that, despite your team's efforts, you were unable to revive the patient and they have died. It is important to be concise and clear. Do not use euphemisms like 'they have passed on', use the term 'died' (Box 19.3).
- Allow the time to process the situation, and answer any questions and offer support. When appropriate, advise them of next steps (e.g. if police have to be called or if the patient's GP is available to sign a death certificate).

If the family asks to see the patient, do not try to prevent them; this is an important part of accepting the death and grieving. Do try to prepare the scene and the patient to reduce distress by (Munoz 2016; Jabr 2021):

- Remove medical equipment from the patient that is not required to be left in place and remove all clinical waste from the scene.
- Aim to make the patient look presentable (e.g. re-dress them, clean up blood or other bodily fluids, and cover patient respectfully, but do not cover their face).
- It can be difficult but, if possible, you can close the patient's eyelids.
- Allow family to say goodbye with privacy; do not put a limit on this time.
- Give the family space but remain on scene and available and approachable to family for any questions they may have.

BOX 19.3   **The Do's and Don'ts of Death Notification**

Do

- Use direct words such as 'dead' and 'dying'.
- Make eye contact.
- Learn the patient's and family members' names and use them when speaking to them.
- Answer questions to the best of your ability but be honest when you do not know the answer and endeavour to find an answer.
- Show your own emotions when necessary. Paramedics are people too and it is OK to be upset by things that are upsetting.

Don't

- Use words such as 'we lost him' or 'he has passed'.
- Rush: rushing the conversation can make the family feel confused, dismissed or unsupported.
- Make assumptions about the family's beliefs or cultural practices; ask about their wishes.
- Apologise: you can be sorry for their loss, but do not say that you are sorry that you could not revive the patient. This could make family think that mistakes were made during the resuscitation which contributed to the patient's death.

Snapshot 19.2

Background

Barry is a 90-year-old man who has a medical history of ischaemic heart disease and chronic obstructive pulmonary disease. He has recently been taken off the majority of his medications by his GP with a focus on maintaining his quality of life and managing his general symptoms. He is frail and spends most of his days at home with his wife, Mary, who is his career.

Pre-arrival Information

At approximately 4.30 a.m. on the 1 June, Mary woke to Barry complaining of chest pain before collapsing in front of her. Mary called for the ambulance immediately and was instructed by the call handler to commence CPR immediately. Mary, being old and frail herself, could not lift Barry off the bed, so she was advised so attempt to perform CPR on her husband on their bed.

On Arrival with the Patient

You and your crew partner and the critical care paramedic arrived approximately six minutes later and ask Mary immediately whether Barry has an advance health decision, to which she replied that they hadn't previously thought about it. Mary said that when she was told to start CPR she thought she had no option. She requests that further resuscitation attempts are made on her husband.

   You move the patient and start resuscitation efforts while the wife stands over her husband crying, overwhelmed and trying to determine what her husband's wishes are. You discover that Barry makes no response to a central stimulus, is not breathing, and has no pulse and is in asystole. Mary begs the crew to continue resuscitating her husband until her daughter arrives.

Questions to Explore

- Are you required to commence resuscitation attempts on this patient?
- Given what you know about Barry, what is the likelihood of a successful outcome? What contributing factors are present that decreases his odds of a spontaneous return of circulation and why?
- How should you proceed if you don't think that resuscitation should be started or if you think it should be ceased?

Discussion

This scene could be handled in a number of ways. There is no one single correct way. The following is a common scenario for how this scene could unfold.

When you arrive at this scene, resuscitation has already been commenced and a family member has requested you to attempt to resuscitate the patient. Therefore, it would be reasonable for you to commence resuscitation. In the absence of a DNACPR or ADRT, and with the family member requesting resuscitation, there is no good justification to withhold or cease the attempt.

If you did not believe that attempting resuscitation was in the patient's best interests, you should discuss your concerns with the family while attempting to resuscitate the patient. Have an open and honest conversation with the family, explaining your concerns. In this case, you might say that Barry has a very low chance of survival given his advanced age, his medical history and his current lack of vital signs. You might explain that a resuscitation attempt carries a high chance of significant trauma and prolonged painful death. Additionally, Barry's GP has begun palliative care management by removing him from his medications and focusing on quality of life for his remaining time.

If the family member then decides that it is not in the patient's best interests and directs you to stop the resuscitation, you can cease.

In this case, if Mary still requests you continue, the most reasonable course of action would be to continue the resuscitation, and so you continue for five minutes, at which point Barry and Mary's daughter, Beatrix, arrives. You explain the situation to Beatrix and explain that, at present, Barry is not responding to the resuscitation and there is a very low chance of survival. Beatrix speaks with her mother and says that she feels that Barry would not want resuscitation. Mary bursts into tears and hugs Beatrix. At this point Beatrix, turns to you and says that you can stop resuscitating Barry. You pause and ask Mary if she is OK with you stopping; she continues to cry but nods her head. You mark the time that resuscitation ceased. While your partner performs a verification of death and cleans the scene of plastic wrappers (leaving all pads and intravenous leads attached to the patient), you attend to the family.

You offer to sit with them and ask if there is anything you can do. Both Mary and Beatrix say they do not want anything. Given the time of morning and being unable to get in contact with the patient's GP, you call the police and explain to the family that this a normal part of the process. There may be some circumstances when death has been imminently expected that the family have preorganised a funeral home and undertaker. In these situations, you do not need to have the police involved and a GP has 48 hours to be contacted and to provide a death certificate. You sit with the family and listen to them talking, answering questions when asked. When the police arrive, you enquire again if there is anything Mary or Beatrix need; they again decline, and you leave them in the care of the police.

Take Home Points

- The body undergoes a series of changes that lead to the eventual cessation of vital functions that take place as three distinct phases: preactive, active and terminal.
- The grieving process is a natural response to the loss of a loved one or significant life change and encompasses a range of emotions, thoughts and behaviours that can vary widely from person to person.
- Palliative care is an individualised approach to end-of-life cares that focuses on improving the quality of life for individuals facing terminal individuals.
- Paramedic management of death and dying revolves around providing pain management, oxygen therapy, fluid therapy, symptom management and emotional support.
- Delivering a death notification requires careful thought and a balance between clear, direct and factual communication and emotional support. Having short but frequent encounters with the family during the resuscitation establishes rapport and primes the family to receiving news of a possibly poor outcome.

Summary

Managing death and dying is an important skill for paramedics. However, given its broad nature, there is often ambiguity around this topic. It is crucial for paramedics to go beyond merely understanding the physiological stages of death and develop the necessary skills and knowledge to address challenges associated with this domain. This includes navigating legal documentation, delivering compassionate death notifications to friends and family, and providing appropriate throughout the grieving process.

Managing incidents involving patients in various stages of dying demands an individualised approach, necessitating flexibility and adaptability in the provision of patient care. The ability to provide pain management and effectively managing symptoms and proving emotional support enables paramedics to provide comprehensive care and support to patients and their loved ones during death.

References

Anderson, N.E., Robinson, J., Moeke-Maxwell, T. et al. (2021). Paramedic care of the dying, deceased and bereaved in Aotearoa, New Zealand. *Progress Palliative Care* 29 (2): 84–90.

Blackmore, T.A. (2022). What is the role of paramedics in palliative and end of life care? *Palliative Medicine* 36 (3): 402–404. https://doi.org/10.1177/02692163211073263.

Boughey, M. (2021). *The Role of Paramedics in Palliative and End of Life Care: Scoping report*. Melbourne: Safer Care Victoria.

Brown, N. (2016). Pre-hospital resuscitation: what shall we tell the family? *Journal of Paramedic Practice: The Clinical Monthly for Emergency Care Professionals* 8 (2): 86–89. https://doi.org/10.12968/jpar.2016.8.2.86.

Good, P., Cavenagh, J., Currow, D. et al. (2006). What are the essential medications in palliative care? *Australian Family Physician* 35 (4): 261–264. 200604good.pdf.

Jabr, A. (2021). Death communication: what we've failed to teach. *EMS World* 1 February. https://www.hmpglobablearningnetwork.com/site/emsworld/article/1225347-ems-death-communication (accessed 14 October 2023).

Juhrmann, M.L., Vandersman, P., Butow, P.N., and Clayton, J.M. (2022). Paramedics delivering palliative and end-of-life care in community-based settings: a systematic integrative review with thematic synthesis. *Palliative Medicine* 36 (3): 405–421. https://doi.org/10.1177/02692163211059342.

Kirk, A., Crompton, P.W., Knighting, K. et al. (2017). Paramedics and their role in end-of-life care: perceptions and confidence. *Journal of Paramedic Practice* 9: 71–79.

Kübler-Ross, E., Wessler, S., and Avioli, L.V. (1972). On death and dying. *JAMA* 221 (2): 174–179.

Martin, E.M. and Barkley, J. (2017). Improving cultural competence in end-of-life pain management. *Home Healthcare Now* 35 (2): 96–104. https://doi.org/10.1097/NHH.0000000000000519.

Munoz, M. (2016). Performing, and emotionally surviving, notifications of death to a patient's family. *Journal of Emergency Medical Services* 8 January. https://www.jems.com/patient-care/performing-and-emotionally-surviving-notifications-of-death-to-a-patients-family (accessed 14 October 2023).

Myall, M., Rowsell, A., Lund, S. et al. (2020). Death and dying in prehospital care: what are the experiences and issues for prehospital practitioners, families and bystanders? A scoping review. *BMJ Open* 10 (9): e036925. https://doi.org/10.1136/bmjopen-2020-036925.

NHS England. (2023). Advance decision to refuse treatment (living will). https://www.nhs.uk/conditions/end-of-life-care/planning-ahead/advance-decision-to-refuse-treatment (accessed 14 October 2023).

Palliative Care Australia (2015). What is palliative care? 8 April. https://palliativecare.org.au/resource/what-is-palliative-care (accessed 14 October 2023)

Rome, R.B., Luminais, H.H., Bourgeois, D.A., and Blais, C.M. (2011). The role of palliative care at the end of life. *Ochsner Journal* 11 (4): 348–352.

Sarbey, B. (2016). Definitions of death: brain death and what matters in a person. *Journal of Law and the Biosciences* 3 (3): 743–752. https://doi.org/10.1093/jlb/lsw054.

Searight, H.R. and Gafford, J. (2005). Cultural diversity at the end of life: issues and guidelines for family physicians. *American Family Physician* 71 (3): 515–522.

Waldrop, D.P., Waldrop, M.R., McGinley, J.M. et al. (2020). Managing death in the field: prehospital end-of-life care. *Journal of Pain and Symptom Management* 60 (4): 709–716.e2. https://doi.org/10.1016/j.jpainsymman.2020.05.004.

Walker, E. (2018). Death notification delivery and training methods. *Journal of Paramedic Practice: The Clinical Monthly for Emergency Care Professionals* 10 (8): 334–341. https://doi.org/10.12968/jpar.2018.10.8.334.

World Health Organization. (2020). Palliative care: key facts. http://www.who.int/news-room/fact-sheets/detail/palliative-care (accessed 21 October 2023).

Further Reading

National Institute for Health and Care Excellence (2015). *Care of the Dying in the Last Days of Life*. NICE Guideline NG31. London: National Institute for Health and Care Excellence https://www.nice.org.uk/guidance/ng31 (accessed 14 October 2023).

National Institute for Health and Care Excellence (2019). *End of Life Care for Adults: Service delivery*. NICE Guideline NG142. London: National Institute for Health and Care Excellence https://www.nice.org.uk/guidance/ng142.

Cameron, C., Lunn, T.M., Lanos, C. et al. (2021). Dealing with dying – progressing paramedics' role in grief support. *Progress Palliative Care* 29 (2): 91–97.

Kübler-Ross, E. and Kessler, D. (2005). *On Grief and Grieving: Finding the Meaning of Grief Through the Five Stages of Loss*. London: Simon and Schuster.

National Institute for Health and Care Excellence. (2023). Prescribing in palliative care. British National Formulary. https://bnf.nice.org.uk/medicines-guidance/prescribing-in-palliative-care (accessed 14 October 2023).

Patterson, R., Standing, H., Lee, M. et al. (2019). Paramedic information needs in end-of-life care: a qualitative interview study exploring access to a shared electronic record as a potential solution. *BMC Palliative Care* 18 (1): 108.

Shaw, J., Fothergill, R., and Murphy-Jones, G. (2015). Does current pre-hospital care for patients at the end of their life reflect best practice guidance? *Emergency Medicine Journal* 32: e13.

Online Resources

NHS Scotland. Scottish Palliative Care Guidelines: https://rightdecisions.scot.nhs.uk/scottish-palliative-care-guidelines
Palliaged. Palliative care and aged care evidence base: www.palliaged.com.au

Glossary

Active dying phase	Occurs within days or hours of death where there is decreased blood flow to vital organs, respiratory system irregularities and decreasing consciousness.
Death	Either (1) the irreversible cessation of circulatory and respiratory functions, or (2) the irreversible cessation of all functions of the entire brain, including the brain stem.
Death notification	Discussions had with friends/family members on scene at an unsuccessful resuscitation where the patient you have resuscitated has died.
Do not attempt CPR order (DNACPR)	A specific type of advance healthcare decision that instructs healthcare providers not to perform CPR in the event of a cardiac arrest.
Mental Capacity Act	If you cannot make decisions for yourself because you do not have the mental capacity to make them, the Mental Capacity Act 2005 sets out what you can do to plan ahead, how you can ask someone else to make decisions for you and who can make these decisions. Applies in England and Wales.
Palliative care	A specialised approach to healthcare that focuses on improving the quality of life in individual's whose conditions are considered incurable.
Preactive dying phase	Occurs days to weeks before death where patients experience decreased energy levels, increased fatigue and gradual decline in overall functioning.
Terminal phase	Final moments before death where vital functions continue to decline until the respiratory system and cardiovascular system no longer function.
Lasting power of attorney	A legal document that allows individuals to appoint a trusted person to make health and welfare decisions on their behalf if they are unable to do so.

419

Multiple Choice Questions

1. Which of the following is an appropriate response when communicating with a grieving family member?
   a. Offering solutions to their problems
   b. Encouraging them to forget and move on
   c. Listening actively and providing emotional support
   d. Distracting them from the topic of death and focusing on better times

2. What is the purpose of an advance decision to refuse treatment?
   a. To assign medical decision-making authority to the healthcare provider
   b. To establish the patient's resuscitation status
   c. To specify the patient's wishes regarding medical treatment
   d. To outline the financial responsibilities of the patient's family

3. Which of the following is an appropriate action for a paramedic to take when caring for a dying patient?
   a. Focus primarily on physical comfort and pain management
   b. Encouraging the patient to discuss their end-of-life fears
   c. Try to convince the patient to accept life-saving measures
   d. Distract the patient from conversations about death and dying

4. When providing care to a dying patient, what is the primary goal of palliative care?
   a. To cure the patient's underlying condition
   b. To prolong the patient's life as much as possible
   c. To administer experimental treatments
   d. To provide comfort and improve quality of life

5. Which of the following is an example of a physical symptoms commonly experienced by dying patients?
   a. Anxiety and restlessness
   b. Delusions and hallucinations
   c. Rapid weight gain
   d. Increased appetite and thirst

6. When discussing end-of-life options with a patient, what is the role of a paramedic?
   a. To make decisions on behalf of the patient
   b. To provide emotional support and empathy
   c. To offer spiritual or religious guidance
   d. To prioritise your personal beliefs

7. What are the five stages of grief?
   a. Irritation, aggression, anger and grief, moodiness, agreeability
   b. Sadness, emptiness, bargaining, acceptance, moving on
   c. Denial and shock, aggression, compromising, sadness, acceptance
   d. Denial and shock, anger and grief, bargaining, depression, acceptance

8. Which of the following best describes a 'do not attempt CPR order?'
   a. An order that prohibits any medical intervention for a patient with a terminal illness
   b. A legal document that designates a healthcare proxy for a patient
   c. An instruction to healthcare providers not to perform cardiopulmonary resuscitation in the event of cardiac arrest
   d. A requirement for all patients above a certain age to forego life-sustaining treatments

9. Which of these is not a common cause of unexpected death in paediatric patients?
   a. Sudden infant death syndrome
   b. Accidental injuries (e.g. suffocation or drowning)
   c. Accidental ingestion or exposure to toxic substances, medications or household chemicals
   d. Myocardial infarction

10. What is not in the scope of management for a paramedic treating a palliative care patient?
    a. Pain relief
    b. Oxygen therapy
    c. Administration of medications used for voluntary assisted dying
    d. Emotional support

Multiple Choice Answers

Chapter 1

1. b
2. c
3. b
4. a
5. b
6. c
7. d
8. d
9. b
10. c

Chapter 2

1. a
2. c
3. a
4. c
5. b
6. c
7. d
8. d
9. c
10. a

Fundamentals of Applied Pathophysiology for Paramedics, First Edition. Edited by Ian Peate and Simon Sawyer.
© 2024 John Wiley & Sons Ltd. Published 2024 by John Wiley & Sons Ltd.

Chapter 3

1. a
2. c
3. a
4. b
5. a
6. a
7. c
8. a
9. b
10. d

Chapter 4

1. b
2. d
3. b
4. d
5. c
6. d
7. a
8. a
9. c
10. d

Chapter 5

1. a
2. a
3. d
4. b
5. b
6. c

7. d

8. c

9. b

10. c

Chapter 6

1. c

2. d

3. d

4. b

5. c

6. c

7. c

8. a

9. d

10. d

Chapter 7

1. d

2. b

3. b

4. d

5. c

6. c

7. d

8. c

9. d

10. b

Chapter 8

1. d
2. c
3. a
4. d
5. a
6. c
7. b
8. a
9. b
10. b

Chapter 9

1. c
2. b
3. d
4. b
5. a
6. b
7. d
8. a
9. b
10. c

Chapter 10

1. b
2. a
3. d
4. d
5. c
6. d

7. c

8. a

9. b

10. c

Chapter 11

1. a

2. b

3. c

4. d

5. b

6. a

7. c

8. d

9. a

10. c

Chapter 12

1. c

2. b

3. d

4. b

5. d

6. d

7. c

8. a

9. d

10. d

Chapter 13

1. b
2. c
3. b
4. d
5. d
6. a
7. c
8. d
9. b
10. d

Chapter 14

1. b
2. a
3. a
4. c
5. d
6. c
7. b
8. b
9. a
10. d

Chapter 15

1. b
2. d
3. a

4. d

5. a

6. a

7. a

8. d

9. b

10. d

Chapter 16

1. b

2. c

3. a

4. c

5. a

6. c

7. d

8. b

9. a

10. d

Chapter 17

1. a

2. d

3. a

4. b

5. d

6. a

7. a

8. a

9. c

10. d

Chapter 18

1. c
2. a
3. d
4. b
5. d
6. c
7. b
8. d
9. a
10. b

Chapter 19

1. c
2. c
3. a
4. d
5. a
6. b
7. d
8. c
9. d
10. c

Index

Fundamentals of Applied Pathophysiology for Paramedics, First Edition. Edited by Ian Peate and Simon Sawyer.
© 2024 John Wiley & Sons Ltd. Published 2024 by John Wiley & Sons Ltd.